RUNNING

The Complete Guide to Building Your Running Program

John Stanton
Founder of the Running Room

PENGUIN
CANADA

PENGUIN CANADA

Published by the Penguin Group

Penguin Group (Canada), 90 Eglinton Avenue East, Suite 700, Toronto, Ontario, Canada M4P 2Y3
(a division of Pearson Canada Inc.)

Penguin Group (USA) Inc., 375 Hudson Street, New York, New York 10014, U.S.A.
Penguin Books Ltd, 80 Strand, London WC2R 0RL, England
Penguin Ireland, 25 St Stephen's Green, Dublin 2, Ireland (a division of Penguin Books Ltd)
Penguin Group (Australia), 250 Camberwell Road, Camberwell, Victoria 3124, Australia
(a division of Pearson Australia Group Pty Ltd)
Penguin Books India Pvt Ltd, 11 Community Centre, Panchsheel Park, New Delhi – 110 017, India
Penguin Group (NZ), 67 Apollo Drive, Rosedale, North Shore 0745, Auckland, New Zealand
(a division of Pearson New Zealand Ltd)
Penguin Books (South Africa) (Pty) Ltd, 24 Sturdee Avenue, Rosebank,
Johannesburg 2196, South Africa

Penguin Books Ltd, Registered Offices: 80 Strand, London WC2R 0RL, England

First published 2010

1 2 3 4 5 6 7 8 9 10 (RRD)

Copyeditor: Lee Craig
Graphic design: Aimee Kozun

Manufactured in the U.S.A.

LIBRARY AND ARCHIVES CANADA CATALOGUING IN PUBLICATION

Stanton, John, 1948-
Running : the complete guide to building your running program / John Stanton.

ISBN 978-0-14-317609-1

1. Running. 2. Runners (Sports)--Health and hygiene. I. Title.

GV1061.S652 2010   796.42   C2010-900603-8

Visit the Penguin Group (Canada) website at **www.penguin.ca**
Special and corporate bulk purchase rates available; please see
www.penguin.ca/corporatesales or call 1-800-810-3104, ext. 2477 or 2474

www.runningroom.com

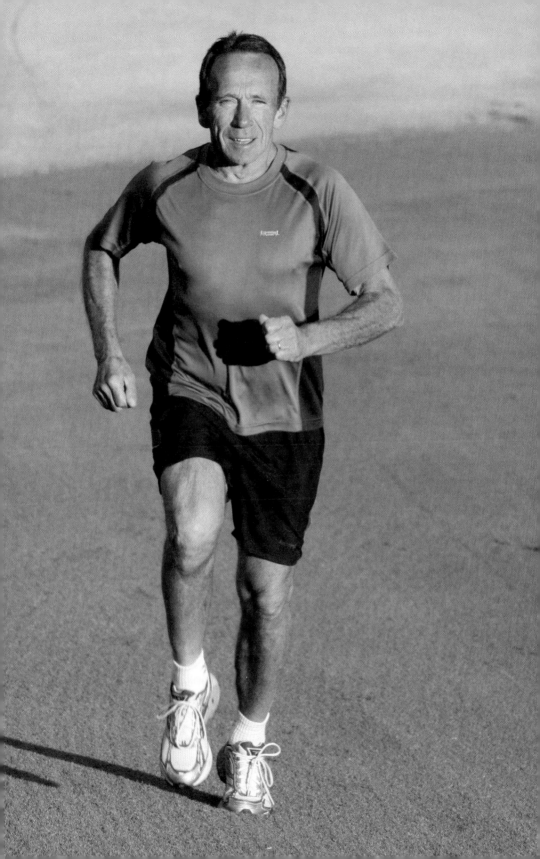

Contents

Chapter 1

Getting Started 16

Chapter 2

Building Your Program 42

Shoes and Clothing 64

Weather 86

Stretching 116

Running or Walking Intelligently 124

Running Form 132

Heart Rate Training 142

Women's Running

Injuries

Chapter 15

5 K & 10 K Events 286

Chapter 16

"The Full" Half Marathon 314

Chapter 17

Marathon 340

The benefits of running can boost the immune system and protect against chronic diseases. This book is for all those people who want to strengthen their bodies, calm and stimulate their minds and soothe their souls. It will improve you mentally, physically and spiritually.

Studies by the American College of Sports Medicine show that exercise lowers the risk of stroke by 27%, reduces the incidence of diabetes by 50 %, reduces the incidence of high blood pressure by 40%, reduces the risk of breast cancer by 50%, color cancer by 60% and Alzheimer's by 40%.

Running burns fat, relives stress, improves your self-esteem and helps you sleep better. It also improves your energy levels, endurance, strength, speed and muscle definition, increases your odds against heart disease, improves your cardiovascular system and helps you relax. Running provides you with a positive attitude: you feel good about yourself and others, increase your metabolic rate, awaken your sex life, work and sleep better and enjoy an improved quality of life. It is a great payback for an investment of playing and having fun for about an hour a day.

Some of your improvements will come fast and easy; others will take time, hard work, discipline and patience. All of the changes will be positive. Running returns you to the basics of life as you take control of your energy, your attitude and your life.

This book will guide you with an intelligent plan, one that is both gentle and progressive in design. Gentle enough to keep you having fun and highly motivated and progressive enough to challenge you to new and improved levels of fitness each day. The secret to running success is to teach the athlete to set new and improved daily, seasonal and dream goals that are both challenging and attainable.

Here in, you will find the motivation, inspiration, training schedules, programs and innovative training techniques that will take you from running a fun run to running a personal best time in a marathon. You will learn about running, goal setting and the sheer joy of good health and good friends.

I want to thank our team of Mike O'Dell, Charlane O'Dell, Aimee Kozun, Lee Craig, Mike Mendzat, John Reeves, Bev Stanton, Jason Stanton, John Stanton, Jr., and our families.

I would like to acknowledge the following individuals for their medical and technical advice: Harvey Sternberg, MD, Richard Beauchamp, MD, Julia Alleyne, BHSc (PT), MD, Jeffery Robinson, MD, Susan Glen, MSc Nutrition, and Heidi M. Bates, BSc, RD.

This book is dedicated to all runners

John Stanton

Introduction

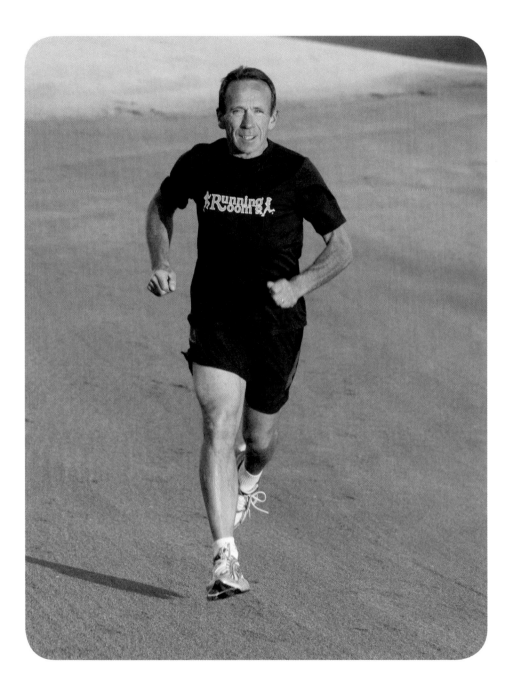

Running was once about the lonely long-distance run; today it is about the social group run, with people laughing and enjoying themselves while reaping the benefits of an active lifestyle. Many of you take up running for very specific goals. Some people run to lose weight, take control of their lives or run a specific distance, from a 5 K fun run to a marathon. Others run for stress relief and the positive feelings exercise gives as a reward for our efforts. Our attitudes towards our personal goals, our family, our career and our community improve as we take charge of life and become more athletic. We learn that life is full of challenges, but with an intelligent plan, a group to share in the journey and the celebration of the finish line, we can achieve success both in running and in life.

Why Run?

Rewards of improved fitness:

+ lose weight
+ take control of your life
+ run a specific distance
+ stress relief
+ healthier eating habits
+ positive feelings
+ improved self-esteem

For many of you running is as natural as brushing your teeth or combing your hair. Running is no longer reserved for those with good genetics; it works for nearly everyone. A look at most healthy living programs and material will show the commonality of some simple recommendations: combine the national food guide for nutritional intake with a regular routine of brisk exercise. Running fits the recommendation perfectly when it comes to brisk exercise. You can run on your own, run in a group and run at a time and place that is convenient for you.

Over the past 20 years running has changed from being a competition to winning at health and fitness through a regular routine of participation. The first step to take is to get a full medical exam—it will give you the encouragement of your medical professional to make this lifestyle change.

Many of you will say, "I am not an athlete. I could never run." I say to you, "Yes, you can. You are an athlete and you can run. With some conviction you can do it!" You will soon adapt to the physical training and feel the benefits. You will learn that the more we exercise the better our nutritional choices. The thought of an evening run reminds us to make the most intelligent choice for lunch. The very thought of how you feel when you run and how your food choices leave you feeling makes you an athlete.

Do not let anyone tell you that you will never be an athlete or runner. I have seen individuals make the decision so many times to take control of their lives and succeed. There are some wonderful examples of these success stories that are shared with you in the last chapter. Take the time to read them; they will inspire you. Do not let your current assessment of your body image be a concern. Running provides an attitude adjustment. The empowerment and sense of self control is the very reason many runners run. Many of our world leaders relish the clarity of thinking, the calming effects and the energy provided by the simple act of placing one foot in front of the other. They know they are better for those they lead by taking care of themselves. If you care about the people important to you, you must first take care of yourself, so you are in a better position to help them.

As we become more athletic, we learn structure and discipline to keep balance in our training and prevent the obsessive compulsive workouts that lead to burnout or injury. Staying highly motivated and injury free provides the consistency of training, the ability to improve and long-term success.

After over 20 years of coaching runners, I have seen many athletes injured from

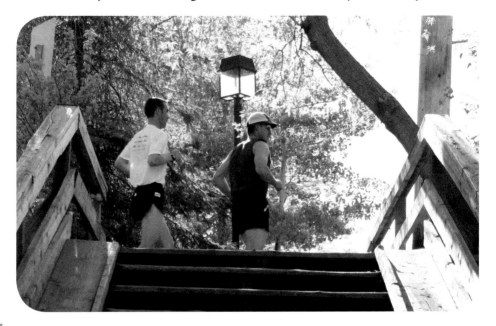

running too fast or too long. Interestingly, I have not seen a single injury from running too slowly. The adage "slow and steady wins the race" certainly applies as you commence a running program. Keep your program gentle while maintaining your motivation and consistency. Getting our butts out the door on a regular basis is often the biggest challenge.

The power of the group run is amazing. Over the years we have encouraged people to meet on Wednesdays and Sundays for a group practice run. Running steadily becomes a way of life. In addition to discovering the many benefits of running, you expand your circle of like-minded friends. This positive peer pressure is a great motivator. The twice-a-week meeting provides the team atmosphere and group commitment. On nonpractice days, the very thought of not keeping up to your practice pace group provides the self-motivation to run.

A question often asked is "What is the absolute minimum amount of training required to run a 5 K, 10 K, half or full marathon?" The answer is to run at least three times per week. All training programs are built on the premise of endurance, strength and speed. The other key ingredient is rest. Rest is a part of every good training program, and you need it for recovery and to improve and be stronger.

Endurance is achieved through your long slow distance training. The combination of running and walking provides stress and rest, enabling you to come back with renewed vigor to each training session. During these long slow runs you should pass the "talk test." Conversation is comfortable during this phase of training. If you experience any huffing and puffing, slow the pace down. If you have a heart rate monitor on, you should be between 60% and 70% of your maximum heart rate.

The next phase of training as a runner is strength training. This you do specifically in the weight room or by running hills or threshold runs. Strength runs are run at about 70–80% of your maximum heart rate. If you are not wearing a heart monitor, run at a pace where conversation becomes labored.

Speed is all about maintaining form and coordination under the stress of higher intensity. Sounds simple enough, but at over 80% effort these sessions must be run in short bursts with adequate rest and recovery periods between each period of high intensity.

The combination of stress and rest and the foundation of endurance, strength and speed will have you arrive at all of your finish lines smiling, and upright.

As you start to run you learn there is an athlete waiting in all of us. Once you are provided with structure and motivation, you discover the benefits of a regular exercise program. You also discover that running is fun!

Staying motivated can be as simple as learning some positive self-talk.

Here are some phrases that work for me:

- I am in control of my own life.
- I can achieve any intelligent goal I set for myself.
- I believe in myself and the people around me.
- I treat every day as a new challenge to improve myself in some way.
- I am strong, fit and a powerful runner.

As your running coach, I provide the inspiration, motivation and information; for real success you must supply the perspiration.

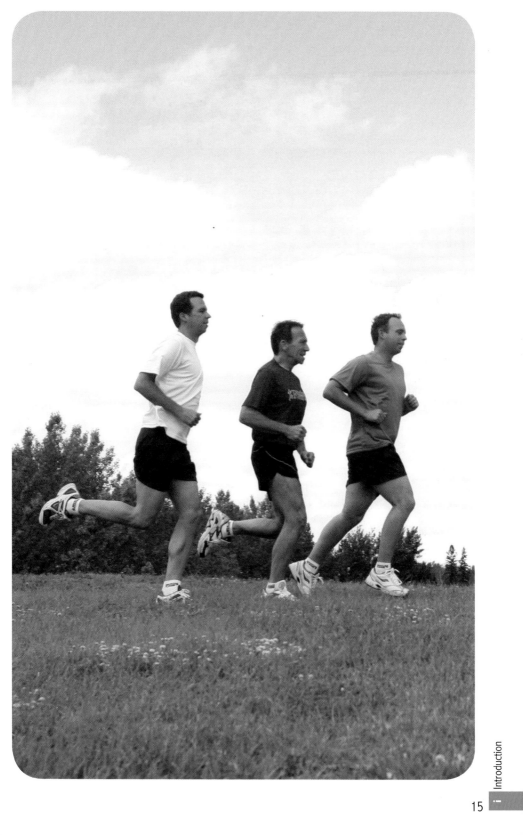

Getting Started

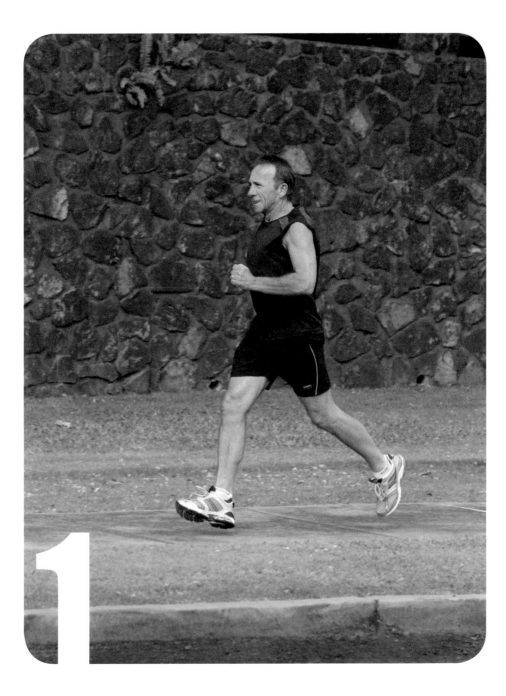

Let's talk about designing your training program. One of the first things to consider is that every runner is unique, so your program must be modified according to your individual requirements, talents and commitment. You recognize that your fingerprints are unique, but so are a number of other factors that you should work around your running program: your distinctive physiological characteristics (body type, resting and maximum heart rates and the basic ability of your body to use oxygen); your individual needs (what you want to achieve through exercise); and the different demands placed on you by your commitments to your family, friends, community and work.

Fitting It All In

All of us are faced with the challenge of fitting a workout into our busy daily schedules. Our friends, families and communities all require time, and in today's marketplace many people have great demands placed on them at work. Our personal time is becoming very precious.

So, just how do we have time to fit it all in? To start with, make a daily appointment with yourself for your own health and fitness. It is not selfish, it is necessary. In order to care about the other people in your life, you must first care about yourself. If not, just how are you going to be any good to them?

One of the more common questions I get asked is, What is the best time of the day to run? Well, here are the answers I have received from thousands of runners over the years. As you will see, there is no best time. There is, however, a best time for you.

I like to get out of bed and run to start my day.

An early morning run works best for some people. It starts their day off and gets them in the right mental shape for the day. They find that they eat less, are more productive throughout the day and then come home to relax without the stress of having to get their run in when they are tired. They also tell me they sleep well at night.

I like to run at noon; it's the perfect time for me.

Runners that run at noon tell me their run breaks up the day, gives them an attitude change for the afternoon and forces them to eat a light lunch.

I like to run right after work, before supper.

These runners say they can come home from work tired mentally, but then go out for a run and come back feeling rejuvenated. They say that the run after work and before supper makes them enjoy their evenings more, and for many of them exercise is an appetite suppressant.

I like to run before I go to sleep.

Some runners tell me that the late-evening run is grand. It relaxes them for the night and is a great time to meditate about life's challenges and find the simple solutions that a run can deliver. They also like to brag that the run revs up their metabolism, which continues to burn fat as they sleep. Sounds like a great deal for those of us looking for a fat-burning advantage.

So, when is the best time to run? Remember that we are each unique and that running is supposed to be adding value to your life, so find the time of day that fits your individual schedule. (For me, an evening run just makes me a bigger fan of late-night television—I return from a late run full of new energy, stay up late and then find myself tired the next day.) Use your runs to improve your mental as well as your physical well-being. Keep your running time as a stress buster—most of us have enough stress in our lives that we do not need to add any more.

Goal Setting

To get the most out of your training program, you should set an ultimate goal and then set several smaller goals to get you there. Your ultimate goal might be to run a particular race, but before you run that race you must first train consistently. It can help to set some smaller, shorter-distance races as targets to test yourself along the way. (Interestingly, many marathon runners will tell you that the true reward comes from the training, not the marathon itself.)

Your goals can be qualitative or they can be quantitative: a qualitative long-term goal might be to make fitness part of your daily routine, just like brushing your teeth or combing your hair; a quantitative long-term goal might be to run a specific marathon when your birthday takes you into a new decade.

Set short-term goals that allow you to savor some of your training rewards. Your first goal might be to run continuously for 20 minutes. One good goal at the start of any program is to run for 30 days without an injury, which will force you to listen to your body.

Stop Procrastinating

+ Plan and schedule your daily workouts.

+ Be flexible within your schedule. Just commit to completing the workout.

+ Be creative in planning your workouts. Use normal down time or waiting time to get in that run, stretch session or cross-training session.

+ Read, listen to or watch something humorous. A good laugh gets rid of most stress. The thought of my good buddy Nick Lees running a marathon in a tutu usually does the trick for me.

+ Vary your workouts. Running the same distance or course every day can soon lead to boredom. A little speed or some hill repeats will put some spring back into your stride.

+ Run with a buddy. You can motivate each other.

+ Imagine yourself in a race leading the pack that is 25 meters behind you. Push just a little.

+ In a safe area, put on headphones and listen to some music, a motivational recording or a comedy.

+ Mix it up: change the time of day you normally run; run in a different direction; run a new workout; or read a great running book.

+ Best yet, run past a hospital to remind yourself how fortunate you are to have your good health. It is a fragile gift you must look after.

+ Savor each run because it is special in its own way.

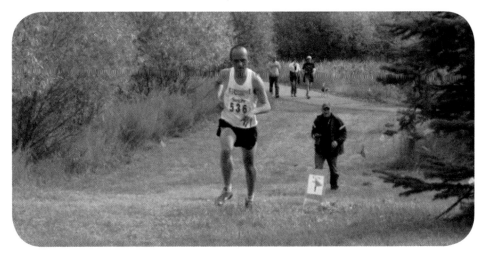

In your program, you will have five kinds of goals:

1. A daily goal to get out the door every day.

2. A self-acceptance goal to condition yourself to the acceptance that daily fitness is part of your lifestyle.

3. A performance goal for a season—either a distance goal, such as running a 10 K , or a time goal, such as breaking 45 minutes for a 10 K.

4. A dedication goal or a special goal for a season—something that will motivate you to continue training throughout the year. Dedicate your year to the memories of a loved one, or dedicate your goal to proving you can do it when others believe you cannot.

5. A dream goal—a big race or special distance that seems just slightly out of reach but achievable.

If your goals are intelligent and realistic, you will be more likely to succeed and not get discouraged partway through your training. There is no special formula for where you should start or the rate at which you should progress, but take care not to let your new-found fitness carry you beyond improvement into overuse. Don't look at the people around, you look at where you are now and start a program of improvement from that point. Set a current benchmark and try to improve by approximately 10% a week. (Keeping a limit of 10% a week allows you to improve while minimizing your risk of injury.)

To help you along the way, in both assessment and encouragement, start a logbook. A daily log will reinforce your progress towards your individual goals. There is a certain pleasure that comes from recording your workouts and assessing the quality of the effort. Record the distance you ran, where you ran and the type of run (e.g., hill workout, long and slow, speed training). Include notes on how you felt, especially if your stress level was above normal, and on abnormal weather conditions.

Be sure to monitor and evaluate your training, adjusting your program and goals to your progress and the other facets of your life. Use your logbook to document any changes in your circumstances and the corresponding adjustments to your short-term and long-term goals. Now, this is not a free-ride ticket that lets you off your training for every little interference, but you should back off if conditions warrant. For example, if the weather becomes extremely hot, you must intelligently modify the program, or if a busy work schedule leaves you tired, and you have bad runs on two consecutive days, you need to progress more slowly.

Remember that sometimes your daily goal will be to have a rest day. Rest is a good four-letter word that lets your body rebuild and get stronger. Sports medicine experts say you need 48 hours to recover from a hard workout, so it should be a scheduled part of every training program.

The setting of athletic goals, the discipline of following a regimented program towards specific goals and the recording of your progress will transfer over into the other parts of your life. Studies continue to prove that people who are physically active are more positive in their approach to challenges, have more energy and eat better. These added benefits and feelings of improved health are some of the reason runners become highly self-motivated over a period of time.

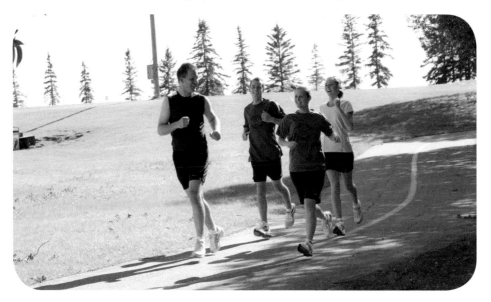

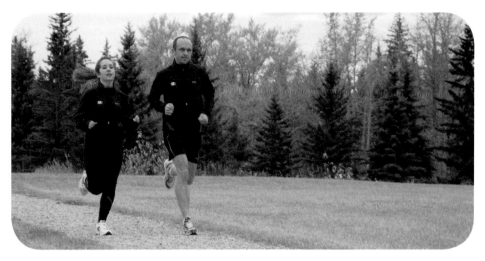

You should decide on a strategy:

A. Determine Your Goals

Try to establish weekly goals for improvement. The more realistic the goals are, the more likely that you will not be discouraged partway through your training. Use a running diary to help evaluate your progress. Always be ready to readjust and reevaluate your goals. For example, bad runs on two consecutive days may indicate a need to back off and progress more slowly.

Short-term goals:

e.g., to complete a 5-km run in the spring.
e.g., to lose 10 lb.

Long-term goals:

e.g., to lose 25 lb. and have fitness as a part of daily routine.
e.g., to complete the Boston Marathon.

Remember!

Your goals can be qualitative (e.g., to get in shape) or quantitative (e.g., run a 25-minute 5 K).

B. Record Your Goals

Commit to your goals by writing them down and reviewing your progress towards these goals on an active basis.

C. Monitor Your Progress by Means of a Logbook

Logbooks reinforce your daily step-by-step progress towards achievement of goals.

D. Modify Your Goals

As you progress in your training, your short-term and even long-term goals may change. Modify your goals according to changes in circumstance and document this change.

Focus on aspects within your control, e.g., skills, preparation. Avoid outcome goals beyond your immediate control, e.g., scores, placing, winning.

How to start:

Step 1
Write down a difficult but achievable ultimate goal.
Long-term dream goal:

_____

_____

_____

_____

_____

Step 2
Write down your dream goal for the next few months that would help attain your ultimate goal.
Dream goal for this season:

_____

_____

_____

_____

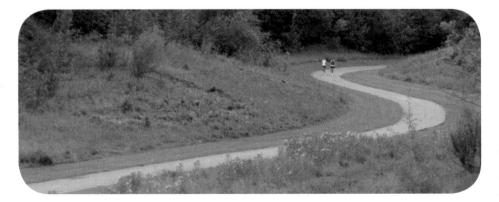

Step 3

Write down your realistic performance goal for this season. It might help to set dates for other goals leading to the performance goal, such as running a distance within a certain time or completing a distance without walking.
Realistic performance goal for this season:

_____
_____
_____
_____

Step 4

Evaluate your progress and consider whether you are aiming too high (you might need more base mileage) or whether you should set yourself a harder target.
Self-acceptance goal:

_____
_____
_____
_____

Step 5

Establish a weekly goal for improvement, remembering that the more realistic you are, the better the chances are of attaining it. Use a logbook, such as the Running Room's Training Log, to record your progress. Use it as a diary to record how you feel and where you ran. Modify your training if necessary.
Daily goal:

_____
_____
_____
_____
_____

For some, running 1 km or running a certain distance without stopping is reward enough. Others may want to lose a certain amount of weight, and yet others may want to qualify for the Boston Marathon. Goals are personal—don't worry about what others strive after. We all compete against ourselves.

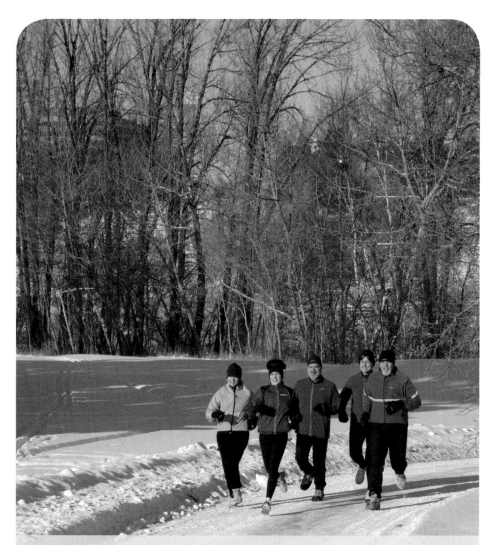

Top 10 Reasons People Take up a Running Program

1. Stress relief
2. Weight control
3. Feeling of well-being
4. To meet people who share similar values of a healthy lifestyle
5. It's a simple fitness program that can be done anywhere, anytime and with little special equipment
6. Low cost of equipment
7. Positive self-motivation
8. Improvement of self-image
9. Pursuit of a specific race goal
10. The group's positive peer pressure to stay motivated

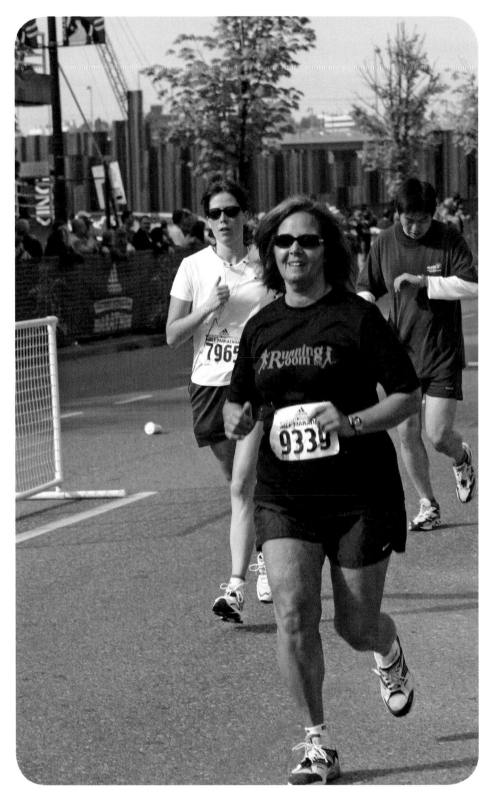

▬Assessing Your Physical Readiness

Running is a strenuous physical activity. Seven questions from the Physical Activity Readiness Questionnaire (Par-Q) will help you assess your readiness to start running.

Questionnaire

1. Has your doctor ever said that you have a heart condition and that you should only do physical activity recommended by a doctor? (Yes | No)

2. Do you feel pain in your chest when you do physical activities? (Yes | No)

3. In the past month, have you had chest pain when not doing physical activities? (Yes | No)

4. Do you lose your balance because of dizziness or do you ever lose consciousness? (Yes | No)

5. Do you have a bone or joint problem that could be made worse by a change in your physical activity? (Yes | No)

6. Is your doctor currently prescribing drugs (for example water pills) for your blood pressure or heart condition? (Yes | No)

7. Do you know of any other reason why you should not perform physical activities? (Yes | No)

If you answered yes to any of the above questions, do not continue until you receive a doctor's clearance. If you answered no to every question, you may be reasonably sure it's safe to increase your physical activity.

Reprinted in part from the 1994 revised version of the **Physical Activity Readiness Questionnaire** (Par-Q and YOU) by special permission from the Canadian Society for Exercise Physiology, Inc. Copyright 1994, CSEP, Inc.

Assessing Your Running Fitness

Unsure of your current fitness level? Where is your starting point? Just how healthy and fit are you?

This self-test checks both your health history and your fitness habits.

Choose the number that best describes you in each of the 10 areas, then add up your score. The results tell you whether your starting-line condition is high, average or low cardiovascular health.

Cardio

Which of these statements best describes your cardiovascular condition? This is a critical safety check before you enter any vigorous activity. (Warning: If you have a history of cardiovascular disease, start the running programs in this book only after receiving approval from your doctor and then only with close supervision by a fitness instructor.)

No history of heart or circulatory problems	3 ○
Past ailments have been treated successfully	2 ○
Such problems exist but no treatment required	1 ○
Under medical care for cardiovascular illness	0 ○

Injuries

Which of these statements best describes your current injuries? This is a test of your musculoskeletal readiness to start a running program. (Warning: If your injury is temporary, wait until it is cured before starting the program. If it is chronic, adjust the program to fit your limitations.)

No current injury problems	3 ○
Some pain in activity but not limited by it	2 ○
Level of activity is limited by the injury	1 ○
Unable to do much strenuous training	0 ○

Illnesses

Which of these statements best describes your current illnesses? Certain temporary or chronic conditions will delay or disrupt your running program. (See warning under "Injuries.")

No current illness problems	3 ○
Some problem in activity but not limited by it	2 ○
Level of activity is limited by illness	1 ○
Unable to do much strenuous training	0 ○

Age

Which of these age groups describes you? In general, the younger you are, the less time you have spent slipping out of shape.

Ages 19 and under	3 ○
Ages 20 to 29	2 ○
Ages 30 to 39	1 ○
Ages 40 and older	0 ○

Weight

Which of these figures describes how close you are to your own definition of "ideal weight"? Excess fat is a major mark of unfitness, but it's also possible to be significantly underweight.

Within 5 lb. of ideal weight	3 ○
6–10 lb. above or below ideal weight	2 ○
11–19 lb. above or below ideal weight	1 ○
20 lb. or more above or below ideal weight	0 ○

Resting Pulse Rate

Which of these figures describes your current pulse rate on waking up but before getting out of bed? A well-trained heart beats slower and more efficiently than one that's unfit.

Below 60 bpm	3 ○
60–69 bpm	2 ○
70–79 bpm	1 ○
80 bpm or more	0 ○

Smoking

Which of these statements best describes your smoking history and current habit (if any)? Smoking is the number one enemy of health and fitness.

Never a smoker	3 ○
Once a smoker but quit	2 ○
Occasional, light smoker now	1 ○
Regular, heavy smoker now	0 ○

Most Recent Run

Which of these statements best describes your running within the last month? The best single measure of how well you will run in the near future is what you ran in the recent past.

Ran nonstop for more than 4 km (2.5 mi.)	3 ○
Ran nonstop for 2–4 km (1–2.5 mi.)	2 ○
Ran nonstop for less than 2 km (1 mi.)	1 ○
No recent run of any distance	0 ○

Running Background

Which of these statements best describes your running history? Running fitness isn't long lasting, but the fact that you once ran is a good sign that you can do it again.

Trained for running within the past year	3 ○
Trained for running 1 to 2 years ago	2 ○
Trained for running more than 2 years ago	1 ○
Never trained formally for running	0 ○

Related Activities

Which of these statements best describes your participation in other exercises that are similar to running in aerobic benefit? The closer they relate to running (as do bicycling, swimming, cross-country skiing and fast walking, for example), the better the carryover effect will be.

Regularly practice similar aerobic activities	3 ○
Regularly practice less vigorous aerobic activities	2 ○
Regularly practice non-aerobic sports	1 ○
Not regularly active in any physical activity	0 ○

Your Rating

If you scored 20 points or more

You rate high in health and fitness for a beginning runner. You probably can handle continuous runs of at least 4–5 km (2.5–3 mi.) or 20 to 30 minutes.

If you scored 10 to 19 points

Your score is average. You may need to take some walking breaks to complete runs of 4–5 km (2.5–3 mi.) or 20 to 30 minutes.

If you scored under 10 points

Your score is low. You may need to start with walking only. Start with 20 minutes of brisk walking, adding 2 minutes each week until you are walking for 40 minutes comfortably.

Fitting It All Together

You're about to embark upon a journey that can positively change the way you look at the rest of your life. You will be joining a dedicated community who are committed to fitness as a regular part of their lifestyles. You will experience a dramatic change in your physical and mental outlook on life. You will have the self-confidence to achieve both your athletic and personal goals. Most people who get into a regular exercise program will eat better food, have more energy, be sick less often and maintain a more positive attitude. You'll find personal resources that you didn't know existed. Above all, you'll have fun, and as you meet the members of the running community, you will share many uplifting experiences.

"A journey of a thousand miles begins with a single step."

Join the Top 10%

Only 10% of the population in Canada, England and Australia do enough exercise to break a sweat.

Visualization/Imagery

+ Imagine yourself in the situations. Imagine yourself responding more effectively to situations that may have slowed or upset you in the past.

+ Imagine yourself in the situations thinking, focusing, believing and acting in more constructive and less anxious ways. Then work on replicating this version of yourself in the real world.

Remember

With persistence you will be successful!

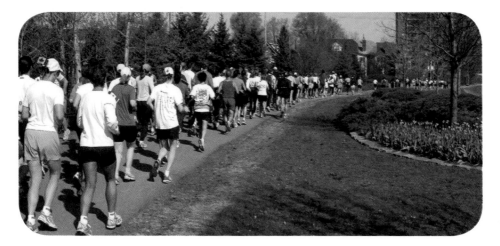

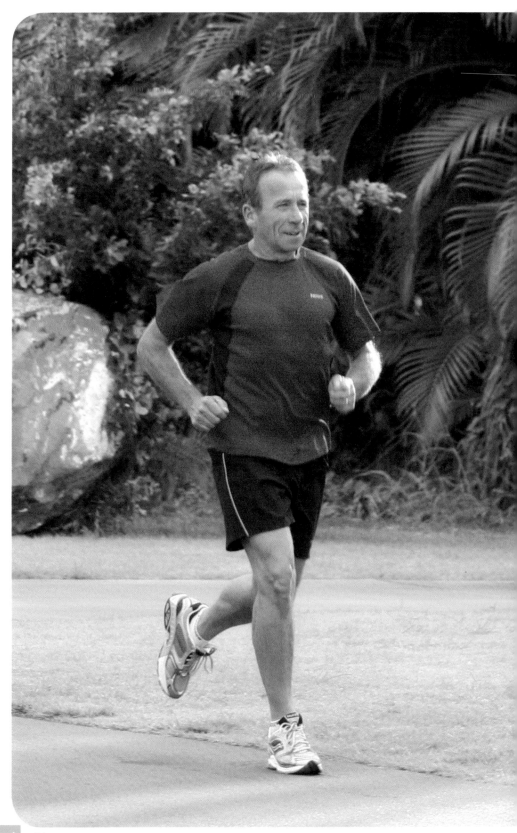

Positive Self-Suggestions

1. I am in control of my thinking, focus and life.

2. I control my own thoughts and emotions, and direct the whole pattern of my performance, health and life.

3. I am fully capable of achieving the goals I set for myself today. They are within my control.

4. I learn from problems or setbacks, and through them I see room for improvement and opportunities for personal growth.

5. Everyday in some way I am better, wiser, more adaptable, more focused, more confident, more in control.

Keeping It Fun

I enjoy my running; it truly is fun. However, there are a few annoyances that can take the fun out of running. I have provided a summary of tips you can use to help stay focused on the "enjoyment" aspect of running. These are general tips, many of which will be addressed later in the book in more detail. Enjoy these tips and stay having fun!

Delayed Onset Muscle Soreness

This general soreness and muscle ache comes from tiny tearing of the muscles as a result of running a longer distance or increasing the speed or intensity of a run.

Ice or a cold water stream on the sore muscles immediately following your run will help provide comfort and recovery. A warm Epsom salt bath and some gentle stretching will make for a more relaxed sleep and speedy recovery.

Skin Chafing

Chafing generally occurs under the arms, between the thighs, along the bra line for women and around the nipple area for men. The culprit is the salt in our sweat, which causes the abrasive chafing in these sensitive areas.

The chafing control product Bodyglide works best. Vaseline also works in a pinch, but it stains clothing, whereas Bodyglide will not. For guys, try NipGuard bandages; they work wonders on preventing raw chafed nipples.

Blisters

Friction between your foot and your shoe is usually the cause of blisters. This can be from poorly fitting shoes, a rib or seam in your sock or, on occasion, running on a slated or uneven surface that causes the shoe to rub on the side of the foot.

The best recommendation is Running Room CoolMax double layer socks—they work. If you do have a blister, cover it with a liquid bandage, which provides protection and helps dry the area—promoting healing while you continue to run.

Black Toenails

You have arrived wearing the badge of the black toe. Most often this condition occurs with an increase in mileage or from running a downhill session for an extended period of time. The repeated tapping of the toe against the front of the shoe causes blood to pool under the toenail.

If there is no pain, leave the nail to fall off by itself, but apply an anti-fungal cream to prevent infection. If you suffer a throbbing toe, then have your doctor (don't do this at home kids) make a small hole in the nail to drain the blood. It sounds far worse than it is; the good news is the relief is instant. The key in the future: make sure you go up from your current shoe size by a half or a full size to prevent a reoccurrence.

Athlete's Foot

Runners with red cracking skin, itching feet and soreness between the toes are nearly always suffering from athlete's foot. This condition usually results from someone using a public change or shower room.

Rule one: always wear sandals in the change room and shower areas of public facilities. Spray your shoes with an anti-fungal product, taking care to remove the insole to give them a good spray.

Muscle Cramps

A muscle cramp during a run is usually caused when the fatigued muscle has become overstimulated and contracts involuntary. Cramping can also result from insufficient electrolytes like potassium and sodium salts or from poor hydration.

Gentle stretching of the affected muscle is one solution. Massage the muscle gently to reduce the cramping effect. Work with isotonic sports drinks to remedy the problem.

Stitches

A stitch is a sharp pain in the diaphragm usually just under the bottom front of the rib cage. There are two theories for the cause. The first is that the discomfort is the result of the dome-shaped muscle of the diagram becoming irritated as it rises and falls to allow the lungs to breathe. The jostling effect of our running irritates this muscle and causes the cramp. The other theory is that the cramp is related to food. Many runners find it helps to avoid foods high in sugar and fat, as well as apples, fruit juices, dairy products and chocolate.

Personally, I think most of the stitch issues are related to breathing techniques. Breath like a swimmer with deep, full and relaxed breaths in rhythm and time with your running cadence. This more relaxed and rhythmic breathing allows for a better run and cuts the risk of the dreaded stitch. Think belly breathing!

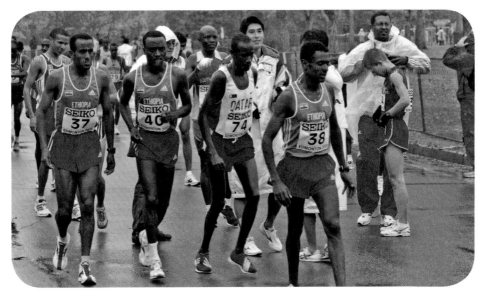

Burping, flatulence, gripping stomach pains and toilet calls

These annoyances can cause considerable discomfort and embarrassment to runners—enough to make some stop running. There is no simple or consistent cause for these calls—nor is there one simple solution. Running activity and the jolting movement of the body cause gastrointestinal disturbances. For some people a cup of coffee will help stimulate the bowels into action prior to the run. Having said this, caffeine and alcohol are stomach irritants, so avoidance may also be the solution. High fiber foods or dairy products prior to a run can also be the culprits. Many of our athletes also find the high sugar content of sports drinks can be detrimental. An easy solution for this is diluting the sports drink with additional water. If you find, as many runners do, that invariably it is at the 10-minute or 15-minute mark into your run that you get a call for the toilet, simply plan a loop around your start point of 10 minutes. Stop, use your facilities and continue your run. Plan your long runs around potential public toilets. If there are none on your route, gyms, health clubs, gas stations, coffee shops, community clubs, fire halls and churches are all generally sympathetic to a runner in need.

Sweating

Sweating is your air conditioning and cooling system. It regulates your temperature and helps eliminate toxins. While running you sweat between 500 and 1000 ml per hour. Sweat by itself doesn't stink; it is when it contacts bacteria that we stink. So start your run clean and with a deodorant. Cotton is more smell resistant, but we know that it runs hot and we chafe. The high technical fabrics are perfect for sweat wicking, and they dry out quickly but retain the sweat odor.

Wash your clothing after each run to avoid stinky clothes. If your sweat smells odd consult your doctor. Sweat odors can indicate a medical condition such as diabetes or liver disease. Your sweat is a sign of your character so don't sweat the sweat— after all you are an athlete.

Urinary Incontinence

Urinary incontinence* affects many runners, particularly woman after pregnancy. This hindrance to running is usually caused by pelvic-floor weakness. These muscles support the pelvis and abdomen and control the emptying of the bladder and bowel.

The best course of action is pelvic floor exercises and lots of them. Done consistently and properly these exercise are very effective in stopping urinary incontinence. If you tried them and they didn't work, you likely did too few or did the exercises incorrectly. Athletes are proactive, so do the exercises and do them often. If they still don't work, see your doctor.

*Urinary Incontinence: Incontinence is the inability to control the passage of urine. This can range from an occasional leakage of urine, to a complete inability to hold any urine. Alternative names—loss of bladder control; uncontrollable urination.

Lacking Motivation

Runners struggle occasionally to get themselves out the door to train. Motivation comes from within us. Do not rely on the coach or the club to motivate you to achieve your lifelong goals. Training tips supply the inspiration—now it is up to you to supply the motivation and perspiration.

Be consistent.
Be gentle and yet progressive.
Set short-, mid- and long-term goals.
Build some rest days into your training.
Mentally prepare as well as physically prepare for every race.
Build long slow distance, strength and speed training into all programs.

Adapt your training to the conditions and take pride in your courage to accept the challenge to run. If you find running boring, it may be you can't stand running with yourself for 30 or 40 minutes, so invite a friend along or join a group for motivation.

I am a Runner, I am an Athlete

As we begin running, we say "I jog." Then, with a little more confidence and not a whole lot more speed, we say "I run." One day we start referring to ourselves as "runners." After running for a while we start to understand the gift of being an "athlete." As an athlete we encounter and celebrate our mental, physical and emotional strengths while discovering the ability to make the impossible possible.

Athletes understand balance in life. Balance in sport, in our careers, in our families and in our communities. Creating this balance is what separates the individual and the athlete.

An athlete can be you, your mom or dad, your children, your family members or your neighbor. An athlete is the ordinary person striving and achieving the extraordinary accomplishment of attaining their personal goal through an intelligent training plan. They also know the importance of having a strong support group to both train with and to celebrate their achievements.

For many runners, we began running to quit smoking, lose weight, or take control of our lives during stressful times—a job change, a death of a loved one or some other personal yet very specific goal. However, we continue to run for a variety of reasons often far different than the ones motivating us to start running. Doing it for fun and learning to play as an adult is the real essence of the athlete.

Running teaches us self-reflection. We discover who we are and occasionally, who we are not. Running teaches us humility. There is always someone better yet we learn to give our best. Some of us love the social aspect of the group practice run, some the solitude and reflection of a solo run. All of us love the feeling and sense of accomplishment that comes from the run, the calming effects it has on our life and the uplifting of our spirits on the completion of the run. Running is a lifelong commitment and running is about who we are.

As an athlete we are aware of our bodies and the effects training, nutrition and rest can have on our personal performance. One good look at yourself and you discover the largest muscle groups are those used in forward motion and running. Our highly engineered cardiovascular system is designed to accept intelligent combinations of stress and rest—we truly are born to run.

Running is pure and simple—a great quality in our complex and occasionally confused and conflicted world. Running is a simple start and finish. Very few rules or guidelines and no luck—just your fitness level matched against the challenge of the day.

Everyone is a winner; there are no losers. Runs and races have a DNF designate for those unable to finish the race. Somehow even our "did not finish—DNF" sounds positive and encourages the athlete to come back and perform better the next time.

Running keeps you in touch with nature. An early morning run with just you and a trail brings you right back to basics of life: the cool morning air, the scrunching sounds of your footsteps on the pathway, the rhythm of your breathing in tune with the bounding of your heart. You cruise over the rolling trail system with its cascade of green colors layered with the dew on the collection of leaves and scrubs. The fresh scent of the air combined with the mist of morning. At times like this thank your body for its good health, thank your self for your diligence to train and savor each and every run as a special celebration of life in its purest form.

Running allows us to play. As adults we need play time to foster creativity and relaxation. Running allows for us to play alone or play in a group. To enjoy play we need to work. An athlete knows their training may be work, but this work allows them to play.

Those who have been on sabbatical from training discover the human body's great ability to adapt and regenerate strong performance through intelligent training. Intelligent training keeps us improving with combinations of stress and rest. For runners this hard-easy approach is orchestrated in hard-easy days and includes hard-easy weeks. Intelligent training also incorporates walk-run combinations on long run days. Intelligent training recognizes one's personal limits and fitness level. We modify the training, keeping it progressive and challenging but not so wimpy we lack improvement. Adopt this "best effort today" attitude. Give yourself the motto of being slightly better each and every day—it will keep you eager to run!

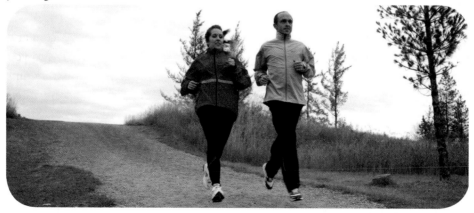

Aging: The 50 Plus Runner

How does aging affect the training schedule of the 50 plus runner?

A sad reality is the one race we all perform at with exactly the same pace is the race against aging!

The primary complaint of the aging athlete is that we simply cannot recover as quickly from high intensity or high volumes. Many runners have adopted a commonly shared choice of running every other day. Treating the aging muscle with respect can allow the athlete to continue to perform near their previous racing targets. Volume and intensity must be reduced as we age. The adaptation phase of your training must be extended to account for this kinder, gentler program.

Between 50 and 60 we see a dramatic fall off and deterioration of skeletal muscles. This is well-documented (F.W. Booth, et al. 1994). About 15% loss of muscle strength per decade up till age 70. After age 70 this decrease jumps to 30% per decade.

We lose our capacity to absorb landing forces, which explains the reason many of us, over 50 years, are always complaining about stiffness in our muscles. Our friend and former Olympian Frank Shorter hobbles when he walks, but he can still run a very respectable marathon. Frank bikes as much as his schedule allows, which takes some of the landing forces away from his training. Combining a routine of swimming and biking with running is an effective way to delay muscle stiffness and progressive joint degeneration.

From my personal incidental experience I often reflect on the runners I used to race against in sub-three-hour marathons; many did not adapt their training and the result was a debilitating injury. For those of us who discovered it is OK to run slow, we are still running and enjoying marathons and the thrill of the finish line. I have coached thousands of runners and have seen many injured and in some cases forced to stop running. One of the major reasons for injuries is running too fast. I have yet to see a running injury from running too slowly. The keys to success in the marathon and in the marathon of life is to stay injury free and to enjoy each run for the sheer joy of running.

Being selective is also a privilege of age. Be selective in your races and selective when you use speed.

Weight training is also fundamental to a runner's career longevity. A factor causing a reduction in V02 max with age is the change in body fat content. Regular weight training can reduce the increase in body fat content with age. Adding weights to your training will improve strength, posture and body composition.

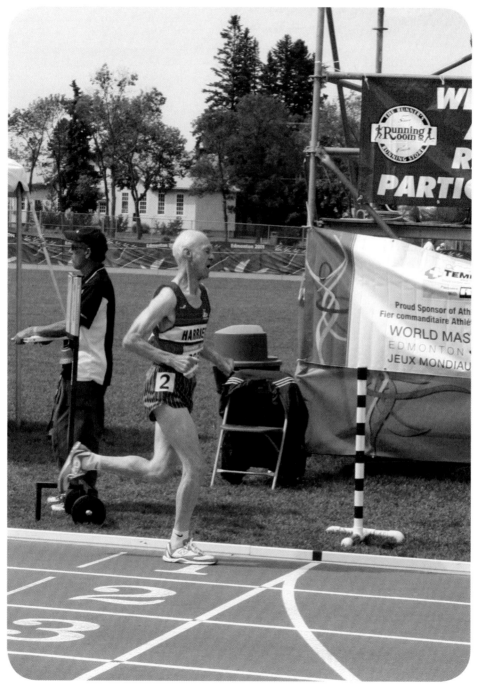

Building Your Program

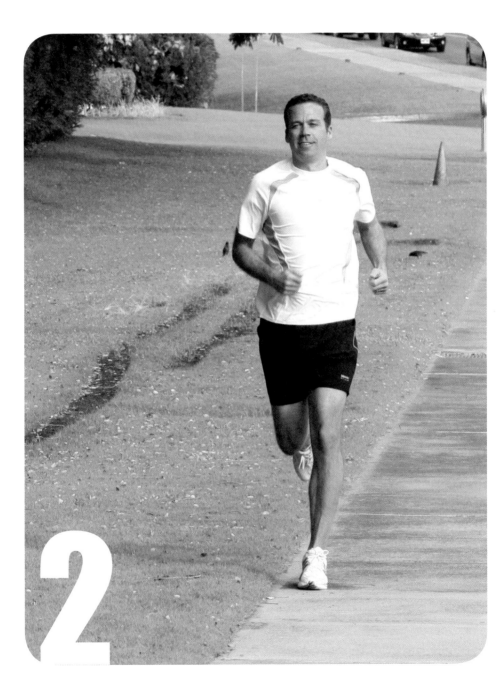

2

Adaptation

Your body will only adapt to unaccustomed stress. In order to stimulate a training response, the stress of a training session must be strong enough to upset the balance of the various functional systems of the body (the cardiovascular system, the skeletal system, the muscular system, etc.). As a result, the body reorganizes the various systems to reestablish a balanced state. This reorganization is the training adaptation, often referred to as supercompensation. The degree of adaptation depends on the degree of imbalance induced: hard training will induce a greater degree of imbalance and a greater degree of adaptation than easy training.

Hard-Easy Principle

The body adjusts to meet exercise induced stresses by enhancing body functions. Excess stress will produce injury and illness. A system of hard (long) runs and easy (short) runs, increasing the distance gradually by 10%, will decrease the likelihood of burnout.

Substitution of alternate aerobic activities or cross-training on one or two easy days a week will also decrease the chance of mental burnout. Rest days are helpful in either case.

Base training constitutes the largest and most important portion of every distance runner's program. For the beginner it should be the sole concentration for at least the first three months. It increases the efficiency of the circulatory system and the strength of the heart muscle. Base training also enhances the ability of the muscle cells to use oxygen when producing energy. Gradually, endurance and speed work are increased. Muscles work more efficiently and withstand the stress of this harder work.

The Foundation of Sport Training

Training principles are the very basic rules that should be followed to ensure a successful training or fitness program and are the foundation from which all programs are developed. At the Running Room, we do not subscribe to the "no pain, no gain" principle of training. This age-old principle doesn't promote a sound training principle. Development of a solid fitness program is determined predominantly by the appropriate implementation of the stress followed by rest principle. This chapter describes the core principles of training that have made the Running Room programs so successful.

Stress and Rest

Stress is another word that can be used for training. In brief amounts, exercise or training stress causes a temporary imbalance in the various body processes (muscular, cardiovascular). In response to this imbalance, the body will react by reestablishing equilibrium and will become stronger and more protected from further imbalance. This is called training. After time, the amount of training stress must become greater and greater to establish an imbalance to promote further training.

Rest should always be combined with training stress, as repair and adjustment to the imbalances can only happen when the body is resting. The rest period should be long enough to allow almost complete recovery from the training session but not so long that you lose the training adaptation. When the rest period is too short, or the stress is too great, the body doesn't have time to repair and adjust, which may cause possible fatigue or injury.

Implementing principles of stress and rest into your program will ensure an adequate training stimulus followed by an appropriate rest period. Even in the early stages of a fitness program, physiological balances can be reestablished in approximately 24 hours. Start out by exercising no more than every other day or a minimum of three times per week.

Practicing the principle of stress and rest will also ensure that the training stress is consistent. If a few days of training are missed, the body may lose some tone and endurance. A day or two of hard training will not make up for what was lost. In fact, it may hurt you in the end by causing undue fatigue or injury. The extra physical strain when trying to make up training will do more harm than just tiring you out, so consistency of training is critical for success. The individual who trains consistently will often see greater improvements than one who trains extremely hard at times and skips training at other times. Think of rest as part of every good training program.

Consistency also has its rewards. As proper training continues, an individual will develop a solid fitness base. A solid fitness base will ensure that when interruption to training does occur for a short time, loss of fitness will be minimal.
The stress and rest principle of training is the foundation of any training program. Its purpose is to ensure an appropriate training stress and adequate rest periods,

thus resulting in the establishment of a consistent pattern of exercise.

Progressive Overload

Running seems to attract hardworking, goal-oriented people who appreciate the fact that the sport rewards honest effort. These individuals have learned that the more they put in, the more they get out. Running is different. Your willpower and your heart-lung machinery can handle much more work than your musculoskeletal system. Beyond a certain point, it's better to relax about your training than to approach every workout in hyperdrive. The following guidelines show you how you can safely enjoy your running without risking injury.

1. Honestly evaluate your fitness level.

If you haven't had a physical exam lately, have one before you begin your running program. Start out running gently and slow to a walk when you feel tired. Remember: you should be able to carry on a conversation as you run. If you're patient with yourself, you can increase your effort as your body builds strength and adapts to the stress of running.

2. Easy does it.

The generally accepted rule for increasing your distance is to edge upward no more than 10% per week. Beginner runners should add just 1 or 2 km per week to their totals. This doesn't sound like too much, but it will help keep you healthy, and that means you can continue building. Start from a base of 20 km per week; you can build up to 40 km per week (enough to finish a marathon, if that interests you) in 10 to 12 weeks. Your long runs are another consideration. To avoid injury or fatigue, these should be increased by only 2 km per week.

3. Plan for plateaus.

Don't increase your distance every week. Build to a comfortable level and then plateau there to let your body adjust. For example, you might build to 20 km per week and then stay at that training level for three or four weeks before gradually increasing again. Another smart tactic is to scale back periodically. You could build up from 10 to 12 to 14 km per week, and then rest with a 10 km week before moving on to 16 km. Don't allow yourself to get caught up by the thrill of increasing your distance every single week. That simply can't work very long.

4. Make haste slowly.

Another cause of injury and fatigue is increasing the speed of your training runs too much and too often. The same is true of interval workouts, hill running and racing. When the time is right for faster-paced running (after you're completely comfortable with the amount of training you're doing) ease into it just once a week. Never do fast running more than twice a week. Balance your fast workouts and your long runs (both qualify as "hard" days) with slower, shorter days. This is the well-known and widely followed hard-easy system.

5. Strive for efficient running form.

You'll have more fun because you won't be struggling against yourself. Poor running form is the cause of many injuries. For example, running too high on the toes or leaning too far forward can contribute to shin splints and Achilles tendonitis. Carrying the arms too high or swinging the elbows back too far can cause back or shoulder stiffness or injury. To run most efficiently, keep your body straight, and concentrate on lifting your knee just enough to allow your leg to swing forward naturally. Combined with a gentle heel landing, this will give you an economical yet productive stride.

6. Turn away from fad diets; go instead with wholesome foods.

Runners function best on a diet high in complex carbohydrates. That means eating plenty of fruits, vegetables, whole-grain products and low-fat dairy foods and avoiding fried foods, pastries, cookies, ice cream and other fat-laden items. Fish, lean meats and poultry are better for you than their high-fat cousins— sausage, bacon, untrimmed red meats and cold cuts. Generally, you're wise to eat three to four hours before running. That way, you're less likely to experience bloating or nausea. Remember: fluids are vital. Aim to drink 8 to 10 glasses of water a day.

7. Hills place an enormous stress on the cardiovascular system, so it's best to warm up for several miles so you raise your heart rate gradually.

When climbing hills, shorten your stride and concentrate on lifting your knees and landing more on the front of your foot. Pump your arms like a cross-country skier. Lean forward but keep your back straight, your hips in, your chest out and your head up. Barreling down a steep hill can multiply skeletal forces several fold, increasing chances of injury. Hold your arms low and tilt your body forward to keep it perpendicular to the slope. Allow your stride to stretch out a little, but don't exaggerate it. Try to avoid the breaking action of landing too hard on your heels.

8. Be smart about injuries.

Runners who interrupt their training programs at the first sign of injury generally recover very quickly. You might not be able to enter the race you're aiming for, but you'll be able to find another one soon. On the other hand, runners who persist in training hard even after they start to break down are courting much more serious injuries. When you develop a persistent running pain, open your eyes and obey the red flag. Stop. Rest. Wait until your body is ready to begin training again. When it is, ease back into your training. Don't try to catch up too quickly: it can't be done.

9. Pay close attention to pain.

It's usually OK to forget mild discomfort if it goes away during a run and doesn't return after. But pain that worsens during a run or that returns after each run cannot be ignored. Remember: pain has a purpose. It's a warning sign from your body that something's wrong. Don't overlook it. Instead, change your running pattern, or if the pain is severe enough, stop running and seek professional help.

"Any Pain, No Brain"

Sport fitness has three basic components:

+ Endurance
+ Strength
+ Speed / Power

Basic Components of Training

Endurance

Endurance must be developed first, for without it most other types of training can not be repeated enough to develop the other components of fitness. In our program, building an endurance base is the primary emphasis. Building a base will train the cardiovascular system to better handle the demands of exercise and will train the specific muscles involved to go the distance. The heart will become stronger and more efficient at delivering oxygenated blood to the muscles and the muscles more efficient at utilizing oxygen for energy and become more resistant to muscular fatigue. These training adaptations lead to enhanced aerobic fitness.

The most common way of developing aerobic fitness is with regular continuous aerobic exercise. Exercise of this nature should be intense enough to raise the heart rate to the 130–150 bpm range (60–70% of your minimum current heart rate) and should be maintained for at least 20 minutes, preferably 30 minutes. The easy test is you should be able to comfortably talk while running. So do the talk test! Muscular endurance is developed somewhat during continuous aerobic training, but is better trained in the weight room by doing many repetitions of low resistance exercise. Circuit training can sometimes be used to combine both muscular endurance and aerobic training.

Strength

Strength can be whole-body strength, as in general conditioning, and specific strength, which is most effective within the range of motion of a given event. Strength is critical to every running event for all athletes. The level of strength has a positive effect on both speed and endurance.

Speed / Power

Speed and power are critical to high level performance. Developing these components of fitness should not be a focus for the first few weeks.

Base Before speed

Before attempting any speed work, you must have built a good base, consisting of the following:

+ Eight weeks of running.
+ At least two months (and preferably three) of aerobic running.
+ Four to 10 weeks of hill training.

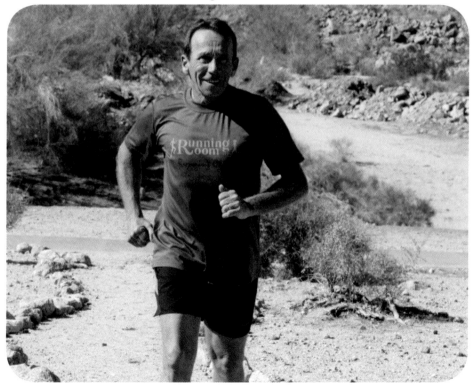

More Is Not Better

There is considerable research which tells us that more is not necessarily better when it comes to exercise. In fact, training to exhaustion does far more to hurt performance than to enhance it. A typical adult can train at far lower levels of intensity than has been traditionally thought and still get fit. Monitoring your heart rate to keep yourself at the right level of exercise intensity has become the training secret of the decade.

Important Tips:

All of us should be able to pass the talk test. The test is simple: if you have difficulty talking then you are running too fast.

Rest:

Walk breaks work! On long runs they are mandatory; they provide many benefits while keeping you highly motivated. During the week, walk breaks are optional. If you are feeling strong on your shorter runs you can run them continuously, but watch the speed. Walk breaks are always optional and a great way to stay highly motivated, minimize injury and improve your recovery. At each group practice run at the Running Room we have a group doing walk-run.

Walking Breaks

The following question is often asked at the end of our Learn to Run Program:

If I can now run continuously for 20 minutes without walking breaks do I need to take them during my long runs? Walking breaks are always optional. They should be incorporated in all long runs. The walk break provides a great platform for the runner to expand the distance of the long run. The key to the running programs developed in this book and in our Running Room clinics is to keep the program gentle and progressive. First, the word gentle. The program is gentle enough to provide the runner with a comfortable, safe system, a program designed to prevent injury and show improvement while keeping runners highly motivated. Second, the word progressive. The program is progressive because it continues to challenge the runner to improve their individual level of wellness and fitness.

The whole purpose of the long run is to build up your endurance training. Endurance training is "Long Slow Distance." This endurance training adapts the runner's fitness to exercising for an extended period of time. The endurance or long run portion of your training is also the fat-burning session. By inserting walk-run combinations we are able to greatly extend the distance we are able to cover on our long run. The added distance has the runner in a fat burning mode for a longer time and challenges the runner to adapt to the rigors of training for a longer period of time. The rest breaks every 10 minutes minimize the risk of injury. The additional stress of an increase of about 10% per week to the long run can be readily added, resulting in a great improvement in the endurance capabilities of the runner. The gradual buildup of distance requires a recovery period after the longer runs. The recovery period can really be enhanced and improved by doing walk-runs during the long run. This improved recovery allows the runner to feel refreshed and ready to run on the shorter midweek runs. By doing the long runs continuously, the runner needs extra rest prior to running again.

The fast, brisk walk provides a gentle and specific stretch to the leg muscles. Sports medicine professionals all encourage and recommend that we stretch our muscles. The stretch provides for more supple muscles with improved range of motion. Strong, flexible muscles will perform better. Think of the walking breaks as "stretch breaks." The stretch can be felt from the hip flexors through the hamstrings, quadriceps, and down into the calves and assorted muscles of the ankle and foot.

The combination of stress and rest is the foundation of any good training program. The rest provides recovery and a rebuilding phase of improvement. The brisk walking breaks provide a phase of active rest. The active rest does two things:

+ The active rest keeps the runner moving forward. Our studies indicate that the average runner will lose less than 15 seconds per kilometer by doing walk-run rather than continuous running. The runner attempting to run continuously will also slow down near the end of the long run. The walk-runner, on the other hand, is able to maintain the pace throughout the long run distance without the dramatic slow down of pace.

+ The active rest helps flush the lactic acid out of our large muscle groups. As we approach our anaerobic threshold, which is 85% of our maximum heart rate, our body starts producing lactic acid. This leaves us feeling heavy-legged with a queasy stomach. The walk-run combinations of active rest will help dissipate this lactic acid build up.

Drop into any of the Running Room's practice runs across North America on a Sunday morning and join in with one of the pace groups doing the walk-run, as well as the long run. There will be a continuous run group heading out, but I highly recommend you join in the larger walk-run group. The walk-run gang are much more social and have a great deal more fun on their long runs. In addition, they break the long run distance into a series of achievable goals while having a fun time. They run 10 minutes and brisk walk for one minute.

Walking breaks work! Try them and you will become a 10 and 1 believer!

Conditioning Program

If you are just beginning, start first with walking and add running later. If you have been inactive for a long time, start with a walking program. Walk before you run. Think of it as a preconditioning program.

Start with a fast walk for 20 to 30 minutes. Slow down if you find yourself short of breath. Don't stop. Keep moving. By pumping your arms as you walk, and really stepping out, you can increase your heart rate to a level nearly equivalent to a slow run. Also, by walking vigorously uphill, you can add to the rigor of your walking workouts.

Once you can walk briskly for 30 minutes, you can start interspersing some easy running into your walking. By slowly exchanging running for walking, over several weeks, you will progress to 20 minutes of running with a one-minute brisk walk at the start and one-minute brisk walk at the end.

The schedule should be run at least three times per week. All running should be done at a conversation pace, and all walking should be done briskly; of course, a proper warm-up and cooldown are required.

Training Rules

1. This program starts conservatively. You can even fall a little behind and still get back on easily.

2. Once you reach the halfway mark, you may find it difficult to keep up unless you run faithfully at least three times a week.

3. If you can't keep up, or lose time from illness or injury, don't panic: stay at the level you can handle or go back a level until you are ready to move on.

4. Remember, it took you a lot of years to get out of shape; take your time getting back into shape.

Your Goal: A program designed to get you running continuously for varying distances. The Running Room Program prepares participants for a long run interspersed with walking breaks.

Seasonal Approach

To build your program using the seasonal approach, start by dividing the year into three major periods, pre-season, in-season and post-season, for example, to give yourself a general focus for your training program. These divisions should help you organize your program according to which activities are the prerequisites to others. In running, for example, base training is the prerequisite to strength training. The progression through the season generally involves a change from predominantly distance training to strength training to higher intensity workouts specific to competition later in the season.

Periodization

If you are currently planning your training around a specific race, you are already practicing a seasonal approach to your training, which is known as periodization. Periodization is a way of structuring your training program using a planned program of base training, strength training, speed training, racing and rest to produce a successful performance without becoming overtrained or injured. This approach to training doesn't mean you have to race, but by planning for peaks in performance it lets you structure your program around the time you would like to be in top shape—like the summer when you might be seen wearing a bathing suit!

Dividing your training into units of time will allow you to structure a progressive increase in training while incorporating rest phases to allow for regeneration and adaptation. Building your intensity or volume progressively requires some rehabilitation, consisting of a rest week or recovery period. A rest week is rehabilitation: it consists of more rest days, and all training sessions are of a lower intensity and volume. You still train but at an adjusted speed and distance.

If you do race, give your body a chance to rest and recover following this peak performance. The distance you ran, the intensity at which you raced and the corresponding muscle soreness determine the amount of recovery you require. If after the race you have no soreness, you can continue training, but do not race or do any speed training during the recovery period. If you have some mild muscle discomfort to the touch, reduce your training for seven days.

If walking is uncomfortable or you are unable to squat with ease, reduce your training for 14 days and do no racing or speed work. If you have pain and discomfort while walking, reduce your training for a full month and do no racing or speed work for a least two months.

How often can we race?

The guidelines I would recommend for racing are: 8 Ks can be run weekly, 10 Ks every two weeks, half marathons once per month, and marathons three times per year. These guidelines will work if you train using a seasonal approach and stay injury free.

The key to increased performance is your body's ability to adapt to the rigors of training and racing.

Building the House

1. Building the Foundation

Building the foundation is usually done with continuous periods of steady effort. In Running Room programs, the continuous effort is sometimes interspersed with short rest breaks. The duration of the session can go from 25 minutes for an easy run to 150 minutes or more for the long sessions of marathon training. With the exception of the short bursts in "fartlek"sessions, the effort is done well below racing speed. The goal is the duration of the session, not the intensity. Walk-run combinations extend the duration of the session. Your heart rate for foundation training is 60–70% of your maximum.

2. Putting Up the Walls

The walls are put up with periods of effort at a pace that is just below the limit of your aerobic training zone. If you like to calculate this effort, use your 10 K race pace: for most people, precise scientific measurements do not come up with anything better. If you wear a heart rate monitor, you will find it showing about 70–80% of your maximum. If you prefer to go "by feel," the pace is the highest you know you can maintain for a longer distance than you are presently covering. With the exception of the short bursts in "fartlek" sessions, the effort is done no faster than this racing speed. The intensity is higher than in the"foundation" session, but the goal is still the duration of the session. At higher levels of intensity, our physiology is designed to slow us down in a short period of time and we are very much aware of this limitation during the effort.

Building Your Program

2

3. Nailing on the Roof

The roof is nailed on with periods of effort that are higher than your race pace. The roof cannot be put on until the walls are built. For an endurance athlete, this kind of training is done only for a short period of time before an important period of competition. If you are not intending to compete, there is little need to enter this high-intensity physiological zone.

Speed Work

The primary benefit of speed work is to teach the body how to run fast when the muscles can't get enough oxygen. To run faster than you have ever run before, you must go beyond your capacity. Speed workouts take you beyond in a regular series of small extensions. By the end speed session, you should have stimulated the demands of the race itself.

Strength Training

Your hill training sessions strengthen the key running muscles in your lower legs, allowing you to shift your weight a bit further forward on your feet and to use your ankles for efficient mechanical advantage-gaining a stronger push-off. Now you're ready for the fast stuff!

Base Period

During the base period, you get your cardiovascular system ready to handle future speed demands. Whether or not you've run speed work before, your base period will improve cardiovascular efficiency.

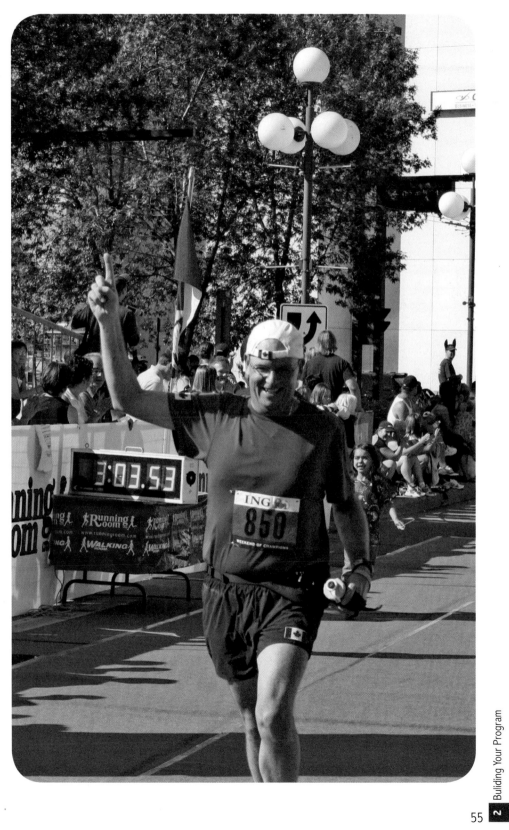

 Building Your Program

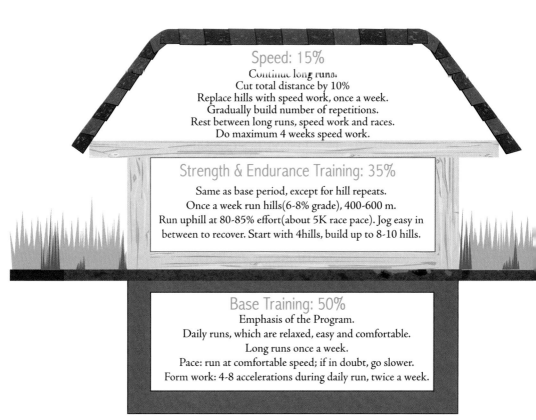

Speed: 15%
Continue long runs.
Cut total distance by 10%
Replace hills with speed work, once a week.
Gradually build number of repetitions.
Rest between long runs, speed work and races.
Do maximum 4 weeks speed work.

Strength & Endurance Training: 35%
Same as base period, except for hill repeats.
Once a week run hills(6-8% grade), 400-600 m.
Run uphill at 80-85% effort(about 5K race pace). Jog easy in between to recover. Start with 4hills, build up to 8-10 hills.

Base Training: 50%
Emphasis of the Program.
Daily runs, which are relaxed, easy and comfortable.
Long runs once a week.
Pace: run at comfortable speed; if in doubt, go slower.
Form work: 4-8 accelerations during daily run, twice a week.

Training Methods

Base

Action

The sum total of the weekly long session and other moderate endurance sessions. Done on easier days.

Purpose

To raise the metabolic rate and anaerobic threshold.

Long Run-Walk

Action

The longest session of your training program, building from 60% to 70% of maximum heart rate.

To build muscular endurance by increasing the capillary network in the working muscles. To raise the anaerobic threshold so that more training is possible in the aerobic zone.

Tempo Runs

Action

Continuous runs at 80% of maximum heart rate for less than race distance. This can be either the entire session or be part of a longer one.

Purpose

To develop stamina and pace judgment.

Tempo Intervals

Action

Repetitions over longer distances than a traditional interval session, with a longer period of recovery in between. Example, 3 X 2000 m near 10 K race pace (80% of maximum heart rate) with 5–7 min. recovery.

Purpose

To develop stamina, consistency and pace judgment.

Rhythm Intervals

Action

A traditional interval session made up of repetitions over shorter distances, with a strict and relatively short recovery. Can be divided into sets if desired. E.g., 10–16 X 400 m (maybe using sets of 4–5).

Purpose

To develop consistent rhythm at race pace. To raise the anaerobic threshold.

Hill Repeats

Action

Repeated efforts up and down a hill with a grade of no more than 10%. Hard up the hill, easy down.

Purpose

To develop muscular strength and raise the aerobic threshold.

Fartlek

Action

A continuous session including changes of pace for various distances of the athlete's choosing. Short bursts at 70–80% effort, plus recovery periods to bring the heart rate down to 120 bpm.

(The nature of fartlek places it in both sections, depending on how the athlete chooses to do it.)

Purpose

To build determination and strength. Fartlek teaches a runner to run at a varied tempo instead of locking into one pace. This will make a runner stronger over a course with varying terrain, and can help a runner learn to stay with their competitors when he or she throw a surge in the middle of a race.

Surges

Action

A more structured form of fartlek. Strictly speaking, this is not true fartlek training; rather it is more of an adaptation of track training used on the roads and trails. Some runners structure their surges runs by timing their hard efforts and rest. This might mean a 2 minute surge followed by a 60 second rest jog, for instance. Others use landmarks as their signals to pick up the pace or ease off. Telephone poles are often used for this purpose. The changes of pace are decided beforehand and can range from 1 min. to several. Surging is a common tactic in marathons during a continuous effort.

Purpose

To develop strength and determination. This will make a runner stronger over a course with varying terrain, and can help a runner learn to stay with their competitors when they throw a surge in the middle of a race.

Speed Intervals

Action

Fast runs over short distances, usually with a relatively long period of recovery to allow the unpleasant side effects of the anaerobic activity to diminish. E.g., 6 X 200.

Purpose

To develop speed endurance, buffer the effects of anaerobic activity and improve coordination.

Overtraining

Overtraining is doing too much too soon. To think that you must have increased your workout or be doing high intensity or have increased distance is a misunderstanding of the term. You can overtrain at any level if you are doing too much too soon. Training is the result of the body adapting to stress. The stress must be regular enough and strong enough to stimulate adaptation, but if it is too strong or too frequent, you will break down—you are overtraining. Rest is the phase during which adaptation takes place, and you become stronger. It is just as important as your workout.

Rest is:

+ Plenty of sleep at night
+ Easy days
+ Days off
+ Alternating activities (e.g., alternating upper-body and lower-body workouts, such as using swimming as a rest from running)

If you do not rest voluntarily, your body will force you to rest—by fatigue, illness, injury, staleness or burnout.

Overtraining is a common cause of poor performance and a common cause of injury. Many personal bests and world records have been set after an injury. This is because an injury is an enforced rest—time for an overtrained body to strengthen and re-establish a balance between stress and adaptation.

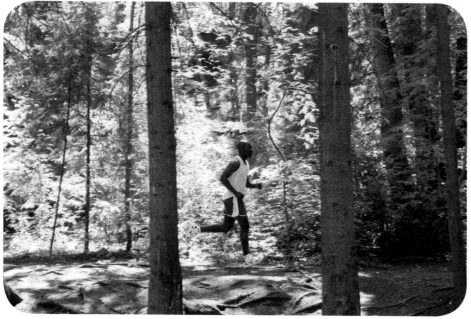

1. Hard Day/Easy Day:

Instead of doing the same workout each day, vary your workouts. Therefore alternate hard and easy days; take days off.

2. The Three 10s:

These may seem conservative but are based on sound training principles:

+ Establish a 10-week training base of endurance before doing any competition, speed work or all out efforts.

+ Increase by 10% per week. That means if you're running 30 km a week you should increase to only 33 km the next week.

+ Make only 10% of your weekly workout high intensity (speed work or competition).

3. Morning Resting Pulse Rate:

When you wake up, rest in bed for 5 minutes and then take your pulse. Any day your pulse is up you haven't adapted to or recovered from your previous day. It should be an easy day or a day off.

If you see a drop in performance your tendency probably is to increase your training. Poor performance is a good indicator of overtraining, so be aware, cut back and apply sound training principles.

Warning Signs of Trouble

The symptoms listed below are warnings that more serious trouble might develop if you don't take immediate preventative action. Develop a sensitive eye to these signals. By quickly interpreting and acting upon these symptoms you can stop trouble at its source.

+ Resting pulse rate significantly higher than normal when taken first thing in the morning.

+ Sudden, dramatic weight loss.

+ Difficulty falling asleep or staying asleep.

- Sores in and around the mouth, and other skin eruptions.

- Any symptom of a cold or the flu (sniffles, sore throat or fever).

- Swollen, tender glands in the neck, groin or underarms.

- Dizziness or nausea before, during or after training.

- Clumsiness—tripping or kicking yourself, for instance—during a run over rather smooth ground.

- Any muscle, tendon or joint pain or stiffness that remains after the first few minutes of running.

Cross-Training

Cross-training can often help you avoid overtraining. Alternate exercises can give your body a break from running if you still want to get in some training.

Treadmill Running

Question:

I was wondering if someone knew how much work the forward motion of a treadmill does for you? How does this affect running outdoors?

Answer:

Treadmill running is slightly easier than outdoor running because of the lack of wind resistance. This enables you to be more efficient in your running on the treadmill. To accommodate for the lack of resistance, increase the treadmill grade to about 2% for all of your workouts. Running on a treadmill is a great way to work on even pacing and to vary the intensity of your workouts. The intensity can be varied using a higher speed or a higher degree of incline for three to five minutes followed by three to five minutes of rest. Long runs can be a social event with a non-running buddy, or your latest TV show can take on a whole new perspective from the treadmill. Safety improves owing to the controlled environment. Like your outdoor workouts, be sure to vary the intensity and duration of the workouts.

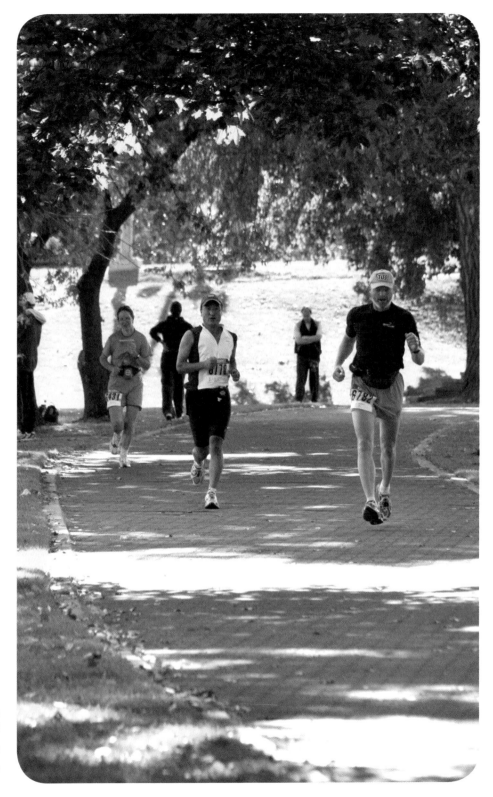

Smoking and Running

I would love to be able to run sometime in the near future. I've always had a strong desire to run and when I've run in the past I have always gotten a rush from doing so. It's a great stress reliever. The unfortunate thing and the source of many of my problems is that I have to quit smoking before I can start running again. Any suggestions? I know that question may sound corny in this day and age of pills, patches, hypnotism, etc.

Answer:

This may sound silly coming from the Running Room guy, but for the time being do not try to stop smoking "cold turkey." You are much better off substituting a positive addiction for a negative one. Try a combination of 20 minutes of walk-run combinations incorporating running for one minute, and walking for one minute. Start with every second day. Each week add one minute of running to each running set.

As an example, in week 2 you will run for two minutes and walk for one minute. As you progress each week and see the benefits of the exercise, you will find the self-motivation to cut back or quit smoking totally. This personal commitment and decision is a much more powerful change of focus and self-improvement than a "patch." Seeing our improvement in appearance and self-esteem drives home the lifestyle change.

Running has a number of marvelous benefits to one's personal life. It's a great stress buster and calorie burner, and, in addition, running with a buddy can be very social. Keep your running and changes fun and positive. Deprivation usually only sets up the urge and desire for the very thing we are trying to do without. A positive change initiates the lifestyle adjustment long term. You can do this. Try the running and enjoy the improvements to the quality of your life. Above all have fun! Think of your new addition as play.

Shoes and Clothing

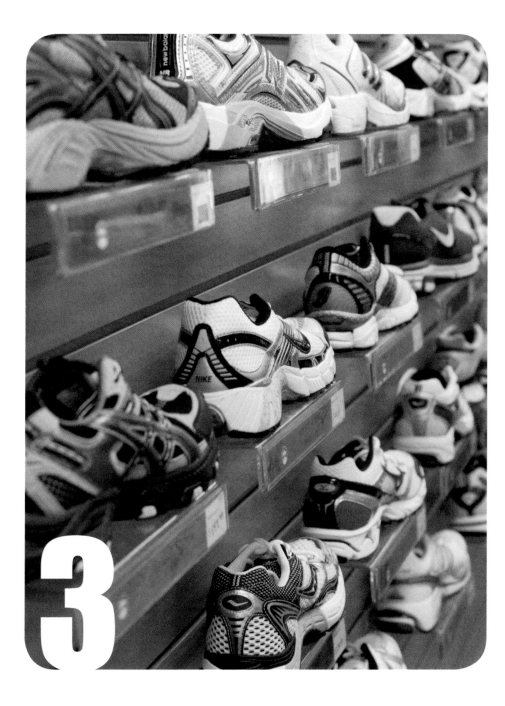

3

Shoes are a runner's most important piece of equipment. The average runner strikes the ground with a force of 3½ to 5 times their weight, which has to be absorbed by the feet and legs. You have to put some thought into which pair you choose. The right pair of shoes can enhance your performance and prevent injuries.

Proper Shoe Selection

Proper shoe selection is an important part of the prevention of injury. Forces greater than three to five times your body weight are placed on your feet and dissipated up your leg when you run. The right running shoes will accommodate your individual needs and can keep you running comfortably.

Determining Your Foot Type

When you run, after your heel strikes the ground your foot pronates by rolling inward and flattening out. Your foot then supinates (rotates outward) after the weight is transferred to the ball of your foot. The foot then becomes a rigid lever so that you may propel yourself forward. Perfect running styles are rare. Over-pronation is more common than oversupination.

The Overpronator

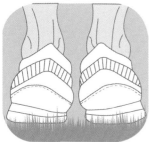

- Feet roll inward too much when running.
- Generally has low arches.
- Knees and kneecaps move towards the inside of the feet when you bend at the knees.
- More susceptible to runner's knee, iliotibial band syndrome, tendonitis, plantar fasciitis.

The Supinator/Under Pronator

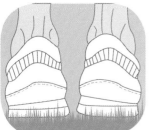

- Lacks normal inward rolling of feet when running.
- Generally has high arches.
- Knees and kneecaps move towards the outside of the feet when you bend at the knees.
- More susceptible to ankle sprains, stress fractures, pain on the outside of the shin and knee, plantar fasciitis.

Reading Old Shoes

Your old shoes reveal many traits about what type of runner you are. If you walk into a Running Room or Walking Room to buy a new pair of running shoes, a salesperson can often put you into the right pair in a matter of moments. Most magicians would never reveal the secrets of their trade, but I can take some of the mystery out of shoe selection with a few tips on how to read your old shoes.

View the upper of the shoe from the rear:
- The shoe's centerline should be perpendicular to the ground.
- The centerline shifts inward, to the medial side of the shoe, if the runner has overpronated.
- The centerline shifts outward, to the lateral side of the shoe, if the runner has supinated.

Check the condition of the midsoles:
- The midsole compresses uniformly if the runner has normal pronation.
- The midsole compresses more on the inside of the shoe if the runner has overpronated.
- The midsole compresses more on the outside of the shoe if the runner has supinated.

Check the wear on the upper:
- The upper retains its shape if the runner has normal pronation.
- The upper sags inward from the toe area if the runner overpronates during push-off.

Shoe Requirements
The Overpronator Category
- Straight or semicurved last.
- Maximum rear-foot stability.
- Substantial extended medial support.

The Stability Category
- Semicurved last.
- Moderate pronation control.
- External counters.
- Durable multidensity midsole material.

The Neutral Category
- Curved or semicurved last.

- Low or moderate rear-foot stability.
- Flexible midsoles.
- Additional cushioning in midsole.

Guidelines to Find the Best Shoe

- Shop in the afternoon to get the right fit.
- Try on both shoes with the same type of sock to be worn during the activity.
- Try on several different models to make a good comparison.
- Walk or jog around the store in the shoes.
- Check the quality of the shoes. Look at the stitching, eyelets and gluing. Feel for bumps inside the shoe.
- The sole should flex only where your foot flexes.
- Your toes should not be pressing against the end of the shoe when standing nor should there be too much room (a centimeter or more). Shoes too big or too small can cause injury to the toenails while running.
- The heel counter should fit snugly so that there is no slipping at the heel.
- Shoes should be comfortable on the day you buy them. Don't rely on a break-in period.
- Consult the staff at the Running Room for help in selecting the correct shoe.

Terms Used by Shoe Manufacturers

Arch Support:

Refers to the inside portion of the shoe directly below the arch of the foot. Most shoes don't have a separate arch support unless it is attached to the removable insole.

Strobel Stitch Lasting:

A new and widely excepted method of stitching the upper of the shoe onto the outer edge of a soft and pliable material, which resembles the shape of the insole. This is then attached to the midsole. The advantage of this method is to provide a softer, lighter and more flexible footbed while providing some torsional rigidity.

Combination Lasting:

A combination of two techniques—board lasting and slip lasting—for joining the upper, last and midsole of a shoe. Usually the back of the shoe is board-lasted for stability while the front is slip-lasted for flexibility. This combination gives stability in the rear-foot with flexibility and cushioning in the forefoot.

Slip Lasting:

A technique for joining the upper, last and midsole of a shoe. The upper of the shoe is placed over the last and sewn together at the bottom, similar to a moccasin. It's then attached to the midsole. Slip-lasted shoes have no boards to cause stiffness. On the other hand, they are less stable than board-lasted shoes.

Curve-Lasted:

Refers to the curvature of a shoe. Curve-lasted shoes have an angle between the rear foot and the forefoot. Most people have moderately curved feet, and shoe companies work with lasts curved about seven degrees. This is comfortable for most runners. The average runner should stay away from severely curved shoes, which can cramp and blister the toes and forefoot.

Straight-Lasted:

As with the term curve-lasted, this refers to the curvature of a shoe. A straight-lasted shoe is constructed on a last with no curve. Theoretically, the shoe could be worn on either foot. Straight-lasted shoes are perfectly adequate for most runners and clearly the best selection for runners with flat feet.

External Heel Counter Stabilizers:

Supports that keep the heel counter from breaking away from the midsole under stress. They're usually designed to help control excess motion, and nearly all of the better made motion-control shoes have some heel counter support.

Heel Counter:

Stiff plastic material that is firmly attached to the rear base of the shoe. An extended heel counter that runs along the medial (inside) edge of the shoe will increase stability and reduce foot pronation and rotation.

Insoles:

Also called sockliners. These line the inside bottom of a shoe and are often removable. If a shoe doesn't come with a good smooth one, replace the insole with whatever insert you need for healthy running.

Last:

The basic form on which a shoe is built. This provides a sculpted profile, which resembles an anatomically correct representation of the foot. Many shoes are now built gender specific as men and women require different configurations.

Midsole Density:

Relates to the firmness of the midsole. A multidensity midsole has materials of different firmness in strategic locations, which can be a big advantage to runners with certain gait patterns. For example, a heavy pronator needs cushioning where the heel strikes, but still needs firmness for stability when the foot starts to roll inward. With a multidensity midsole, the lateral (outer) part of the shoe, where the heel strikes, is soft for shock absorption, and the medial (inner) side is firm for increased stability.

Outsoles:

The undersurface of a shoe. Outsoles can be divided into two major categories: they are more aggressive (lugged); or more sculptured and road friendly (herringbone). If you're going to be running on grass or dirt trails, lugged shoes provide excellent traction. The more road friendly sole is better suited for asphalt or cement. The longest-lasting outsole material has more carbonized blown rubber in the forefoot along with added flez grooves to help heel to toe transition.

Uppers:

The top covering of a shoe. Mesh Nylon is the best material for the uppers, because it puts little abrasive force on the foot and allows it to breathe.

Three Types of Shoes

1. Motion Control

You quickly break down midsoles, overpronate and need a firm midsole with a sturdy heel counter.

Motion Control Features

- Straight or semicurved last.
- Maximum rear-foot stability.
- Substantial extended medial support.

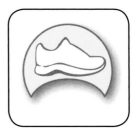

2. Cushioning

You need cushioning, a flexible forefoot and no motion control features.

Cushioning Features

- Curved last.
- Low or moderate rear-foot stability.
- Soft midsoles.
- Additional cushioning in midsole

3. Stability

You need extra cushioning and some degree of stability, and you are not an excessive pronator.

Stability Features

+ Semicurved last.
+ Moderate pronation control.
+ External counters.
+ Durable, multidensity midsole materials.

A Visual Breakdown of Your Shoe

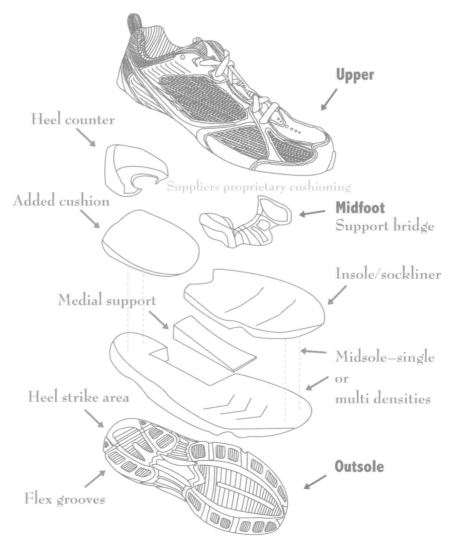

Upper

Heel counter

Added cushion

Suppliers proprietary cushioning

Midfoot
Support bridge

Insole/sockliner

Medial support

Heel strike area

Midsole–single
or
multi densities

Outsole

Flex grooves

Foot Characteristics for Each Shoe Type

1. Motion Control Foot Characteristics

+ Feet and ankles roll inward (excessive, medial).
+ Low/flat arches.
+ Knees move towards middle when bending.
+ Injuries: knee pain, IT band, plantar fasciitis.

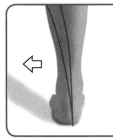
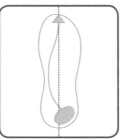
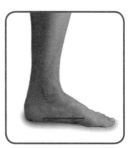

2. Stability Foot Characteristics

+ Ankles roll inward (moderately).
+ Normal-sized arch, semi-flexible arch.
+ Knees slightly roll in when bent.
+ Injuries: knee pain, IT band, plantar fasciitis.

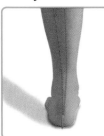
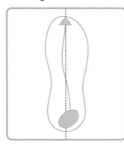
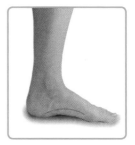

3. Cushioning Foot Characteristics

+ Ankles roll to the outside (lateral).
+ High and/or rigid arches.
+ Underpronates.
+ Injuries: stress fractures, pain on outside of shin or knee.

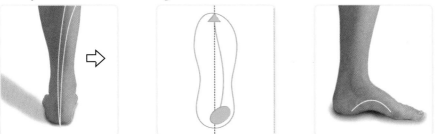

3 Shoes and Clothing

How to Determine Your Foot Type

1. Wet footprint

All you need for this one is a piece of paper and water. Wet your foot and make an imprint with your foot on the paper. Look in the arch area, if you see a dry space between the heel and the ball of your foot, that would indicate you have a high, rigid arch, which means you have a neutral foot type or belong to the cushion category (yellow). If you see a portion of the area between the heel and the arch filled in, that would indicate your arch is lower and may in fact collapse, which means you are a normal pronator foot type or belong to the stability category (blue). If the area between the heel and the ball of your foot is completely filled in, that means you belong to the overpronator foot type or motion control category (red). This an easy way to get an idea of your foot type.

2. Feet shoulder width apart

Bend at the knees and hold in that position. You will want to look at where your knees line up in respect to your big toe. Try to imagine a plumb line from the top of your knee to the top of your foot. If your knee is to the inside of the big toe, that would indicate that your feet have an inward/medial roll. You would want to look at the stability category or the motion control category depending on how much to the inside the knee comes. The farther to the inside the knee comes the more support you will need. If the knee lines up more to the outside/lateral side of the big toe, that would indicate that your arch is more rigid and you would want to look at the neutral category. This is an easy step that you can do to get a good idea of how much support you will need.

3. Lunge forward

Lunge forward and hold in that position. You will again be able to see where the knee is in comparison to the big toe (same as above). This will also work better if you have another person watching from the front. The person watching from the front should be looking at the knee position and also the arch and ankle. If the arch and ankle look very straight then that would indicate more of a cushion category foot type. If the arch looks like it is starting to flatten and the ankle looks like it is starting to role inward/medial then that would indicate more of a stability category foot type. If the arch is flat to the ground and the ankle looks like it is rolled inward/medial side more excessively, that would indicate more of a motion control foot type.

4. Old shoes

If you have a pair of worn athletic shoes, you can use them to read the wear pattern on the sole to get an idea of your foot type. Pick up your right shoe and look at the sole. You will most likely notice that there is some wear on the left side of the heel. This is normal wear. If you look more towards the front of the shoe or the forefoot you will be able to get a really good idea what category you belong to. If you see wear on the far left/lateral side of the forefoot or more to the center, this would indicate that you belong to the cushion category. If you notice wear more to the right/medial side, that would indicate you belong to the stability category. If you notice that the wear is on the far right/medial side, that would indicate you would need more of a motion control shoe.

5. Have someone watch you run

If you are able to get a friend watch you run as normal as possible in bare feet or in socked feet then they will want to look for some key characteristics such as ankle movement and knee movement. If you see the knee lining up with the top of the big toe and the ankle rolling in a straight position from heel to toe-off or movement to the outside or lateral side then this would indicate a more cushion category foot type. If you see the knee rolling inward/medial past the big toe and the ankle also rolling inward/medial then this would indicate more of a stability foot type. If you notice the knee rolling excessively past the big toe and the ankle rolling inward in an excessive way then this would be more of a motion control foot type. With this exercise I would suggest to run towards and away from the person to give them a chance to see you from both directions.

Steps in Selecting the Best Shoe

If you visit your local Running Room every six months, you will seldom find the same model of your most trusted running partner: the running shoe. Even when the model is still in existence, production changes often leave it fitting or working like a different shoe from the one with which you had success. Most runners have made their share of shoe buying mistakes and consequently have a closet of little-worn shoes to show for it. With the advent of discount shoe stores, the number of shoe mistakes seems to be increasing. The constant search for a bargain leads most runners to a highly rated shoe at a great price from a discount store or a mail order outfit at least once. Most of these bargains, however, have disappointed their owner. The best advice for your purchasing decision is to get the best advice and solicit the advice of a grassroots specialty running store. These folks use the equipment daily and are trained to find a shoe that best fits

Shoes and Clothing

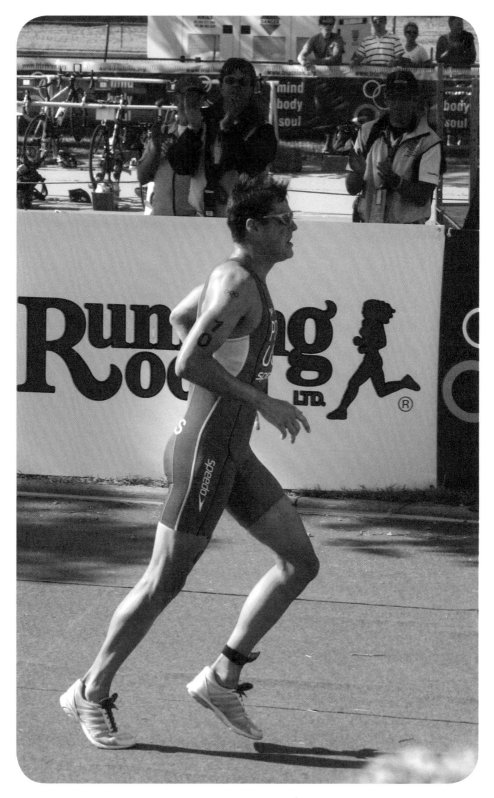

the needs of the customer. Moreover, they are in touch with the shoe gossip grapevine. They can often steer you away from a costly bargain.

Tips for Shoe Buying

1. Spend Time.

Set aside up to an hour for your running shoe purchase. Don't go if you are in a rush. There are lots of little problems that appear only when you have time to compare products. You must walk and run in the shoe. Do not be rushed into a shoe decision.

2. Don't Pick Someone Else's Shoe.

Just because it worked well for a friend does not mean it will work for you. The best shoe for one runner can actually be injurious to another. More than other sport shoes, running shoes are designed to accommodate specific types of feet. You must find out what works for you.

3. Bring Your Worn Out Shoes.

Your current running shoes and socks will help your shoe expert determine wear and fit. Experienced shoe salespeople can collect vital information from a pair of worn running shoes. They can "read" your wear pattern and determine how your needs have been met by your current shoe. You will need socks to simulate the exact fit you desire. If you wear orthotics or use a foot device of any type, bring them along too.

4. Sales Questions.

Your store staffperson should ask you about your running history, upcoming goals, terrain, past injuries, etc. The more information, the better your chance for a good fit. A knowledgeable sales person can help you avoid problem shoes and cut down the searching time.

5. Foot Exam.

The staffperson should examine your foot for width and foot type. Whether your foot is floppy or rigid will determine what type of shoe will work for you. Shoes must be fitted to the shape and function of your feet. The care taken by a trained salesperson can result in a better shoe for you.

6. Fitting to the Shape of Your Foot.

Common sense will lead you to a good fit. Places where the shoe causes pressure on your foot are susceptible to blisters, which can produce pain while you are running. Avoid them! A loose fit, however, will allow the shoe to slip on your foot, which can also cause blisters. When the foot slides excessively, you will lose energy on the push off.

7. A Snug Fit.

Your foot should feel secure on the heel and across the breadth of your foot (the widest part). It is fine to pull the laces so that the shoe is snug, but do not pull it until it hurts or puts pressure on any part of the foot. A snug fit will give your foot a feeling of security without discomfort. How and where you tie the shoe-lace will determine how snugly it will fit your heel. You can adjust the laces on a normal shoe so that you can tie the shoe tight and yet provide room for your foot by loosening other laces. Many of today's shoes have an optional lace hole at the top which gives you an option of even tighter lacing.

8. Selecting the Right Last.

The shape of the shoe is determined by the "last" or form around which the shoe is made. Today shoes are built on varying degrees of curved and straight lasts. A perfectly straight right shoe will look the same as a perfectly straight left one. A very curved shoe by contrast, bends strongly to the inside. If you have a curved foot and you wear a straight shoe, you will feel pressure on the inside of your big toe and will tend to roll off the outside. There are so many shoes with different configurations that your chances of finding one that matches your foot are excellent. Do not buy one that pinches or rubs against your foot. On the other hand, a larger size will not support your foot and will cause it to slide around inside the shoe.

9. The Selection Process.

First, select two to three shoes that work best for your foot function, rigid or floppy. Once you have narrowed down the candidates, you are ready to compare the fit of each shoe. Finally, stand around, walk around and run in each shoe to see how it actually performs. Spend some time in the shoes and you'll tend to get a much better fit.

10. Running in Cross-training or Aerobic Shoes.

A common asked question is, "Can I run in cross-training or aerobic shoes?" The simple answer is no. Shoes for running are designed for the forward motion and for cushioning the impact of running, whereas cross trainers are designed for some other specific use and support more lateral movement. Aerobic shoes are designed for lateral support and toe flexibility. Running shoes are built for a particular style of running and cushioning. They are also built for forward motion and support the foot from heel to toe transition.

11. Where to Start.

The very best way to determine what you require in a shoe is to do an analysis of the runner's gait and foot-strike.

12. How Do I Know When I Need a New Shoe?

The average life of a shoe, based on the manufacturer's and the sports medicine testing, is approximately 800–1000 km (500–600 mi.). Many times the shoe's upper will still be in great shape, but the cushioning and supportive features have been lost. A good test is to drop in when you have 800 km on your shoes and compare a run around the block in a new pair to the old ones. Specialty stores like the Running Room will let you do just that. The key to staying off the injury list is to keep your shoes in good shape, so they can keep you in good shape. Happy, healthy running!

13. Lightweight Training or Racing Shoes.

You're training hard, feeling good and ready to run your goal event in your goal time. This is when you may want to look at purchasing a lightweight shoe to be used only on race day. They are extremely light and comfortable, providing you the feeling that you can "fly." Putting on a pair of lightweight shoes on race day is the final stage in your preparation. When you put them on you put yourself into a mental framework for running. Lightweight shoes may be light shoes, but they do provide very good cushioning for racing. Some shoes come with additional support and stability for those who tend to overpronate or need a little more arch support.

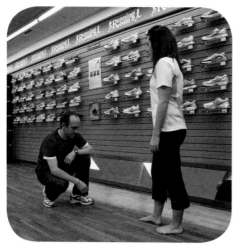 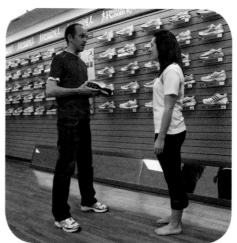

Running Gear and Accessories

Besides shoes, there's an almost endless variety of clothing and accessories that can make your running more enjoyable. Below you will find a summary of basic clothing and accessory needs, what to look for and why. For a more detailed review of clothing needs related to weather, look in Chapter 4, Weather, Warm-Weather Clothing, page 96 and Winter Clothing, page 113.

Socks

Socks are important. After all, if your feet aren't comfortable, your walk won't be either. Socks have a range of thickness: thin, midweight and cushioning. They can be made with a single or double layer of fabric and all synthetics and wool that wick moisture away and help cushion your feet. Some socks have reflective lettering or markings on the ankle to help keep you visible after dark. Take along your shoes if you plan to buy socks, so you'll know exactly how they'll feel out on the road.

Outer Layer

A good jacket can take you from fall through to spring, when it's layered properly. Most importantly, you want a fabric that is windproof and breathable. Water resistant is also good. Vents along the back, zippered vents under the arms and adjustable sleeve cuffs allow you to control the amount of moving air flow you want on a particular day. Reflective strips are great for those winter walks when the daylight disappears long before your walk is over. Some jackets have a panel in the back that can drop down and cover your posterior, warding off the wind and rain, and a drawstring waist helps keep the wind out.

Zippered pockets are also helpful to hold keys and cell phone for an emergency phone call.

For all your walking gear, think fit, function and fashion. You want to look good, feel good and walk your best.

Base, Inner or Single Layer

Forget cotton. It absorbs moisture, which causes chafing on longer walks. Look for a synthetic fabric designed to wick moisture away from the body. A snug fit will allow the fabric to perform the wicking action. By doing so, you stay dry and cool in the heat and warmer in colder conditions.

Pants, Capris and Shorts

Look for fabric that wicks moisture away from the body. You want protection according to the seasons from the various elements like wind and rain.

Outer Layer

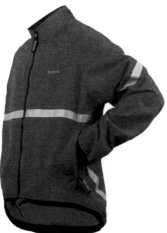

Inner Layer

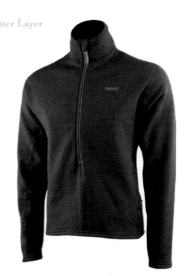

Capris

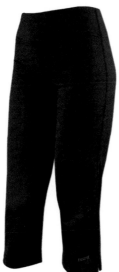

Pants

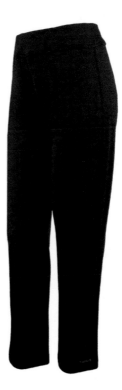

Socks

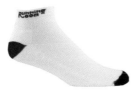

Socks

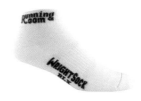

3 Shoes and Clothing

Mid Layers

Look for fleece with the similar performance and functionality as the jacket. Typically, it should be a heavier weight fabric than your base layer. A multifunctional piece that can be worn on cold days or as the outerwear piece of a base layer. Look for a front zipper to allow for temperature control and small pockets to carry the essentials.

Underwear

Look for a technical fabric that will help carry the moisture from your skin to the next layer.

Women: A supportive bra is essential for comfort during your workout. Different features are needed to accommodate different shapes and sizes. Look for these items in high support bras:
+ Encapsulated Cups
+ Compression
+ Adjustable Straps
+ Hook and Eye Back Closure
+ Non-Stretch Molded Cups

Men: For maximum protection during cold weather, especially in the wind, look for a boxer or brief with a wind panel.

Hats

A good percent of your body heat can be lost through the head, so a hat that covers the ears is needed in winter, and the face cover in very cold temperatures. Depending on the temperature, a band over the ears can do. In summer, a walking cap with a broad rim made of breathable fabric can protect from harmful UV rays and rain.

Mittens and Gloves

Your hands do very little work to generate heat during walking, so it is important to protect them from the cold. Look for windproof and wickable fabric. For colder conditions mittens are warmer than gloves.

Hats

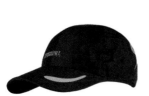

Underwear

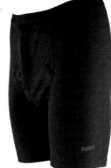

Mid Layers

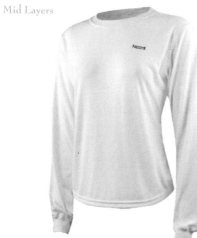

Underwear

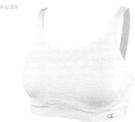

Mittens and Gloves

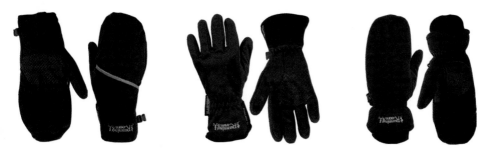

Speed, Distance and Heart Rate

One of the biggest challenges for runners has been to monitor the intensity of workouts, pace and distance. You will find lots of walking speedometers—odometers that claim they can tell you how far and how fast you are running. However, many speedometers can be tricky to get calibrated for walking and rely on input of your stride length. They will always vary by 10% or more on distance, and therefore on speed. Technology now allows for the extremely simple and accurate speed and distance monitors to work right out of the box. Let's review what's available.

There are a number of methods of calculating running speed, pace and distance. Some of these units use GPS like the Garmin® products. The GPS devices can be used for any outdoor sport, and most will download collected data to your computer. Every runner should have one. A single wrist unit uses GPS satellites to trace your outdoor workout. Displays speed, distance, pace, time and laps in large display. Chart your route as you run, and it can point you back to start. Pace alerts and a virtual partner can pace your workout. You can download all data to a computer with the provided serial interface. It generally has free logbook software, or uses free online GPS Visualizer programs that come with the units. Many models are available with or without a heart rate monitor to help you make the most out of your training. Train in a certain heart rate zone to improve your fitness level or compare your pace and heart rate to past performance on the same workout.

Others use a highly accurate and sensitive accelerometer device that discreetly attaches to the shoe laces, Nike®, Polar® and adidas® miCoach PACER. These footpod devices are not like the basic pedometer we are most familiar with. They are highly accurate and they do not rely on the user to set stride length, etc. The Polar® Footpod accurately measures your running speed/pace and distance. This essential piece of kit attaches to your laces and will be with you every step of the way. With the Nike® Sports Kit you put your sensor in your shoe, and you're ready to run. The receiver connects to your iPod Nano, collecting workout data with every step. This pedometer sensor transmits data wirelessly to an iPod nano where you can view it and have it spoken to you over your music mix. It uses an accelerometer rather than GPS, so accuracy varies if your stride varies. It works indoors or outdoors. The adidas® miCoach PACER measures heart rate, distance, pace, stride rate, calories burned, and elapsed time. It works with any MP3 player (if you like to listen to music while you run) and syncs to adidas.com/micoach where you can track your progress, see detailed analysis of your run and receive online coaching feedback.

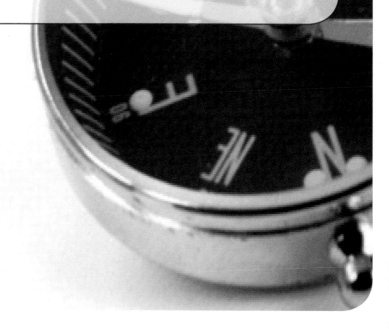

What is GPS?

Global Positioning System (GPS) is the core technology behind many new products that track your training and wirelessly sends your data to your computer. Each walk is stored in its memory, so you can review and analyze the data to see how you've improved. Monitor your time, distance, pace and calories.

Originally developed in 1973 by the U.S. Department of Defense for military purposes, the NAVSTAR GPS network consists of 30 satellites orbiting the earth every 12 hours, and five ground stations that monitor the satellites' position in space and operational status. To determine your location and other data accurately, such as current and average speed, pace, directional heading and elevation, GPS devices use a receiver to acquire signals from at least four of these satellites to calculate the location within 10 meters. The device uses four simple data points (latitude, longitude, altitude and time) collected every few seconds.

Running Gear and Accessories Checklist Before the Race

Cap

A breathable, lightweight cap that will help keep you cool and keep the sun's damaging rays off of you during the race is a good choice.

Water bottle

Most good races will have adequate water along the course. If you're unsure of the frequency of the water stations, wear a torso pack to take you own water with you.

Bodyglide / Slick Stick

Will keep you from chafing.

Pedometer

Pedometers are adjustable to your stride length to measure the distance run. Some have a stopwatch.

Shirt

Pick one that gives you both comfort with sun and wind protection.

Gel Flask

Holds up to five gels and can be carried on a torso belt.

Watches

A runner's watch is essential in gauging the intensity and duration of your workouts. It also gives the run/walk ratio. Be sure to get one that is waterproof and readable in the dark. Sometimes a watch, pedometer and heart rate monitor can all be found in the same device.

Shorts/Tights

There are some great technical fabrics that will keep you dry and chafe-free in a variety of conditions.

Race number

Make sure you have it and make sure you pin it on the singlet or shirt that you will be wearing in the race. Take a few extra pins or race belt.

Duffel Bag

Keeps all your workout essentials organized in 3 separate compartments, shoes, dry clothes, and wet clothes. Features a side pocket with a detachable key chain and waterproof pocket, adjustable strap and sidereflectivity. 45L Capacity.

Water belt

Look for a light, snug fit around the waist so your bottle won't jiggle uncomfortably, even with an angled bottle. Some have pockets for keys, food and change, and are insulated for your water to stay cold.

Shoes

The best shoes to race in are the ones you trained in. Some folks like racing flats for shorter races, but with improved shoe technology making high-quality, lightweight trainers available, most opt for their training shoes.

Socks

Choose a comfortable pair that you have used in training.

Gel

A must have for long runs, giving you the extra energy to keep going.

Reflective Clothing and Accessories

Working out after dark or early in the morning? Make sure you can be seen. Reflective clothing and accessories adds a measure of safety to your workout without adding a heavy layer. Reflective arm bands can be added to any running outfit.

Heart rate monitor / GPS

Very complex monitors show heart rate, intensity, distance, repeats, GPS, memory and more. Monitors have become a tool for the modern runner.

Timing Chip

The new timing systems sometimes sell individual timing chips to racers. If you have one of these, be sure to take it along with you.

Weather

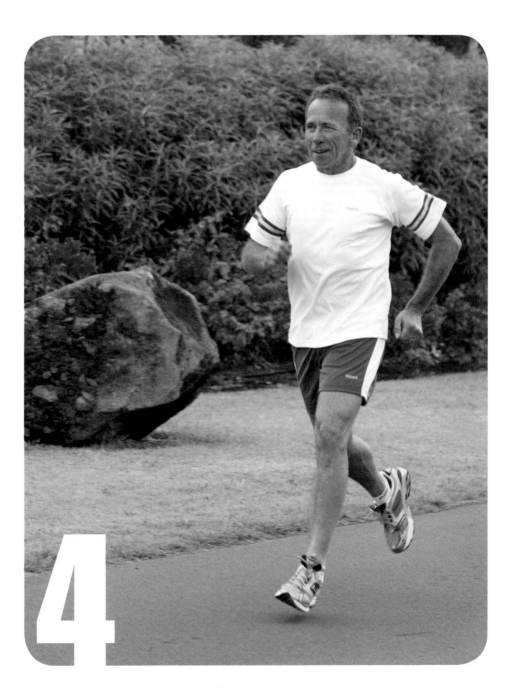

4

Hot Weather Training

In most cases we are not often exposed to consistently high temperature conditions. However, we are often exposed to dramatic temperature changes. This presents us with the challenge of being sure that we are properly prepared for hot weather running. You'll know from your winter holiday that a certain amount of acclimatization to hot weather occurs in a few days. The heat that blankets you as you leave the plane does not seem so bad when you head home. Acclimatization is not immunity: it simply means that your body is automatically taking precautions.

Heat is the one of the endurance athlete's greatest enemies. Heat stress does not need to progress very far before it becomes a medical emergency. It may be unpleasant to contemplate, but heat works on the protein in the body in much the same way as it does on any other protein—it starts to cook! Luckily we have defense mechanisms that protect us. Distance athletes may not like the slowing down that these mechanisms produce, but they are there for our protection. At the first sign of any symptoms, stop, cool off and seek help. Your cooling mechanism operates on water. In hot conditions, you need to drink frequently before, during and after exercise. If you feel thirsty, you are already dehydrated. For the length of normal fitness activities, plain water is your most effective drink. Sports drinks work best immediately after you have finished.

Symptoms

Symptoms come in degrees of severity. Heat stress is followed by heat exhaustion which is followed by heatstroke, a life threatening condition. These levels are reached as your cooling mechanisms reach and go beyond their capacity.

Heat Stress

Under heat stress, your cooling system is working at the upper limit of its capacity. You will not be able to exercise as vigorously as you can under cooler conditions (but, if you're in a race, neither will any of your competitors). You will be sweating profusely and you will likely not be enjoying the effort as much as you otherwise might. You will likely feel muscle cramps.

Heat Exhaustion

Heat exhaustion means that your cooling system is overloaded. It is still working, but it is not able to keep up with the cooling demands. Danger is mounting. The body defends you by slowing you down even more, actually trying to make you stop, so that the production of body heat does not continue. Your pulse grows weak, you look pale, and you may actually feel chills. You begin to feel dizzy and disoriented; speech slurs and muscle control is lost. With rest, fluids and external cooling, the heat exhausted athlete will recover quite quickly. But the body keeps up its protection as you recover. It doesn't want you to exert yourself for a while. You become very tired and will doze off, your rest often interrupted by bouts of vomiting. Finally, you will be able to sleep off your experience, likely waking with a wicked headache as a reminder of the stress you were under.

Heatstroke

Heatstroke is when your cooling system simply gives up. If you get heatstroke, you won't remember much about it. You will wake in a hospital bed some time afterwards with an IV in your arm putting fluids directly back into your body. After a short rest, you will be able to go home. You may wonder what all the fuss was about. In the meantime, people worked furiously to keep you alive. You stopped sweating. You collapsed and remained unconscious. You were rushed to the hospital and packed in ice, because your body no longer had a way to cool itself. Your body temperature was so elevated that your brain was in danger of being permanently damaged. You were lucky to wake up at all.

Precautions

There are some precautions you can take that will make your hot-weather running safer.

1. Drink at least two cups of water before and a cup for every 15 to 20 minutes during your run.

2. Water is the best drink for exercise lasting less than three hours; over three hours we suggest a sports drink because it will replace lost electrolytes and provide some fuel (sugar) for exercise. If you are going to use a commercial sports drink, be sure to try it in training prior to a race.

3. Wear a vented cap, sun visor, sunglasses and protective sunscreen. If you are sun-sensitive or concerned about sun exposure, wear some of the new long-sleeve CoolMax or Fit-Wear shirts. They are both safe and cool.

4. Lubricate your underarms and inner thighs. Gentlemen, Bodyglide your nipples and ladies, the bra line. This will reduce chafing, a common problem in the summer months.

5. Avoid the use of alcoholic beverages. They will only make you feel warmer

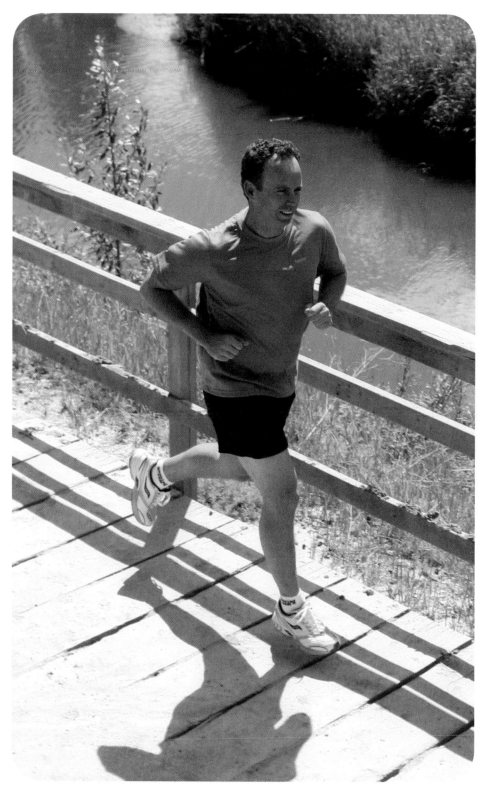

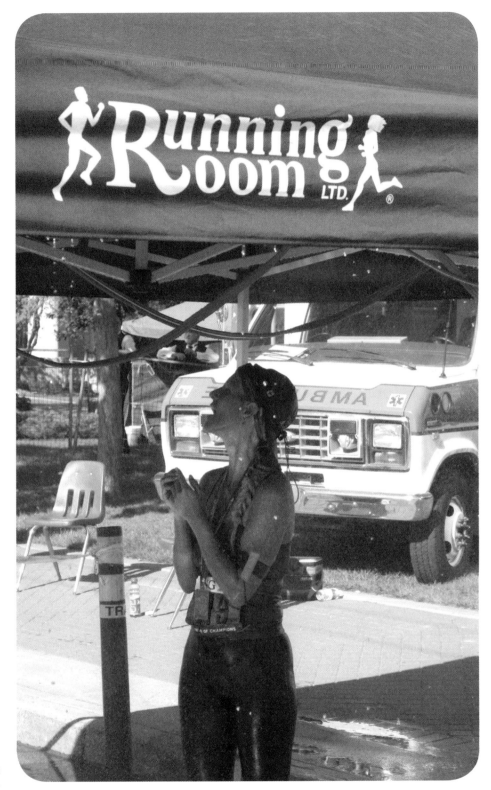

as their calories are burned quickly, raising your metabolic rate and body temperature. Alcohol is a diuretic, bringing a risk of dehydration.

6. Adjust your intensity to the temperature. In extreme conditions, slow down your pace.

7. Increase your intake of vitamin C. It is a natural and effective defense against heat stroke, cramps, prickly heat rash and exhaustion.

8. Let someone know your route if you are running alone. Better still, run with a buddy—you'll run with less intensity and it will be more social.

9. If you plan to race on a hot-weather holiday, give yourself four to five days to adjust to the heat.

10. Early mornings are the best time to run. Sunset runs can catch you out in the dark.

11. Water running can be very social and a cool, high-quality workout.

12. Include lots of fruit in your diet. Watermelon, oranges, bananas and strawberries are a good way to take in vitamin C and potassium, two nutrients that are lost when we sweat.

13. Take a fresh change of clothes with you if you are running out of a park so you don't get chilled after the run.

14. Savor the odd low-fat frozen treat to reward yourself for keeping the daily workout fun!

15. Skim milk is also a great cool drink. It contains a very low fat content.

Warm-Weather Clothing

This is the time when all you want to do is take it off, but putting something on may keep you cooler and protect you from the sun's harmful rays.

What to wear when the temperature rises:

Despite what you have been told, cotton is not the best. Cotton holds moisture, and a lot of it.

• Exercising in a sweat-soaked cotton shirt on a hot day reduces the ability of water to evaporate from your body. This reduces cooling, particularly in a humid environment.
• Cotton loses its soft texture when wet, which can often cause chafing in places where it comes into contact with the skin.

What to look for:

Surprisingly enough, look for garments made of synthetics, such as polyester or nylon, CoolMax and Supplex. These are special weaves that enable them to repel moisture and enhance evaporation. The more evaporation, the greater the cooling effect on the body.

Remember:

+ Light-colored garments absorb less light and therefore keep you cooler.
+ On a bright day, covering up reduces heat accumulation brought on by direct sunlight.
+ Wearing fabrics such as CoolMax and Supplex keeps you cooler and dryer and may help reduce summer chafing.
+ Wear a hat. Protect your head from the heat and direct sunlight (especially men who are a little thin on top).

Is It Safe Out There?

Many factors influence your decision to exercise in hot weather. Acclimatization and hydration aside, there are days, or at least hours during those days, when you shouldn't even try to exercise. When deciding if conditions are safe for strenuous exercise you should refer to the heat index shown on page 98, which combines two conditions, humidity and temperature, to give you the "apparent temperature," or what the heat feels like to your body. If the temperature is 29°C (84°F) and the humidity is 60%, then the apparent temperature is 32°C (90°F). It's something like the wind-chill factor in reverse. But be warned that sunlight is still an important issue. If the air temperature is 29°C (84°F) that means it's 29°C whether it's overcast or sunny. If the sun is out, your body will soak up electromagnetic radiation and heat up much faster than on an overcast day. Treat the figures in the chart as guidelines. It's possible to get heat exhaustion on a 21°C (70°F) day, particularly if you're used to working out in 10°C (50°F) weather.

No matter what climate you're used to or what you're wearing, when the apparent temperature goes over 41°C (105°F), which can happen, it's probably best to stay at home—or flee to the nearest air-conditioned movie theater.

Summer Running Surfaces

Come summer we have a choice of running surfaces. While the grass may seem greener, there can still be holes or soft spots in the long grass that you need to be aware of. Flat, even and manicured grass, such as on a golf course, is the ideal running surface; random speed sessions while avoiding the golf course groundskeeper can also be fun. But trespassing charges are not fun, so make sure the golf course is runner friendly, or find a park to run in.

Your three main choices for running surfaces in the summer are concrete (sidewalks), asphalt (roads) or packed dirt trails (pathways and trails). Of these three, concrete is the hardest surface, and it absorbs very little shock of impact. Avoid concrete sidewalks as much as possible. The shock of landing on the hard surface causes trauma to the body and can delay recovery times or lead to injury.

Asphalt is more absorbent than concrete. Run on the sidewalk on a hot summer day and then run on the side of the road. You will readily feel the additional absorption of the asphalt.

Dirt paths are the best choice for running because they are relatively soft. Be careful of your footing, so that you don't trip over a rock or tree root.

Varying your running surface improves the physiological and psychological benefits of running.

Outdoor Exercise During Heat and Smog Alerts

Exercising outdoors during a smog or heat alert can be dangerous. A smog alert is issued when smog conditions reach dangerous levels and a heat alert is issued when the combination of heat, humidity and other weather conditions can be very dangerous.

Health risks may increase during high smog or heat levels for those who walk or run outdoors.

How air pollution and heat affect your body

When you exercise you breathe harder than normal, bringing dirty air deeper into your lungs. You also breathe mostly through your mouth, bypassing the filtering actions of the nose. If you exercise when it is very hot, your body temperature will get very high and your body has to work extra hard to keep cool.

When exercising outdoors during a smog alert, even healthy people may:
+ Cough and/or wheeze
+ Feel irritation in their throat
+ Have difficulty breathing
+ Inflame and damage lungs cells (short and long term)

- Reduce the immune system's ability to fight off respiratory bacterial infections
- Have difficulty performing their best (the lungs can't work at full capacity).

People exercising outdoors during a heat alert may:
- Get heat cramps (muscle pains in the legs, arms or abdomen)
- Have a very high body temperature that could damage vital organs
- Suffer from headache, nausea, dizziness, confusion and/or weakness due to heat-related illness.

For people who have lung or heart conditions, exercising outdoors during a smog or heat alert could worsen their conditions.

Protecting Your Health During Heat and Smog Alerts

Reschedule your run, etc., if possible, to another time when the smog or heat alert is over. Or you could work out indoors in an air-conditioned area.

If you're going to be active outdoors:
- Drink plenty of water before, during and after exercise (during exercise, drink water every 15 to 20 minutes).
- Wear loose-fitting clothes that allow for evaporation of sweat.
- Wear a hat and use sunscreen (at least SPF 15).
- Take lots of rest breaks.
- When running, avoid busy streets, especially during rush hours.

Being overcome by smog and/or heat while exercising can be serious. Stop exercising and seek medical help as soon as possible if you or someone else has the following symptoms:

- difficulty breathing
- weakness or fainting
- feeling more tired than usual
- nausea
- headache
- confusion

Help a sick person by:

+ calling for medical help
+ removing excess clothing from the person
+ cooling the person down by patting or sponging with lukewarm water
+ moving the person indoors to a cooler place
+ giving the person sips of cool water (not ice cold water) or a sports drink

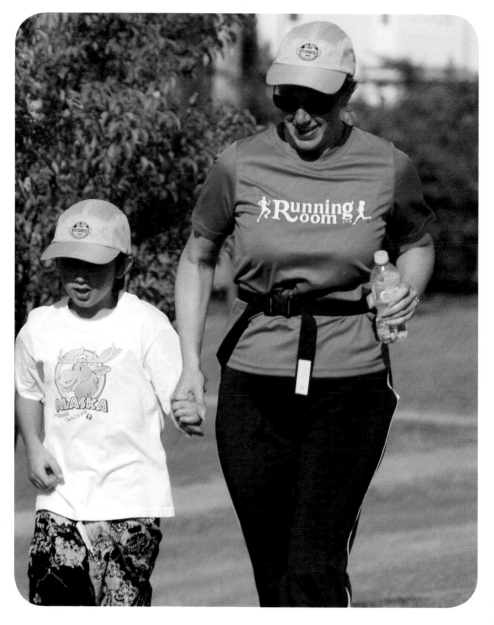

Heat Index

Relative Humidity	Actual Air Temperature (°C)										
	20	23	26	29	32	35	38	41	44	47	50
	Apparent Temperature										
0%	17	20	22	25	28	31	33	35	38	40	43
10%	17	20	23	26	29	32	35	38	41	45	48
20%	18	21	24	27	30	34	37	41	45	50	55
30%	18	22	25	28	32	36	40	45	51	58	65
40%	19	22	25	30	34	38	44	51	59	67	
50%	19	23	27	31	35	42	49	58	67		
60%	20	24	27	32	38	46	56	66			
70%	20	24	29	33	41	51	63				
80%	21	25	29	36	45	58					
90%	21	25	30	38	50						
100%	21	26	32	42							

Heat Index

Relative Humidity	Actual Air Temperature (°F)										
	70	75	80	85	90	95	100	105	110	115	120
	Apparent Temperature										
0%	64	69	73	78	83	87	91	95	99	103	107
10%	65	70	75	80	85	90	95	100	105	111	116
20%	66	72	77	82	87	93	99	105	112	120	130
30%	67	73	78	84	90	96	104	113	123	135	148
40%	68	74	79	86	93	101	110	123	137	151	
50%	69	75	81	88	96	107	120	135	150		
60%	70	76	82	90	100	114	132	149			
70%	70	77	85	93	106	124	144				
80%	71	78	86	97	113	136					
90%	71	79	88	102	122						
100%	72	80	91	108							

Apparent Temperature	Risk from prolonged exercise and /or exposure
18° to 32°C (64° to 90°F)	Fatigue, dehydration possible
32° to 41°C (90° to 105°F)	Heat cramp or heat exhaustion possible
41° to 54°C (105° to 130°F)	Heat cramps or heat exhaustion likely; heatstroke possible
Above 54°C (above 130°F)	Heatstroke very possible

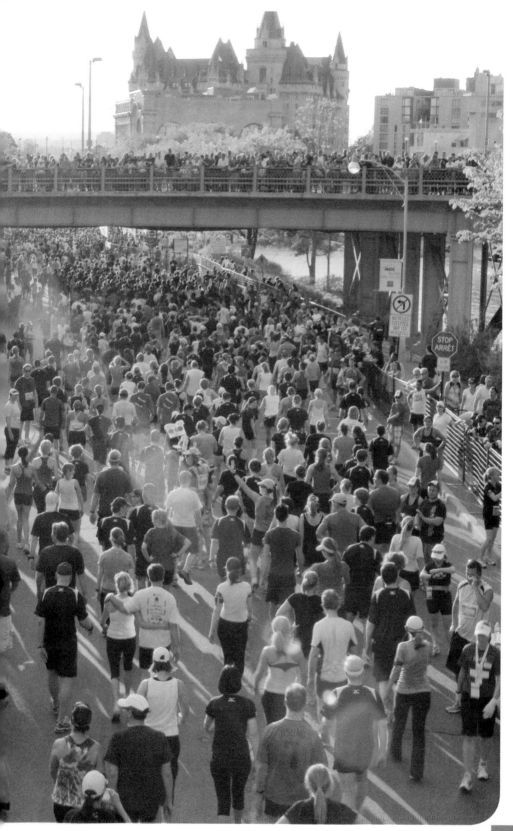

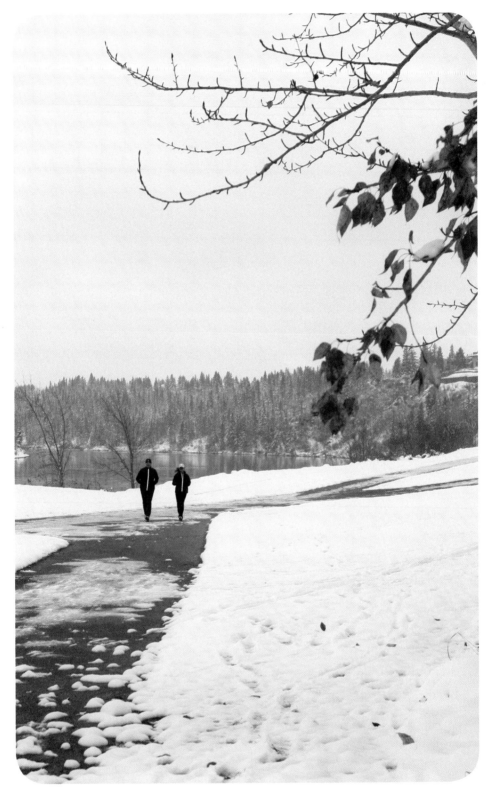

Winter Running

The ABCs (and D) of suiting up for winter running

There is a special joy in being the first to make fresh footsteps in the snow, so don't pass up the excitement of a crisp sunny run through the early morning or the delight of an evening run through the darkness as large snow flakes float through the stillness of the evening. Building a snowman in the fresh snow can add a new cross-training regime to your winter workout, so loosen up and enjoy the winter. It's a fact those cold winter days build character—the kind you can use in the late stages of a long run. If you are feeling rough at 32 km, think back to the challenges you overcame during those long winter runs.

Winter Running Tips

The following are some cold-weather running tips. Most of the tips involve some good common sense in the severe conditions.

1. Adjust the intensity of your workout.

2. Up to 50% of body heat is lost through the head, so keep it covered.

3. Warm up properly, start your runs at a comfortable pace and slowly build up the pace to a pace slower than your normal training pace.

4. Shorten your stride to improve your footing on icy roads. Wear Ice Joggers over the soles of your shoes for greater traction.

5. Carry a cell phone so you can make a call or carry cab fare in your shoe or pocket.

6. Wind chill does not measure temperature, it measures the rate of cooling. On a day with high wind chill, prepare for the wind. Take a look at our wind chill charts on page 118 as they will help you assess your risk of frostbite.

7. Run into the wind for the first part of your run and with the wind on the return portion.

8. When running by yourself, run in a loop in case you need to cut the run short.

9. On your first few runs on snow or ice, you may experience slight muscle soreness in the legs. That is because your supporting muscles are working harder to control your slipping.

Weather

4

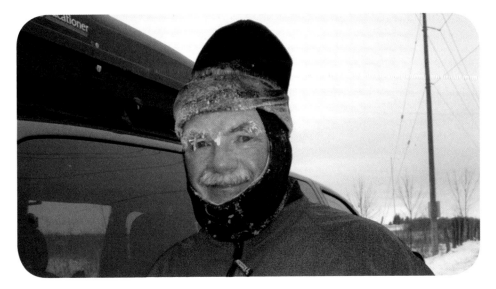

10. Cover all exposed skin with clothing or skin lotion. If you or your running partner have exposed skin, be aware of each other to prevent frostbite.

11. In the winter it's dark, so wear reflective gear and run facing the traffic in order to be more visible.

12. Mittens are warmer than gloves.

13. Drink water on any run over 45 minutes.

14. Use a lip protector (like a lip balm such as ChapStick) on your lips, nose and ears.

15. Gentlemen, protect your future generation—wear a wind brief.

16. Our beauty tips for those dry hands: petroleum jelly on the hands helps keep them warm and makes a great moisturizer.

17. Do speed work indoors on dry surfaces.

18. Be aware of hypothermia for both yourself and those running with you. Hypothermia is a drop in your core body temperature. Signs of hypothermia include incoherent, slurred speech, clumsy fingers and poor coordination. At the first sign, get to a warm, dry place and seek medical attention. You are more likely to experience difficulty on a wet and windy day.

19. Do not accelerate or decelerate quickly in the cold weather

20. Make sure your changes in direction are gradual to avoid slipping or pulling muscles that are not properly warmed up.

21. Freezing your lungs is just not possible. The air is sufficiently warmed by the body prior to entering the lungs. If you find the cold air uncomfortable, wear a face mask; it will help warm the air.

22. No need to get out the wool socks or double up on your regular pair. Wear a single pair of thermal socks to stay warm.

23. Take your wet clothes off and get dry ones on as soon as possible.

24. Wear your water bottle under your jacket to keep it from freezing.

25. Review runner safety. Safety is even more important in the winter with less light and far more ice and other obstacles on the running paths and roads.

Weather and Running

We know that not every day will be a nice fall morning or a brisk spring evening, so we need to prepare. What do you wear? How do you alter your training schedule? How do you protect yourself from the elements? These are some of the issues we will deal with.

Cold-Weather Running Tips

With the temperatures such as they are I wanted to point out a few simple rules to keep in mind if you are going out in this weather.

First, if it is -30°C (-22°F) or colder, you do not have to be a hero. Find an alternative to running outside. This could be a great day for cross-training.

1. Wear three layers: base layer, insulating layer and windproof shell. Some clothing is quite efficient, such as Fit-Wear, and if you have this then two layers will suffice.

2. Do not expose too much skin. Keep all extremities covered, i.e., ears, hands, wrists, ankles and neck. Your respiratory area (nose and mouth) will stay warm because of the breathing business going on.

3. Apply Bodyglide or another type of body lubricant to any exposed skin to help protect it from the wind and drying effects of the cold.

4. Run in small loops close to your home base. If you find it is getting unbearable, you will not be too far away from shelter.

5. Bring cab fare, cell phone and I.D.

6. Tell someone where you are going (route map) and give that person an idea of your approximate time of arrival.

7. If you start to detect frostbite, seek shelter immediately and warm up. **Do not stay out any longer.**

How to Know if You Have Frostbite and What to Do if You Get It

Frostbite is nasty stuff. Once you have been frostbitten, you can be scarred for life and you can have circulation problems in the effected areas for the rest of your life.

You get frostbite when you have skin exposed to severe cold temperatures for a period of time (the amount of time depends on body type, size and other factors) and your body stops sending blood to that area to save the rest of the body. Once this happens, freezing is not long off.

You know when you have frostbite because the effected area is numbed or deadened to feeling. The area becomes white and can have blotchy patches. If you pressed into the effected area the flesh will not come back into shape immediately. There will be a depression from where you pressed in.

When you come into the warmth and you start to thaw, there will be a tingling sensation and then you can have some pain. It can vary from mild to excruciating. Severe frostbite can result in the affected parts having to be amputated.

The best method for bringing back warmth to the affected area is to use warm (not hot) water. Soak or rinse the area until feeling comes back.

If you get frostbite, seek medical attention.

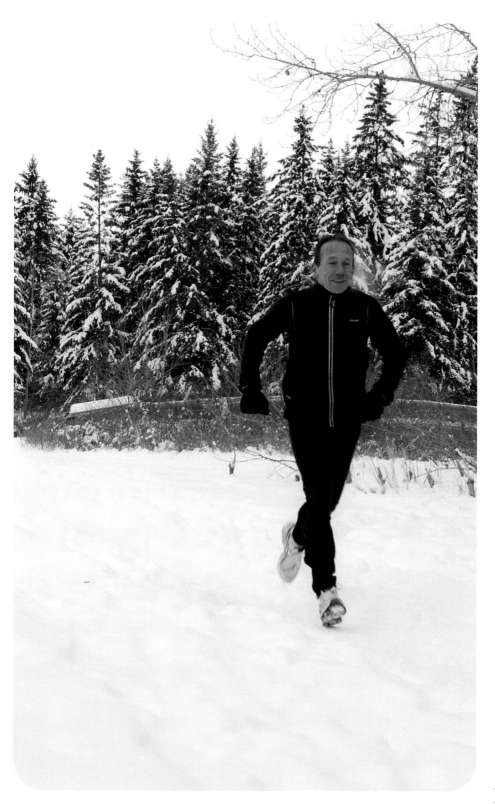

Hypothermia

Hypothermia occurs when the core temperature of your body drops and your equilibrium can be sent out of balance. It can be very dangerous. Symptoms are incoherence, slurred speech, clumsiness and poor coordination. Extra caution is necessary on cold, wet, windy days. At the first sign of hypothermia, get yourself or your training buddy to a warm, dry place. Seek medical advice and do not let the person fall asleep.

Most of all, though, be smart and listen to your body.

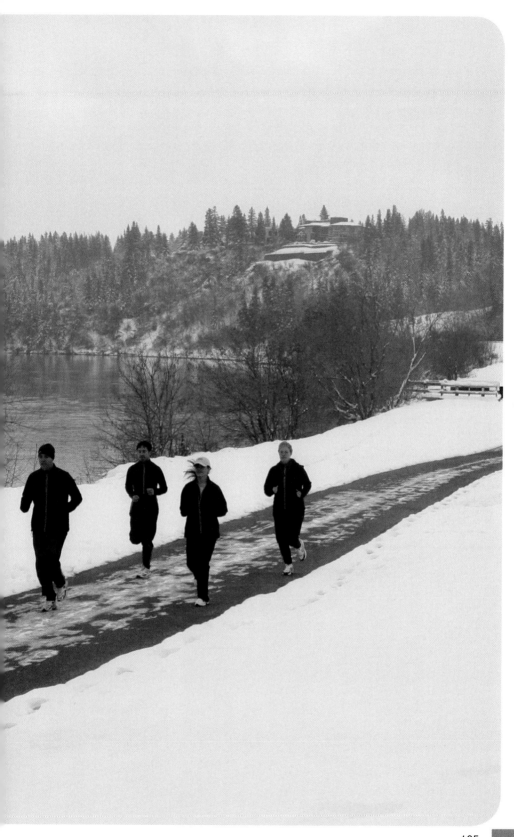

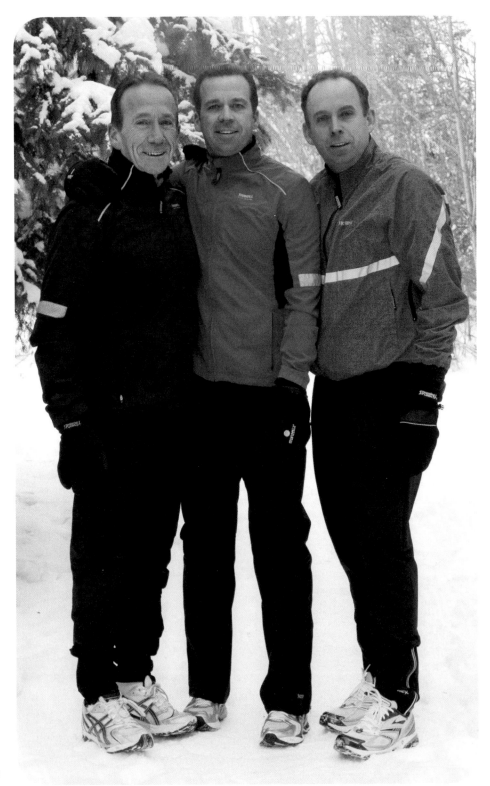

Winter Clothing

Tips for Dressing in Winter:

The key to comfortable cold-weather running is to dress in layers. Air between the layers provides the warmth you feel. Normally the top half of your body needs three layers and the bottom half two layers to provide warmth.

1. Base Layer

2. Thermal Layer (optional, especially on bottom half of body)

3. Outer Shell

1. Base Layer:

This is by far the most important layer. If it is doing its job properly this layer should keep you both warm and dry. Look for form-fitting long-sleeve shirts and long underwear made of technical fabrics that wick moisture and allow evaporation. Cotton is definitely out for this layer as it holds moisture. Keeping warm in the winter means staying dry.

Products to look for: Fit-Wear, ThermaStat, X-Static

2. Thermal Layer:

This layer is optional. Not everyone will feel they need the added warmth of this layer. In recent years the development of Polar Fleece and Arctic Fleece have made this an additional layer for warmth and not weight, which may be a problem when wearing thick cottons and wools. Try not to defeat the purpose of your base layer by using nonwicking material. Arctic Fleece is a great example of the triple layer fabrics that can act as your base and thermal layers in one.

Products to look for: Dryline, Fit-Wear

3. Outer Shell:

Probably not a necessity everyday but definitely an asset on the colder, windier days. A proper shell should prevent the cold winter wind from reaching your damp base layer as well as allowing moisture and some heat to escape from inside. A windproof, breathable shell is your best bet. Waterproof is an added feature that will allow you to utilize your investment throughout the entire year.

Products to look for: WindPro, Power Shield, Fit-Wear

Winter Running Products

The following products will help keep you warm, dry and safe:

1. X-Static/ThermaStat base layers

2. Dryline top

3. Dryline bottom

4. Power Shield/WindPro jacket/pants

5. Balaclava

6. Double layer ThermaStat socks

7. Reflective materials or battery-powered lights

8. Reflective vest

9. Power Bar

10. Angled water bottle carrier

Winter Running Surfaces

Reflecting on winter training; we have to learn a new sense of discipline. Just getting our butt out the door for a run and sticking to our training program is in itself a major victory. We strengthen our character and provide a valuable resource to draw on come the summer racing season.

Running outdoors in the winter burns up to 12% more calories and 32% more fat than doing the same run indoors. We burn calories to maintain core body temperature as well as to run. Daylight exposure increases vitamin D intake and lessens our chances of suffering seasonal affective disorder. Running on a tree-lined trail along a lake or river is certainly more calming and provides a better feeling of well-being than running in the crowded artificial light of a sweaty and loud indoor facility.

Icy, slippery winter days expose the runner to additional risk of injury. On icy surfaces the tendency is to run with a shorter stride and a wider stance for balance. Arm movements become those of an athlete on a balance beam. Hard-packed, firm snow can be a great surface to run on as it absorbs shock. However, fresh, deep snow and uneven winter ruts can lead to strained calf muscles, Achilles tendonitis and injury. Run smart by adjusting the intensity of the workout to the running conditions and surfaces.

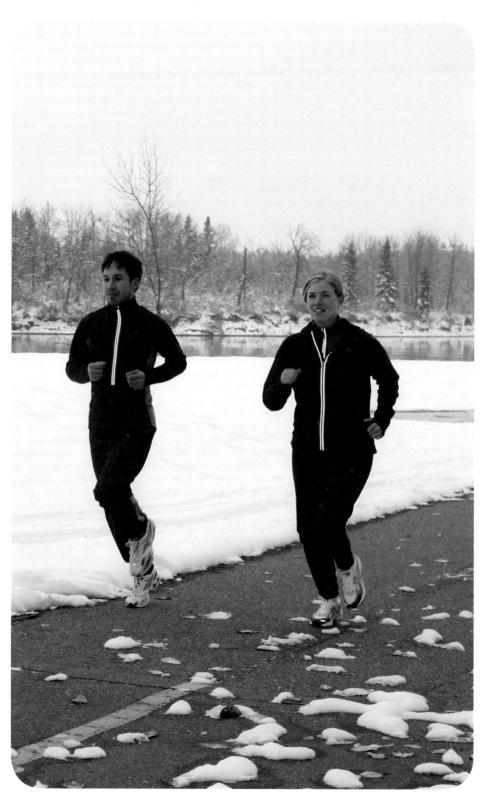

Indoor tracks offer an alternative during inclement weather conditions. Most indoor synthetic running tracks have marvelous shock absorption; they are designed to provide suction and rebound at the same time. Be careful of the tight turns on some of the smaller indoor tracks. Added stress is placed on our lower legs when we run the turns. Most of us are used to running outdoors, and the repetitive turning can present some injury risk. Often, indoor tracks switch directions on different days. A fun workout is to run a few easy warm-up laps and then cruise the corners and run fast on the straight-aways. This workout provides some high intensity and low intensity while minimizing some of your risk of injury.

Summary:

Remember, your body generates a lot of heat all on its own while running. Dressing too warmly can cause you to be chilled or cold in the long run as the increased sweating results in wet clothing. You should be leaving for your run feeling chilly. Start out slow and you'll find yourself warm in no time.

Our Running Room clinic programs have seen many long runs done under severe conditions with a temperature of -40 with a wind. Our successful members have enjoyed those runs because of a commonsense approach and dressing for those conditions.

Remember the warmth of a smile—use it!

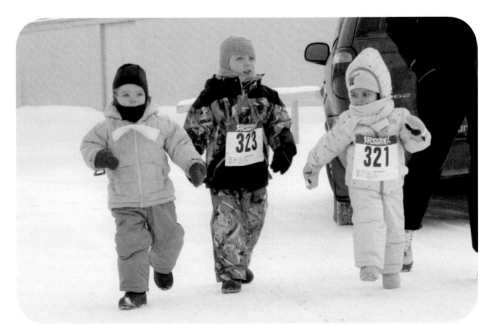

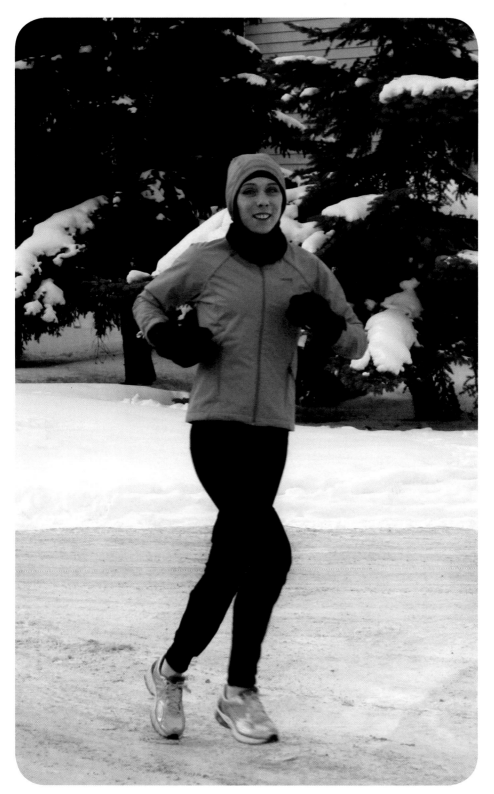

Wind Chill

Actual Air Temperature (°C)									
Calm	4	-1	-7	-12	-18	-23	-29	-34	-40

Wind Speed (km/h)	Equivalent Chill Temperature								
8	2	-4	-9	-15	-21	-26	-32	-37	-43
16	-1	-9	-15	-23	-29	-37	-43	-51	-57
24	-4	-12	-21	-29	-34	-43	-51	-57	-65
32	-7	-15	-23	-32	-37	-46	-54	-62	-71
40	-9	-18	-26	-34	-43	-51	-59	-68	-76
48	-12	-18	-29	-34	-46	-54	-62	-71	-79
56	-12	-21	-29	-37	-46	-54	-62	-73	-82
64	-12	-21	-29	-37	-48	-57	-65	-73	-82

Wind Chill

Actual Air Temperature (°F)									
Calm	40	30	20	10	0	-10	-20	-30	-40

Wind Speed (mph)	Equivalent Chill Temperature								
5	35	25	15	5	-5	-15	-25	-35	-45
10	30	15	5	-10	-20	-35	-45	-60	-70
15	25	10	-5	-20	-30	-45	-60	-70	-85
20	20	5	-10	-25	-35	-50	-65	-80	-95
25	15	0	-15	-30	-45	-60	-75	-90	-105
30	10	0	-20	-30	-50	-65	-80	-95	-110
35	10	-5	-20	-35	-50	-65	-80	-100	-115
40	10	-5	-20	-35	-55	-70	-85	-100	-115

Apparent Temperature	Risk of Frostbite
Above -30° C (-20° F)	Little danger
-30 to -57° C (-20 to -70° F)	Increasing danger — exposed flesh may freeze within 1 minute
Below -57° C (-70° F)	Great danger — exposed flesh may freeze within 30 seconds

Note: Winds above 64 km/h (40 m.p.h.) have little additional effect

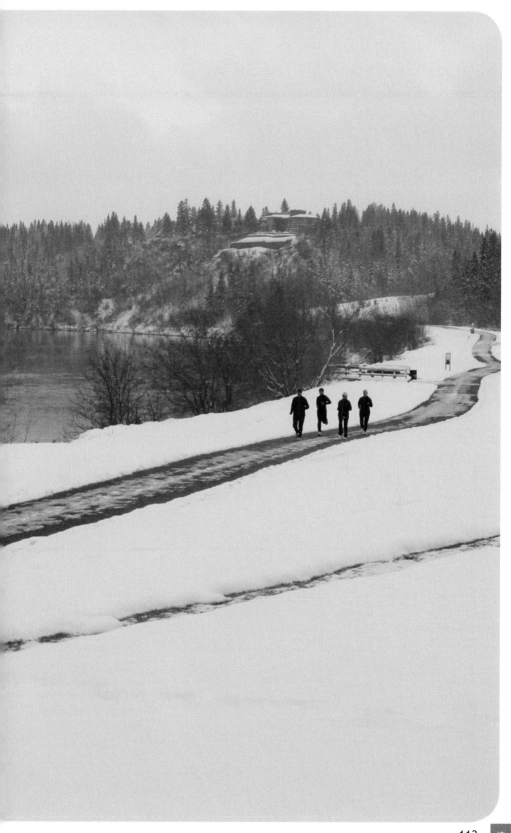

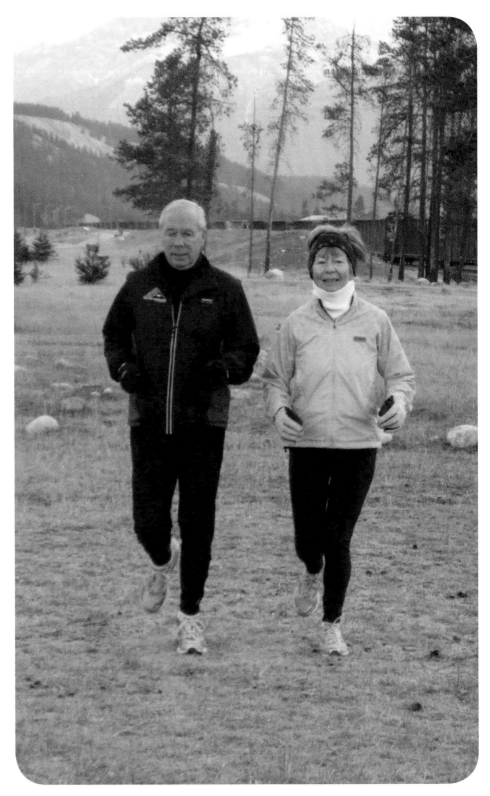

High-Altitude Training

As we increase the altitude above sea level the oxygen content of the air is reduced. The number of oxygen molecules is reduced and under resting conditions the individual can increase their rate of breathing to compensate for the limited amount of oxygen. The higher the altitude the more profound the effect. On a good note, your maximal breathing capacity is greater at altitude than at sea level.

There is also less air resistance at altitude. The air is also cooler and drier at a high altitude. This is good from a heat exchange standpoint but can also promote respiratory water loss. Another thing to consider is that solar radiation is higher, so the use of sunscreen is even more important.

During the first few days at high altitude you may be less tolerant to lactate productions, but through a few days of adaptation and staying well hydrated you should notice little difference in your overall performance.

My advice is to arrive a few days in advance and stick to your current training program. If you are fit and healthy to run a marathon at sea level you will do equally well in a marathon of 3,000 ft.

Stretching

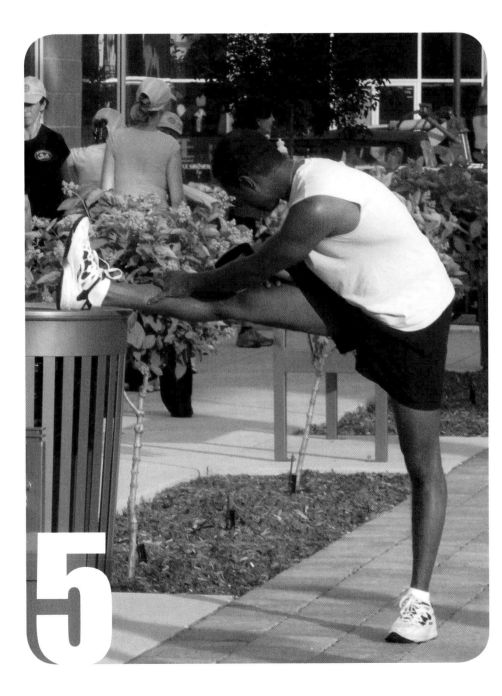

5

Why Stretch?

"Stretching? Well, maybe to get that last chocolate chip cookie on the far side of the table, but not for running."

A lot of runners will give you this kind of response when you ask about stretching. The debate on the benefits of stretching has been going on for a while, between runners who follow a regular routine and runners who only do the occasional stretch as they blink away the previous night's sleep.

Studies by the sports medicine experts tell us that there is a correlation between injuries and stretching habits. They have found very little difference in injury rates between runners who stretch on a regular basis and runners who do not stretch at all, but runners who stretch occasionally have the highest incidence of injuries. In looking for a reason for their higher injury rate, they concluded that sporadic stretchers often stretch incorrectly and at the wrong time.

So, why stretch, you ask, when you can drop into a major road race and see some of the elite runners who can barely touch their toes without bending their knees? Well, remember that most of the elite runners did a good job in selecting their parents. Pure speed has a lot to do with genetics. The rest of us need whatever other advantages we can find.

The thing I have found as I have aged from a runner to a coach is that maintaining flexibility is a real factor in maintaining some semblance of speed. Think of the two ways we run faster: a faster leg turnover and a longer stride. As we age, if we do not work at maintaining our flexibility, the stride length of your youth will soon leave us. Even if you are able to maintain your leg turnover, a shorter stride length means slower times.

The repetitive action of running causes the two major muscle groups, the hamstrings on the back of the high thigh and the quadriceps on the front, to tighten up when put through the relatively limited range of the running motion. Stretching is integral to maintaining a full range of motion at the ankle, knee and hip.

Warm-Up, Stretching and Cooldown

Along with aerobic fitness and strength, flexibility is also an important component of total body health and wellness. It has been traditionally believed that performing warm-up exercises that include stretching can help avoid injury during the subsequent activity. Although this may not be completely true, a well-planned warm-up, cooldown and stretching regimen are important aspects of every training session.

The Purpose of Warm-Up

The main purpose of warm-up is to ready the body for the subsequent activity. It assists the heart, lungs and muscles to prepare for the intensity of exercise and to ease the body through the transition from rest to exercise. There are many forms of warm-up. Calisthenics, stretching and other forms of stationary exercise are popular. The best form of warm-up is doing your planned exercise activity, only much more slowly for the first few minutes of the session. For example, you may want to start your run with a brisk walk and a slow jog. Tennis players often warm-up playing at the service lines rather than using the full court. Start your activity, only on a smaller scale. How do you know if your warm-up has been long enough? Are you sweating yet? Perspiration is a sure sign that warm-up can end and your exercise session can begin.

The Purpose of Cooldown

The purpose of cooldown is the exact opposite of warm-up. Incorporating a planned cooldown at the end of your exercise session assists the body in the transition from exercise to rest. It allows the heart to adjust to the decreased intensity more slowly and can prevent labored breathing at the end of higher intensity exercise sessions. Blood flow can slow more naturally with a cooldown, which will prevent the pooling of blood in the exercising muscles and thus any dizziness or nausea that can result from suddenly stopping a particularly high-intensity exercise. The optimal length of the cooldown period is dependent on the intensity and duration of the prior exercise, with long, more intense sessions requiring an extended cooldown. A cooldown period of 5 to 10 minutes should suffice for almost every workout. Like warm-up, the bulk of the activity done during the cooldown should be the same as the exercise session, only slower or on a smaller scale. Finish your run with a slow jog or a walk.

Stretching

Stretching is always best done when the muscles are warm. If your preference is to stretch before you work out, then be sure to do a full warm-up first (10 minutes). On the other hand, stretching can become a part of an extended cooldown. If improved flexibility is your goal, then stretching while your muscles are cooling from a training session will give the best results. Never sit down and stretch too soon after your workout. Stretching is only recommended after an appropriate cooldown.

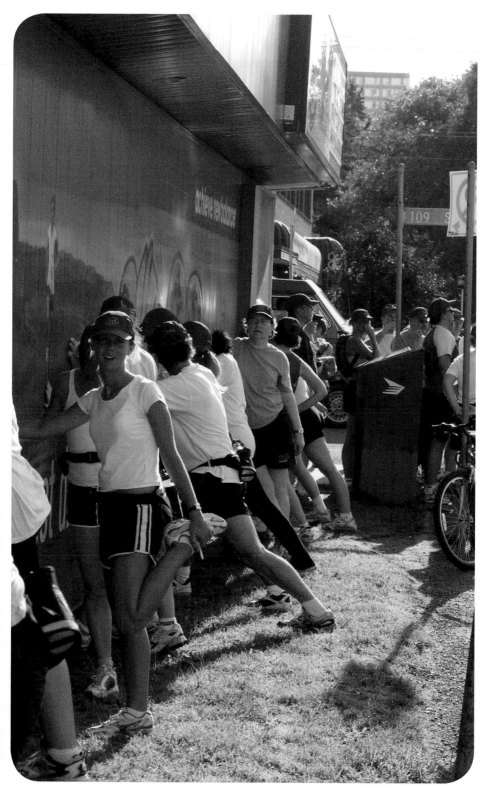

How to Stretch

Stretching should be done slowly without bouncing. Stretch to where you feel a slight, easy stretch (not pain). Hold this feeling for approximately 20 seconds. As you hold the stretch, the feeling of tension should diminish. If it doesn't, ease off slightly into a more comfortable stretch. This easy first stretch readies the tissue for the developmental stretch. After holding the easy stretch, move slightly farther into the stretch until you feel mild tension again. This is the developmental stretch, which should be held for 20 to 30 seconds. This feeling of stretch tension should slightly diminish or stay the same. If the tension increases or becomes painful, you are overstretching. Again, ease off to a comfortable stretch.

The developmental stretch reduces the risk of injuries and will safely increase flexibility. Hold the stretch at a tension that feels comfortable to you. The key to stretching is to keep relaxed while you concentrate on the area to be stretched. Your breathing should be regular. Be sure not to hold your breath. Don't worry how far you can stretch in comparison to others—increased personal flexibility is a guaranteed result of a regular stretching program.

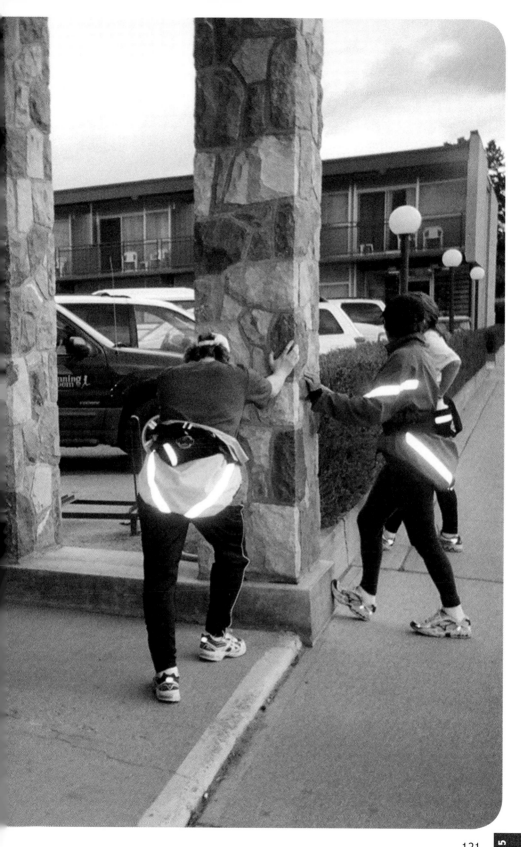

The Stretches

The following are recommended stretches for beginner and novice runners.

Calf

Stand about 3 ft. (1 m) from a wall, railing or tree with your feet flat on the ground, toes slightly turned inward, heels out and back straight. The forward leg should be bent and the rear leg should be gradually straightened until there is tension in the calf. (figure 1-a) Finally, bend the straight leg at the knee to work closer to the Achilles tendon. (figure 1-b)

Hamstring

Lie down on your back with one knee bent and foot flat on the ground. Slip a Thera-Band under your other foot, and grab the ends in your hands keeping your knee bent. (figure 2-a) Slowly straighten this leg. (figure 2-b) Feel the stretch. Repeat with the other leg.

Quadriceps (also known as "quads")

Place one arm on something handy to balance yourself and use the other hand to pull the foot back when one leg is bent at the knee. The bent knee should touch the other knee. Don't push it forward or pull it back. While this stretch is being executed, the belly button should be pulled up under the rib cage, which is called a pelvic tilt. The tilt protects the back. (figure 3-a)

Iliotibial Band Stretch

With one leg towards a railing, bench or wall and the other leg slightly bent, cross the leg to be stretched behind the bent leg. Shift your hip towards the wall to stretch the iliotibial band. You should feel the stretch over the hip area. (figure 4-a)

Buttock Stretch

Sit up straight with one leg straight and the knee of your other leg bent, with the foot of the bent leg on the outside of the straightened leg. Slowly pull the bent leg towards the opposing shoulder. (figure 5-a) The buttock of the bent leg will be stretched.

Hip Flexor Stretch

Kneel on one knee and place the other leg forward at a 90-degree stance. (figure 6-a) Keep the back straight and maintain the pelvic tilt while lunging forward. (figure 6-b) The rear knee is planted to stretch the hip in front.

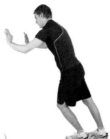

(figure 1-a)

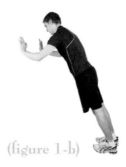

(figure 1-b)

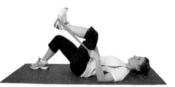

(figure 2-a)

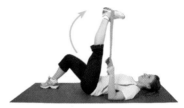

(figure 2-b)

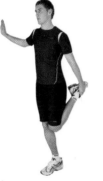

(figure 3-a)

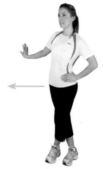

(figure 4-a)

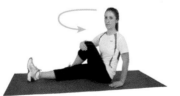

(figure 5-a)

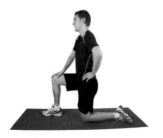

(figure 6-a)

(figure 6-b)

Running or Walking Intelligently

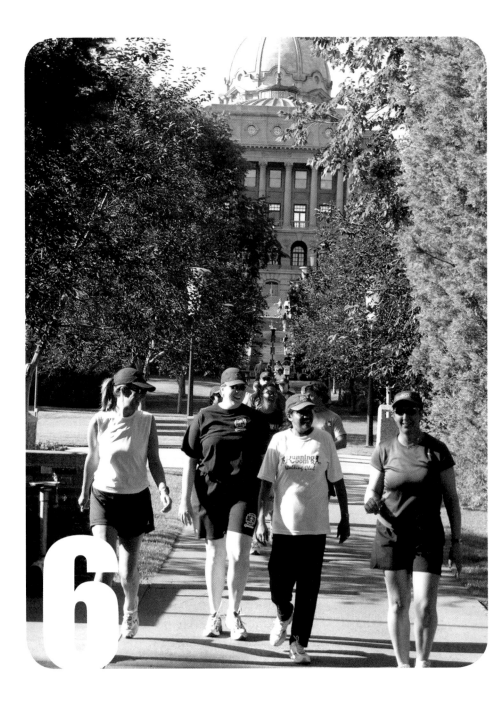

Introductory Training Program

So you've decided to take up a healthier lifestyle and you've chosen running as your means of getting there. Making that decision is a big step, but the hardest part of getting started is making the initial commitment to yourself. The real secret to staying committed is to make your program gentle enough for current physical condition and yet challenging enough that you will see some progress.

Fitness is a lifetime goal, so be easy on yourself to start with and keep the intensity gentle.

This program is measured out in minutes to help you manage a low-intensity workout. Sports medicine experts tell us that as little as 20 minutes of activity, three times a week, is a good way to get started and is also a good way to maintain cardiovascular fitness.

The chapter on nutrition goes into details about how to fuel that athletic body you're going to have, but for now just focus on these key points:

+ Drink 8 to 10 glasses of water each day.
+ Cut down on the amount of fats and oils in your diet.
+ Increase the amount of complex carbohydrates in your diet.

Walk Before You Run

Just how do you get started if you've been a sedentary adult who has done nothing in the way of physical activity? The following walking program is a gentle way to get started and is normally acceptable to most people. The mistake that most people make in getting started is going too far, too fast and with too much intensity. Fitness is a lifetime goal, so be easy on yourself to start with and keep the intensity gentle.

Preconditioning Phase

During this phase, concentrate on time, not intensity, in your walks.

Preconditioning Program							
	Mon	Tues	Wed	Thurs	Fri	Sat	Sun
Week 1	Off	Off	Walk 25 min	Off	Walk 20 min	Off	Walk 25 min
Week 2	Off	Off	Walk 25 min	Off	Walk 20 min	Off	Walk 30 min
Week 3	Off	Off	Walk 25 min	Off	Walk 20 min	Off	Walk 35 min
Week 4	Off	Off	Walk 25 min	Off	Walk 20 min	Off	Walk 40 min
Week 5	Off	Off	Walk 25 min	Off	Walk 20 min	Off	Walk 45 min
Week 6	Off	Off	Walk 30 min	Off	Walk 25 min	Off	Walk 45 min
Week 7	Off	Off	Walk 35 min	Off	Walk 30 min	Off	Walk 45 min
Week 8	Off	Off	Walk 40 min	Off	Walk 35 min	Off	Walk 45 min
Week 9	Off	Off	Walk 45 min	Off	Walk 40 min	Off	Walk 45 min
Week 10	Off	Off	Walk 45 min	Off	Walk 45 min	Off	Walk 45 min

Congratulations! You are now into some real fat-burning exercise. In just 10 weeks, you have progressed from being a sedentary person to being an athlete who gets in three, 45-minute fat-burning sessions a week. Now you will really start to see an improvement in your fitness.

This is a good time to talk about the scale. Many people become slaves to weighing themselves when they start a fitness program. My suggestion is to only weigh

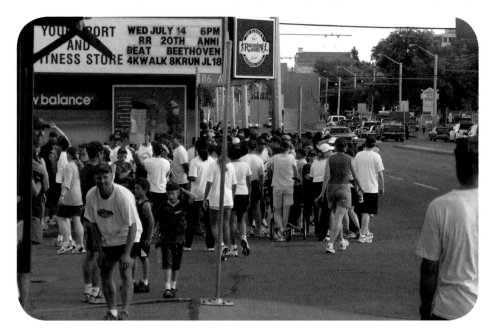

yourself at the start of the program, so you know your starting point. Rather than using weights as a measurement of your progress, it is better to use the fit of your clothing. Take a pair of pants and a shirt that fit before you start your program, and try them on each week to see how they loosen up as your fitness improves. Watching your clothes slowly become baggy can be very motivating, and it keeps you away from the scale, which sometimes only shows how much water you've been drinking.

Endurance Phase

Now that you are comfortable walking for 45 minutes, three times a week, it's time to combine some faster walking with slow, recovery walking. This is not power walking or race walking, but a series of timed intervals: intensive phases where you simply walk faster, followed by recovery phases where you walk slower.

Endurance Program

	Mon	Tues	Wed	Thurs	Fri	Sat	Sun
Week 11	Off	Off	10 min warm-up; 3 min fast; 3 min slow; 3 min fast 3 min slow; 3 min fast; 3 min slow; 10 min cooldown	Off	Walk 45 min	Off	Walk 50 min
Week 12	Off	Off	10 min warm-up; 3 min fast; 3 min slow; 3 min fast; 3 min slow; 3 min fast; 3 min slow; 10 min cooldown	Off	Walk 50 min	Off	Walk 60 min
Week 13	Off	Off	Walk 60 min	Off	Walk 60 min	Off	Walk 75 min
Week 14	Off	Off	Walk 70 min	Off	Walk 80 min	Off	Walk 90 min

Wow! Now you're up to 1½ hours of calorie-burning exercise. As an athlete, you've learned how much fun and enjoyment you can get from an intelligent training program. Now you're probably ready to start training as a runner.

Beginer's Conditioning Program

If you are just beginning, start first with walking and add running later. If you have been inactive for a long time, start with a walking program. Walk before you run. Think of it as a preconditioning program.

Start with a fast walk for 20 to 30 minutes. Slow down if you find yourself short of breath. Don't stop. Keep moving. By pumping your arms as you walk and really stepping out, you can increase your heart rate to a level nearly equivalent to a slow run. Also, by walking vigorously uphill, you can add to the rigor of your walking workouts.

Once you can walk briskly for 30 minutes, you can start interspersing some easy running into your walking. By slowly exchanging running for walking, over several weeks you will gradually progress to running for 10 minutes and walking for 1 minute.

The following schedule should be run at least **three times** per week. All running should be done at a conversation pace, and all walking should be done briskly. Of course, a proper warm-up and cooldown are required. Start and end all sessions with a one-minute walk.

Training Rules

1. This program starts conservatively. You can even fall a little behind and still get back on easily.

2. Once you reach the halfway mark, you may find it difficult to keep up unless you run faithfully at least three times a week.

3. If you can't keep up or lose time from illness or injury, don't panic— stay at the level you can handle or go back a level until you are ready to move on.

4. Remember, it took you a lot of years to get out of shape; take your time getting back into shape.

Your Goal: The Beginning Runner Program is designed to get you running using the run-walk approach for varying distances.

Beginner Conditioning Program

Week	Training Session	Total Exercise Time Running	Walking
1	walk 1 min; run 1 min, walk 2 min x 6 sets; run 1 min, walk 1 min	7 min	14 min
2	walk 1 min; run 1 min, walk 1 min x 10 sets	10 min	11 min
3	walk 1 min; run 2 min, walk 1 min x 6 sets; run 2 min, walk 1 min	14 min	8 min
4	walk 1 min; run 3 min, walk 1 min x 5 sets	15 min	6 min
5	walk 1 min; run 4 min, walk 1 min x 4 sets	16 min	5 min
6	walk 1 min; run 5 min, walk 1 min x 3 sets; run 2 min, walk 1 min	17 min	5 min
7	walk 1 min; run 6 min, walk 1 min x 3 sets	18 min	4 min
8	walk 1 min; run 8 min, walk 1 min x 2 sets; run 2 min, walk 1 min	18 min	4 min
9	walk 1 min; run 10 min, walk 1 min x 2 sets	20 min	3 min
10	walk 1 min; run 10 min, walk 1 min x 2 sets	20 min	3 min

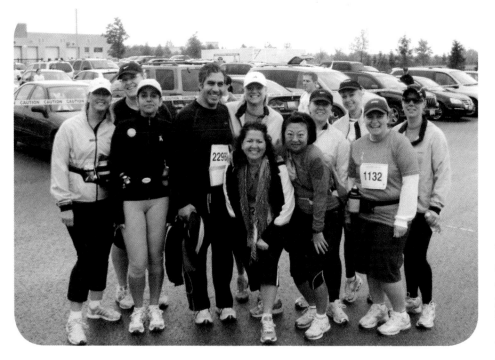

Intermediate Running Conditioning Program

After you can run five minutes nonstop, you are ready for the intermediate program. This phase of training requires that you stay at the level of running for five minutes but do it three to five times a week, for three to four weeks.

Note: When you have reached 30 minutes, three times per week, pause. Hold your running at this level and concentrate on gradually bringing your running time up to 30 minutes on the other days that you are running. You are progressing well, and you don't want to risk injury, fatigue or boredom.

Intermediate Conditioning Program

Week	Training Session	Sessions per Week	Total Exercise Time Running	Walking
1	walk 1 min; run 5 min, walk 1 min x 4 sets	3	20 min	5 min
2	walk 1 min; run 7 min, walk 1 min x 3 sets	3	21 min	4 min
3	walk 1 min; run 10 min, walk 1 min x 2 sets	3	20 min	3 min
4	walk 1 min; run 10 min, walk 1 min x 2 sets	3	20 min	3 min
5	walk 1 min; run 10 min, walk 1 min x 2 sets	3	20 min	3 min
6	walk 1 min; run 10 min, walk 1 min x 2 sets; run 2 min, walk 1 min	3	22 min	4 min
7	walk 1 min; run 10 min, walk 1 min x 2 sets; run 4 min, walk 1 min	3	24 min	4 min
8	walk 1 min; run 10 min, walk 1 min x 2 sets; run 6 min, walk 1 min	3	26 min	4 min
9	walk 1 min; run 10 min, walk 1 min x 2 sets; run 8 min, walk 1 min	3	28 min	4 min
	walk 1 min; run 10 min, walk 1 min x 2 sets	1	20 min	3 min
10	walk 1 min; run 10 min, walk 1 min x 3 sets	3	30 min	4 min
	walk 1 min; run 10 min, walk 1 min x 2 sets	1	20 min	3 min

The Advanced 5 K Conditioning Program

If you can currently run 20 minutes or longer on a consistent basis, you are ready for the advanced 5 K program. This program focuses on safely increasing your total running time or distance as well as adding in extra days of training.

After you have reached week 10, when you are running five times a week, hold your longest runs up to 30 minutes and concentrate on gradually bringing your other runs up to 30 minutes as well. You don't want to risk injury, fatigue or boredom.

Advanced Conditioning Program

Week	Training Session	Sessions per Week	Total Exercise Time	
			Running	Walking
1	walk 1 min; run 10 min, walk 1 min x 2 sets	3	20 min	3 min
2	walk 1 min; run 10 min, walk 1 min x 2 sets; run 2 min, walk 1 min	3	22 min	4 min
3	walk 1 min; run 10 min, walk 1 min x 2 sets; run 4 min, walk 1 min	3	24 min	4 min
4	walk 1 min; run 10 min, walk 1 min x 2 sets; run 6 min, walk 1 min	3	26 min	4 min
5	walk 1 min; run 10 min, walk 1 min x 2 sets; run 8 min, walk 1 min	3	28 min	4 min
6	walk 1 min; run 10 min, walk 1 min x 3 sets	3	30 min	4 min
	walk 1 min; run 10 min, walk 1 min x 2 sets	1	20 min	3 min
7	walk 1 min; run 10 min, walk 1 min x 3 sets	3	30 min	4 min
	walk 1 min; run 10 min, walk 1 min x 2 sets; run 2 min, walk 1 min	1	22 min	4 min
8	walk 1 min; run 10 min, walk 1 min x 3 sets; run 3 min, walk 1 min	3	33 min	5 min
	walk 1 min; run 10 min, walk 1 min x 2 sets; run 2 min, walk 1 min	1	22 min	4 min
9	walk 1 min; run 10 min, walk 1 min x 3 sets; run 3 min, walk 1 min	3	33 min	5 min
	walk 1 min; run 10 min, walk 1 min x 2 sets; run 4 min, walk 1 min	1	24 min	4 min
10	walk 1 min; run 10 min, walk 1 min x 3 sets	2	30 min	4 min
	walk 1 min; run 10 min, walk 1 min x 2 sets; run 5 min, walk 1 min	2	25 min	4 min
	walk 1 min; run 10 min, walk 1 min x 2 sets	1	20 min	3 min

Running Form

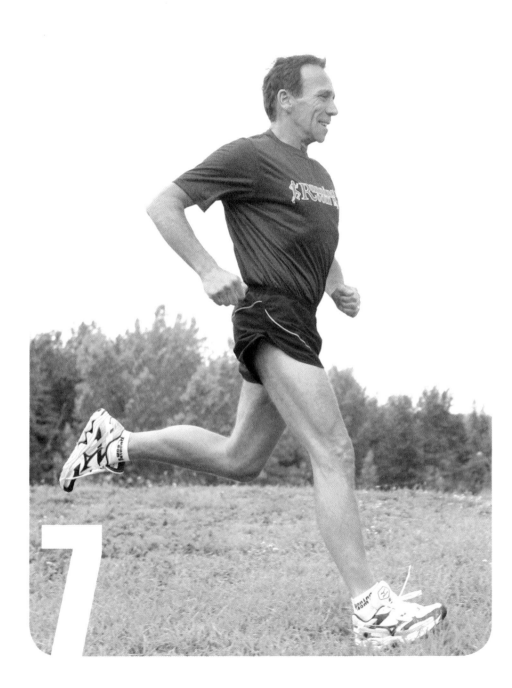

7

How can I improve my form? This is one of the most frequent questions coaches hear. Before getting into a discussion of form or giving advice to a trainee, I usually suggest that they come with me to the finish area of a local road race, so they can watch the lead runners come in. It is always very apparent that in the lead pack, as in the whole pack, there are some runners with great-looking form and then there are some with butt-ugly form. What I ask the trainee to look at is not the display of form as much as the degree of relaxation. The lead runners are certainly fast, after all they are in the lead at the finish, but if you study their concentration, you can see that they maintain a more relaxed form even under race conditions.

Another thing to do is to go down to a local track area and listen to the advice of the running coach. The number one thing you will hear the coach say during a workout is, Relax. The coach will be making all kinds of points to the runners, but the basic thing the coach wants the runners to do, no matter how hard they are pushing, is to relax.

So relax, and let's take a look at how to improve your running form.

Posture

Have a buddy videotape your running—both at the start of a run and near the end of a long run. You will end up with a valuable tool to assess any running posture problems. Here are some of the most common problems as well as some tips on how to improve them.

Overstriding

Increase the rhythm of your arm swing and concentrate on shortening your swing. Think of running on hot coals to shorten your reach with each foot stride forward.

Tightness in Shoulders

Learn to relax the palms of your hands by gently touching your thumb to the middle finger. Your fingers should be loose, so make sure you do not grip a fist as you run. Practice running with a couple of soda crackers held in your hands. Cup your hands with thumbs up top.

Knee Lift

Your knees should be lifted just high enough to clear the ground. Too high a knee lift causes wasted energy—most runners are training for a forward-motion sport.

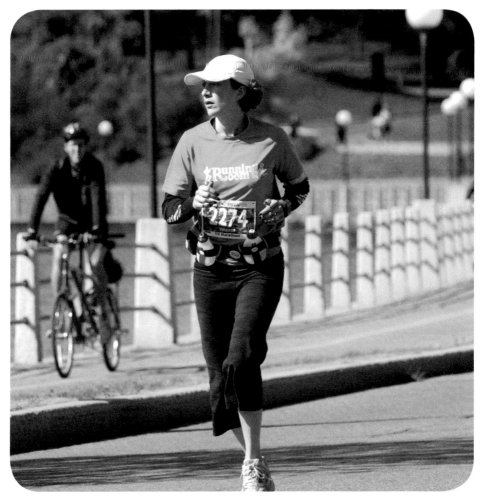

Arm Carriage

Holding the palms of your hands inward and slightly upward will keep your elbows near your sides. Think of your arm swing being in the general area of your heart. Too high an arm swing results in your heart having to pump uphill. Think of the words relaxed and rhythmic. An increase in your arm swing can help increase the turnover rate of tired legs.

Too Much Bounce

Look at the horizon and concentrate on keeping the head in the same plane. Do some accelerations with an increased body lean, stressing lower knee lift and try to think of reaching with your arms rather than pumping them.

Perfect Form

There really is no perfect form. Check out the top finishers at some local races:

you will see some gazelle-like form alongside some butt-ugly form. The important thing to remember is to stay relaxed, stay rhythmic and push hard. Much of your running form is a gift from your parents, but you can make the most of your gift with some attention to fine tuning your individual form.

Form Tips

1. Stay Upright

Good running posture is simply good body posture. When the head, shoulders and hips are all lined up over the feet, you can move forward as a unit, with a minimum amount of effort.

2. Chest Forward

Many runners let their chest sag into a slouch. In such a position, the lungs won't maximize their efficiency. Before starting your run, relax and take a deep breath, which moves the lungs into an efficient position. After you exhale, maintain the chest in this beneficial alignment. The most efficient way to run is to have your head, neck and shoulders erect. When you run leaning forward, you're always fighting gravity.

3. Hips Forward

One of the most common form of errors is letting the hips shift back and the butt stick out behind you. Taking a deep breath often pulls the hips forward also, into an alignment which allows easier running.

4. The Foot Plant

There is a difference between what should happen and what you may be able to control. First, let your shoe professional fit you with a couple of pairs of shoes that are right for you. Then just start running! Your personal stride is the result of your shape, your physique and the strength and balance of your muscles at least all the way up to your waist! Please don't try to change your foot plant as you train: you will not be running naturally and you are very likely to cause more problems than you solve. Changes to your gait only happen as a result of longer-term changes elsewhere. As you gain fitness and strength, you may well notice that many irregularities resolve themselves. Modern training shoes are designed to accommodate biomechanically different feet. Maybe the problem you thought you had will turn out to be not so much of a problem after all. But if you really do have a problem that continues to affect your activity, you may have to seek the advice of a therapist or coach to assess and deal with your particular situation.

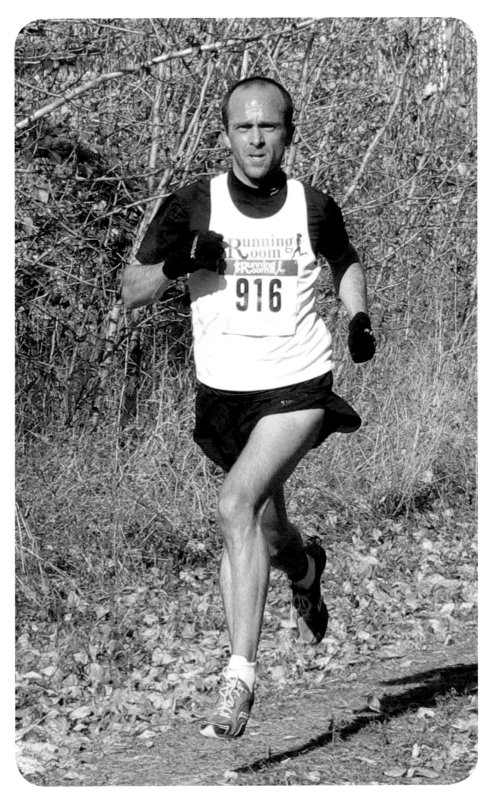

5. Arms

Arm position can vary widely from one runner to the next. In general, the arms should swing naturally and loosely from the shoulders. Not too high and not too low. This usually means staying relaxed. Staying relaxed will prevent the arms from being carried too high and too rigid, which will expend more energy than needed. Your hands should never cross the center of your chest. Remember you want your body to go forward and not side-to-side, so your arms should, too. Keep your hands in a relaxed position and try not to clench or make fists.

6. Stride Length

As a coach, my experience has shown that as runners get faster, their stride length shortens. Leg turnover rate, the cadence of the runner's legs, is the key to faster and more efficient running. Staying light on your feet with a more rapid leg turnover rate will keep many of the aches, pains and injuries away, providing injury-free training.

Sprinters have a high knee lift. The long-distance runner, anyone running more than mile, needs to minimize knee lift. If your knees go too high, you are overusing the quadriceps muscles on the front of the thigh. This overstriding leaves the runner with sore quadriceps at the end of their run. Keep your leg turnover light and rapid—more of a shuffle than the sprinter's stride.

Stay relaxed with a low, short stride while lightly touching the ground. This will prevent tightness in the shin, behind the knee or in the back of the thigh in the hamstring. Kicking too far forward tightens up the lower leg and hamstrings.

Do short accelerations while staying light on your feet. Keep your foot strike quieter with each stride, keeping your foot close to the ground to prevent any negative forces of gravity from excessive bounce.

7. Head and Neck

Your torso will normally do what your head is doing. So if you are dropping your head right down, your torso will probably follow and lean too far forward. Keep the neck and shoulders relaxed. Try not to hunch your shoulders, which will cause undue fatigue to that area. Your eyes should be looking somewhere about 20–30 m ahead of you.

8. Practice Your Technique

Once or twice a week, a little technique work is really helpful. After your warm-

Running Form

7

up, run some accelerations of 50–150 m. Pick one of the elements of good form and feel yourself executing it well during the acceleration. Rehearse each element at least four times, and keep to one or two elements at most in each session. A change in technique may feel a little awkward at first, but you'll know when you've got it right it feels so good! You can follow the lead of athletes in events like sprinting and hurdling, where effective technique is a vitally important ingredient of success. Their warm-up is actually designed so that their technique (they often call it "skill") is rehearsed every time they prepare for training or competition. Your warm-up consists of a period of jogging and stretching. Build in some technique accelerations, too. They take very little extra time. You'll get the most effective "motor learning" by focusing on one point of technique for a short period of time and repeating it several times. When you're moving your body in a new way, your body gets tired, and quickly! You'll feel it and there will be a noticeable loss in your coordination and motor skill. It's temporary; the short break between accelerations will give you the recovery you need.

Look Ma, No Arms!

"When I'm running, I'm never sure just what to do with my arms."

If you hear yourself in that statement, you're not alone. Take a look at a group of runners, and you will notice that everyone has a different arm carriage and arm swing: some runners carry their arms up high like a shadow boxer; others carry their arms low and have little arm swing; some arms are loose and relaxed; others are tight. Proper arm carriage is more efficient, so it will allow you to run faster with less effort. The key to efficient arm movement is the same as for many other aspects of running form: stay relaxed.

Let's start with your hands. To relax them, try touching your thumb and middle finger lightly. You will notice that this relaxes the palm of your hand. Now think about keeping your wrists loose and relaxed. Keep the palm of your hand down as you run. And don't clench your fists. One trick to teach you to relax your hands is to run holding saltine crackers in your hands. They should still be whole at the end of the run.

If you can keep your hands relaxed and as loose as possible, you will find that your forearms and upper arms also stay relaxed. We have all seen people running along with their arms dangling trying to loosen up their shoulders. The reason that most of them end up with tightness in their shoulders is that they have been running with clenched fists. The tightness that starts in your hands and forearms

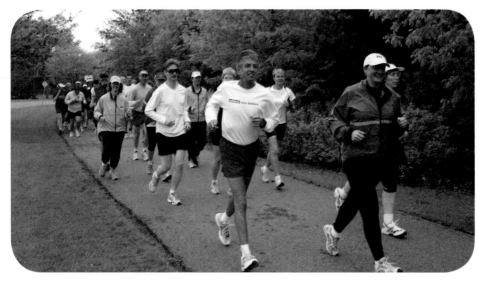

works its way up the arms into the shoulders. Staying relaxed can easily prevent this discomfort.

The next thing to consider is arm swing. Think about your heart. It has to pump blood to all parts of your body, and all the major muscle groups are looking for additional blood during running. As far as your hardworking heart is concerned, the most efficient place to carry your arms is in the area of your heart, so keep your arms bent at about 90 degrees. If you carry your arms too high, the blood has to be pumped uphill; if you carry your arms too low, the heart has to pump the blood a further distance.

Remember that running is a forward-motion sport; try to keep all your movements in the same direction as your running. I like to think of my arms as a metronome that keeps the timing and rhythm of the run smooth.

Your body type and running gait also govern your arm motion. You will see elite runners who sometimes have one arm with a flick of outward motion. It is because one of the legs is slightly shorter than the other. Our bodies adapt very quickly to irregularities, and arm flex is its way of compensation to keep our running form efficient.

Track coaches work hard with their athletes to keep their arms under control and efficient; if you think your arm carriage needs some work, here are a couple of arm drills that might help. (Some runners find these drills awkward; they prefer to just focus on keeping their arm and hand movements smooth and rhythmic when they run, and not to cross the centerline.)

Apple Pocket Drill

Think of reaching for an apple, placing the palm of your hand over it, pulling it back and putting it in your pocket. The palming motion of your hand over the imaginary apple gets you to relax your hand. Bringing your hand back towards your pocket keeps your movement in your line of motion. Work at keeping your hands really loose, and practice clipping your hip with your thumb on the way.

The tightness that develops between the shoulders in many runners is often the result of running with clenched hands and tight forearms. The tension travels up the arms and settles in between the shoulders. This drill will help keep you relaxed and loose in the upper body.

Hands and Arms Drill

This drill is one you have likely seen track athletes working on, running and slicing the air with their hands. Think of a line drawn through the center of your head and body down between your legs; you want to keep your arms from crossing over this line. If your arms cross over too far in front of your chest, the lateral motion causes your lower back to tighten up. Try standing on the spot and work your arms in a running motion. If you exaggerate the crossover motion you will feel the stress that it puts on your lower back. Think of running as a forward-motion sport; keep your movements efficient by concentrating on this in all your motions. Relaxed arm swing keeps your upper body relaxed while improving your form and ease of breathing.

How to Breathe

Question:

I am looking for a recommended way to breathe. I have the "Runner's Stitch." I have tried lots of stuff and found that exhaling all the air from the lungs seems to work. The thing is that I would actually like to run without getting it! I believe it's my whole approach to breathing: long ins and outs from the mouth! Should I try in from the nose out from the mouth or the other way around? Should I follow some sort of pattern?

Answer:

Breathing, the simple act of inhaling and exhaling, can be complicated. Much like running, the act of putting one foot in front of the other, is a lot more complicated than one would expect. Watch the super talented singer who has mastered breathing. This mastery allows them to hit and hold the long high notes.

Better yet, the swimmer has mastered breathing, if for no other reason than they do not want to get a mouth full of water. As runners we occasionally get caught up in our sport and forget some basics like breathing. We start our runs in a race or group environment and the excitement causes us to breath high in our chest, rather than "belly" breathing. The short, high breathing can cause us to hyperventilate or get the dreaded "runner's stitch." Here are some tips that will make your stitch go away and get you more relaxed in your breathing, thereby allowing you to run faster.

Stand up tall, shoulders back and put one hand on your belly. Purse your lips and fully exhale. When we fully exhale we do not need to think about breathing in, as nature does this as part of our survival technique. We breathe in relaxed and "belly breathe" when we fully exhale. This deep breathing is both more relaxed and more efficient in the use of oxygen. Keep your breathing relaxed, deep, rhythmic and in time with your running stride by concentrating on fully exhaling. Inhale in a relaxed, full, deep breath. So now as you run, concentrate on the upper body being relaxed and rhythmic with the power of your running focused on your hip down. The initial power is coming from the push off of the ankle and the glide and relaxed lift of the knee coming from the hip flexors. Save the huffing and puffing for the big bad wolf stories. Now you know why one of the most common things a coach gets the athlete to concentrate on is to relax. The more relaxed we are the higher the level of performance.

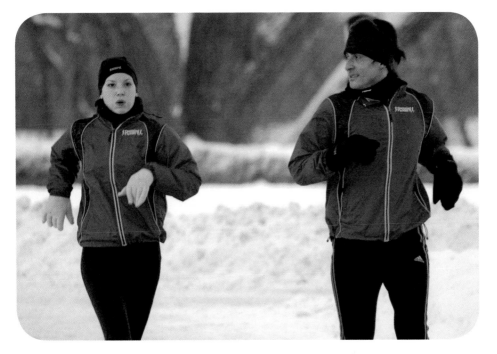

Heart Rate Training

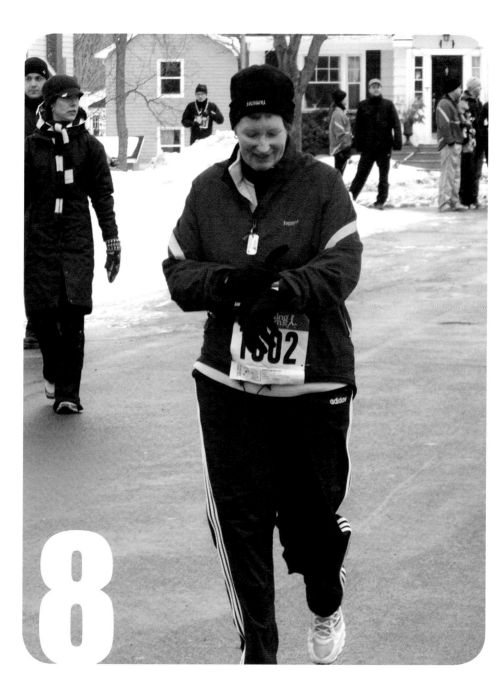

8

Understanding Exercise Intensity and Target Zones

Different training workouts require you to exercise at different intensities. As your training intensity increases, so does your heart rate, and monitoring your heart rate is probably the most widely known method of determining your training intensity. The development of wireless heart rate monitors has given many athletes, from beginners to experts, an easy, effective way to gauge their training intensity.

You can't always predict how your heart is going to respond to exercise. Fatigue, illness and overtraining can have profound effects on heart rate, so always listen to your body. Don't be a slave to your heart rate monitor; you should look at it about every 10 minutes, not every minute, especially during a race.

Objectives:

After completing this chapter you will:

+ Understand what exercise intensity is and why it should be measured or tracked during activity.
+ Determine your estimated maximum heart rate and your personal target heart rate zone for exercise.
+ Be able to measure how your body responds to cardiovascular activity.

The New Tools of the Trade

With a heart rate monitor (HRM), you have at your disposal a powerful control tool for making your workouts more effective and time efficient, safer and—equally important—much more fun.

The Heart Rate Window

Your HRM gives you a physiological window—through accurate heart rate measurement—into your body's response to the moment to moment rigors of physical activity. This precise view of what's happening inside your body allows you to make immediate adjustments in your exercise intensity to the level most appropriate for your body and your particular needs. Far more accurate than any other measure of physical activity—how fast you're going, or how far you've gone, for example—your heart rate reflects exactly how your system is functioning, and provides a measure of how hard you're working. (It's like watching a car's tachometer: The tach tells you how hard your engine's working in revolutions per minute, while your HRM tells you how hard your heart is working in beats per minute).

More Is Not Better

There is a considerable body of research that tells us that more is not necessarily better when it comes to exercise. In fact, training to exhaustion does far more to hurt performance than to enhance it. A typical adult can train at far lower levels of intensity than has been traditionally thought and still get fit; even reducing dress or slack sizes. Monitoring your heart rate to keep yourself at the right level of exercise intensity has become the training secret of the decade.

Benefits of Proper Training

Some basic exercises and training goals are universal. For example, strengthening the heart muscle through aerobic activity helps the heart pump more blood with each stroke. As total blood volume increases, the blood becomes better equipped to transport oxygen. Lung capacity increases, blood pressure decreases, and the entire cardiovascular system functions more efficiently. Some well-known benefits of aerobic training are better performance, better general health, improved muscle tone, weight loss and relief from stress and insomnia.

Training Smart

Monitoring your heart rate will take the guesswork out of training and ensure that your training intensities are optimal. If your heart rate during exercise is too low, you aren't working yourself hard enough to do yourself much good. If your heart rate is too high, you will most likely fatigue before the exercise can be beneficial. Monitoring your heart rate ensures that you stay within your optimal target heart rate zone, optimizing the benefits of your workouts and eliminating uncertainty about safety.

The Benefits of Monitoring Heart Rate

Heart Rate Monitors and Motivation

Statistics show that over 70% of the people who start an exercise program will quit within the first six months—and many within the first few weeks. What makes it so hard for individuals to stick with an exercise program? Why do they give up so quickly? One of the primary factors affecting adherence to exercise is a loss of motivation.

Most people start an exercise program with a specific goal or need in mind that becomes the driving force or motivation behind their desire to exercise. However, many individuals run into common obstacles that cause them to lose sight of these goals and begin to lose their motivation to keep going.

Fortunately, a heart rate monitor can provide the solution to many of the obstacles that stand in the way of success in an exercise program.

Keeps You in Your Zone

If you want to reach your exercise goals, it's important to stay in your target heart rate zone during workouts. A heart rate monitor is your constant reminder of the intensity and quality of each workout session. Nothing keeps you in your zone more accurately than a Heart Rate Monitor. The Polar™ brand of Heart Rate Monitors are some of the best monitors available.

Heart Rate Monitor Shows Your Progress

It takes four to six weeks of consistent exercise before you begin to see any external changes to your body. Although you can't see them, internal improvements begin to take place immediately. Your heart rate is an efficiency rating for your entire body. As your fitness level improves, your heart rate improves along with it. A heart rate monitor gives you a physiological window into your body's response to the daily improvements in your physical health.

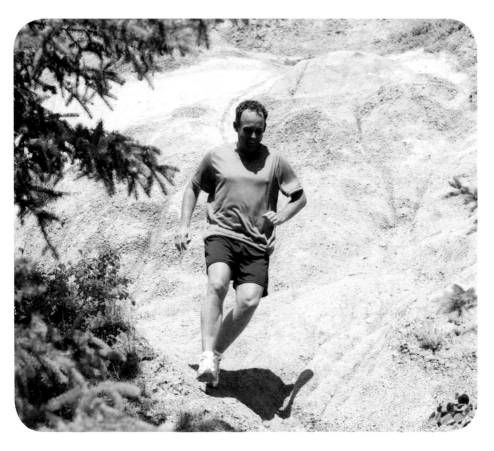

A Heart Rate Monitor Eliminates Frustration

If your heart rate is too low during exercise your body reaps little or no benefits. This means you're not likely to see the results you want, like weight loss or increased endurance. If your heart rate is too high during exercise you may tire too quickly and become frustrated, or even run the risk of injury. In either case, you're likely to quit exercising because you're not getting the results you want or because it's simply too difficult. A heart rate monitor keeps you exercising by showing you results that you otherwise would not see.

Keeps You Safe

Exercising too hard can put you at risk for injury. A heart rate monitor reminds you of the safe and effective heart rate intensity in which you should exercise and warns you when you leave that safety zone.

Exercise Intensity and Heart Rate Monitors

To understand exercise intensity and how a heart rate monitor helps achieve fitness goals, our friends at *Polar Heart Rate Monitors* provided these rules—be familiar with Three Keys to Success:

1. Working out at the correct exercise intensity is the only way to achieve your fitness goals.

   Too hard = injury, muscle soreness = can't finish workout.

   Too easy = no improvement or results = will not reach fitness goals.

2. Heart rate is the only accurate measurement of exercise intensity.

3. HRMs are the easiest and most accurate way to measure continuous heart rate.

The continuous display of heart rate is what makes your workout effective. This is because your heart rate is guiding you during your whole workout, just like a coach. As the speedometer in your car tells you how fast your car is going, your heart rate tells you how fast and hard you are going.

What Is Exercise Intensity?

Exercise intensity is simply a measurement of how hard you are working at a given time during exercise. The American College of Sports Medicine (ACSM), the world's leading medical and scientific authority on sports medicine and fitness, recommends that every individual involved in an exercise program should know how hard their body is working during exercise.

Your heart provides key information for determining how intensely you are working during exercise. Your heart rate (how many times your heart beats per minute) is really an efficiency rating for your entire body. The number of times your heart beats during each minute of exercise is a measurement of the intensity of the exercise. If your heart rate is low, exercise intensity is low; if your heart rate is high, your exercise intensity is high.

Why Should Exercisers Monitor Exercise Intensity?

Your heart is the most important muscle in your body and, like all muscles, must be exercised regularly to remain strong and efficient. According to fitness experts, exercise is more effective when you work out in a specific heart rate range or zone. (This is referred to as your Target Heart Rate Zone (TZ)). This zone can vary greatly depending on your age, fitness level and various other factors.

Example

Debby and Thomas are at the same cardiovascular fitness level and plan to run 5 mi. Debby decides to jog and Thomas decides to sprint. Whose exercise intensity level will allow them to maintain their speed for the entire 5 mi.? The answer is Debby. Thomas will be too tired to sprint the entire 5 mi.; he cannot maintain an exercise intensity that high.

Monitoring exercise intensity helps you stay at a level of exercise that allows you to accomplish your goals. In fact, the ACSM recommends that, in order to get the most benefits from your cardiovascular exercise, you should work within your Target Heart Rate Zone for at least 20 to 60 minutes per workout, three to five times per week, at an intensity of 60–80% of your maximum heart rate. Knowing your exercise intensity (heart rate) will allow you to work at the right level of exercise to accomplish this.

What is Maximum Heart Rate?

Maximum heart rate (MHR) is the maximum attainable heart rate your body can reach before total exhaustion. True maximum heart rate is measured during a fatigue or "stress" test. This test must be done in a clinical setting and is not practical or accessible for most people. Fortunately, your maximum heart rate can be estimated with a high degree of accuracy using the following simple formula:

Heart Rate Training

8

Male Estimated Maximum Heart Rate = 220 - Your Age
Female Estimated Maximum Heart Rate = 226 - Your Age

If John is 30 years old, what is his estimated maximum heart rate?

John's Estimated Maximum Heart Rate = 220 - 30
John's Estimated Maximum Heart Rate = 190

John's heart can beat an estimated maximum of 190 times per minute before his body would fatigue or "max out." This number is extremely helpful because it tells us the absolute highest exercise intensity John can handle before his body wears out. What this means is that during exercise, John should keep his heart rate below his maximum so that he will not become exhausted and have to quit. In fact, this gives John a specific percentage range of his maximum heart rate to exercise in known as his Target Heart Rate Zone (TZ).

How Do I Determine My Target Heart Rate Zone?

Your Target Heart Rate Zone (TZ) represents the minimum and maximum number of times your heart should beat in one minute of exercise. The ACSM recommends that all individuals should work within a TZ of 60–80% of their maximum heart rate (MHR). This means that your heart rate during exercise should not fall below 60% or rise above 80% of your maximum heart rate. Let's look at John from our earlier example.

John is 30 years old, so his estimated maximum heart rate is 220 - 30 or 190 beats per minutes (bpm). The ACSM says that John should exercise between 60% and 80% of 190 bpm to stay in his TZ. Let's determine John's TZ:

John's Estimated MHR	=	190 bpm
190 bpm (MHR) x 0.60 (60%)	=	114 bpm
190 bpm (MHR) x 0.80 (80%)	=	152 bpm
John's TZ	=	114–152 bpm

John will want to keep his heart rate in the range of 114–152 bpm during exercise in order to achieve his goals. If John is a beginning exerciser, he'll want to stay at the low end of his TZ. If John is a more advanced exerciser, he may want to work at the higher end of his TZ to challenge himself more.

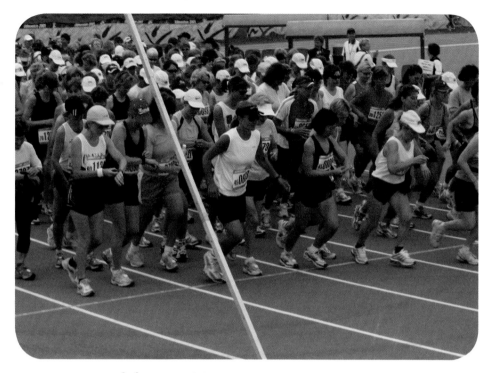

In summary, to define your TZ:

- The level that your heart rate needs to get to = lower limit
- The level that your heart rate should not exceed = upper limit.
- Keeping your heart rate between the lower and upper limits = staying within your TARGET ZONE.

The formula to find your target zone:

220 minus your age = maximum heart rate (MHR)

MHR x 60% = lower target zone limit

MHR x 80% = upper target zone limit

The Importance of Target Heart Rate Zone (TZ) in the Workout

Staying within your TZ is critical to meeting your exercise goals. However, the question becomes, "What is the correct TZ?" Before that question can be answered, you must know what your exercise goal is, because the most effective TZ is matched with your exercise goal.

- Maintain or lose weight, your TZ is 60–70% of MHR
- Reach cardiovascular fitness, your TZ is 70–80% of MHR
- Increase athletic performance, your TZ is 80% + of MHR

ANAEROBIC

Speed Training

80% Plus Max Heart Rate

+ 5 K to 10 K Race Pace
+ Speed Intervals
+ Increase athletic performance

AEROBIC

Threshold Training

Hill Training/Tempo/Fartlek
Done at 70 - 80% Max Heart Rate

+ These runs should be at a pace where you can talk, but not easily
+ Approaching anaerobic threshold but staying just below it
+ Reach cardiovascular fitness

RECOVERY/ENDURANCE

Base Training

Steady Runs & Long Slow Distance (LSD) Runs
Done at 60 - 70% Max Heart Rate

+ These runs should be easier, and you are still able to carry on a conversation
+ Maintain or lose weight

Heart Rate Training Made Easy

Base Training (Recovery/Endurance):

Typically you should find it difficult to keep your heart rate below the limits you have set for yourself. Don't cheat! Strict training in this area will prevent you from losing steam the last few kilometers of your long run. All training at this level is done at 60–70% of your maximum heart rate.

Threshold (Aerobic) Training:
Building the Walls

A good guideline in most cases is to run at your 10 K race pace. The purpose of this type of training is to work on proper form, strength and endurance. Hill training qualifies in this part of the house. Like hill training, you are not going to do this type of run every day. Any more than a couple times per week will over-fatigue your legs and compromise your long run. All training at this level is done at 70–80% of your maximum heart rate.

Speed Training (Anaerobic):
Putting on the Roof

Remember, owing to intensity, runs of this nature are best done as interval training. Your intervals should be no longer than a few minutes. Your hear rate should recover to approximately 120 bpm (one to two minutes of rest) before starting the next interval. Like hills, start off with only a few (two to three). Vary the distances of each interval and the total distance covered from week to week. Build slowly from there. With this type of training, a warm-up and cooldown are critical. Warm-up with a couple of kilometers of easy running and a stretch. All training at this level is done at a range of 80% plus of your maximum heart rate.

Aerobic or Anaerobic? That is the Question.

These terms are thrown around quite loosely in the gyms and on the track these days. Here's the low-down on what they really mean. Aerobic means "in the presence of oxygen." What makes an activity aerobic or not is its intensity. Energy for low-intensity exercise can be supplied by aerobic metabolism. Although aerobic metabolism can supply a lot of energy (from birth to death), it can only do so quite slowly. Aerobic metabolism is very efficient and has very few by-products such as lactic acid. Only very small amounts of lactic acid are produced during aerobic exercise, and this can normally be removed by the body before we feel any adverse effects.

During high-intensity exercise there is a quick and high demand for energy at a very fast rate. Since aerobic metabolism is too slow to supply the energy, our body must shift gears and produce energy at a faster rate. Although anaerobic metabolism can produce a lot of energy in a very short time, the chemical reactions involved create a great amount of lactic acid. So much lactic acid is produced that we cannot get rid of it fast enough, causing it to accumulate in the muscles and blood. Lactic acid accumulation to a high level causes that burning feeling in the legs and queasy feeling in the stomach. If anaerobic exercise persists, lactic acid interferes in the energy making process. Exercise intensity will have to slow in order to continue or come to a complete halt. This is why predominantly anaerobic exercise can be done for no longer than approximately two minutes. Yes, only two, even for highly trained athletes. For most of us, it's less!

Examples of predominantly aerobic exercise:
+ Walking
+ Running easy
+ Cycling easy
+ Swimming

"Anaerobic" means "in the absence of oxygen"; when the intensity of exercise is too high for the body to get enough oxygen, and aerobic metabolism is too slow to supply energy at such a fast rate, the body must shift gears and produce energy by anaerobic metabolism. Such high-intensity exercise is called "anaerobic exercise."

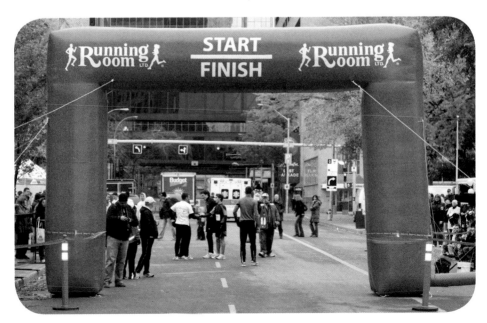

Examples of predominantly anaerobic exercise:

+ Speed work, as outlined in *Chapter 9, Types of Running*

No one activity is only aerobic or only anaerobic. Most activities that we participate in day to day require both types of metabolism.

Glossary of Heart Rate Terms

Resting Heart Rate:

This is the number of times your heart beats per minute during complete uninterrupted rest. It is usually taken upon waking in the morning, before you lift your head from the pillow.

Maximum Heart Rate:

This is the highest number of times your heart can contract in one minute. It can only be measured accurately by taking a stress test in which you exercise until exhaustion. Predictive formulas are most commonly used.

A more practical test for maximal heart rate without a stress test is the maximal hill run. To perform this test you need the following:

1. A hill (6–8% grade, approx. 400–600 m in length)

2. Heart rate monitor

3. A healthy dose of determination

After an appropriate warm up of at least 10 minutes that includes stretching, make your way to the bottom of the hill you have chosen. From there you run as hard as you can without stopping, to the top. At the top check your heart rate monitor. You should be pretty close to your maximum heart rate. Don't stop at the top. You have just run really hard and taxed your anaerobic system, so there will be a lot of lactic acid in your blood and muscles. An active recovery of walking or slow running will speed your recovery and help remove lactic acid from your muscles and blood. Be sure to do a proper cooldown including some stretches.

Anaerobic Threshold:

This is the point (intensity, heart rate, speed) at which aerobic metabolism is not able to supply energy fast enough to keep up with the demands of the activity. A shift to anaerobic metabolism takes place and, if continued, exercise will cease (whether you want it to or not).

VO 2 max:

This is the maximum amount of oxygen our muscles can use for exercise. Our bodies are able to take in much more oxygen than our muscles could ever use. What we do by endurance training is train our heart, lungs and blood to deliver more oxygen to the exercising muscles. We also train our muscles to use more oxygen more efficiently. VO2 max occurs at the intensity of exercise that corresponds to maximum heart rate. We are usually able to exercise at this intensity for only a few minutes.

Anaerobic Threshold Heart Rate (ATHR):

This is the heart rate that corresponds with the change from aerobic to predominantly anaerobic metabolism. The threshold is often known as OBLAS: onset of blood lactate accumulation.

Heart Rate Recovery:

This is the time after you exercise that is used to measure the reduction in your heart rate. Total Heart Rate Recovery is the time between cessation of exercise and return to normal heart rate. A common recovery time is two minutes.

Calculate HR Zones:

Using Heart Rate Reserve (HRR) to calculate your Heart Rate training zones is also referred to as the Karvonen method. The formula is HRR x Intensity% + HRmin (resting heart rate).

To calculate your HRR take your HRmax (Maximum Heart Rate)— 226 minus age for women or 220 minus age for men—and subtract your resting heart rate. You can then use that in the formula above to calculate the following zones:

Zone 1: 50–60%
Zone 2: 61–70%
Zone 3: 71–80%
Zone 4: 81–90%
Zone 5: 91–100%

Remember, the best time to measure your resting heart rate is just as you wake or just before you go to sleep. Your heart rate (both at rest and in training) can be elevated by many factors, including:

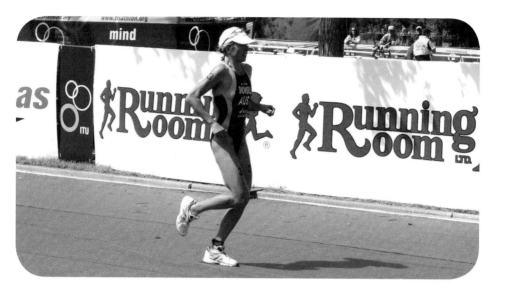

- Nutrition, especially hydration levels, will also greatly influence your HR. Dehydration will skyrocket your HR.
- Heat will also increase HR until your body adapts to it usually in 7 to 12 days.
- Altitude will affect your HR as well. You will have a higher HR for the same level of intensity at higher elevations, so give your body three weeks or so to adapt.

Warning Signs Of Trouble:

The symptoms listed below are warnings that more serious trouble might develop if you don't take immediate preventative action. Develop a sensitive eye to these signals. By quickly interpreting and acting upon these symptoms, you can stop trouble at its source.

- Resting pulse rate significantly higher than normal when taken first thing in the morning.
- Sudden, dramatic weight loss.
- Difficulty falling asleep or staying asleep.
- Sores in and around the mouth, and other skin eruptions.
- Any symptom of a cold or the flu (sniffles, sore throat, or fever).
- Swollen, tender glands in the neck, groin or underarms.
- Dizziness or nausea before, during or after training.
- Clumsiness—tripping or kicking yourself—during a run over rather smooth ground.
- Any muscle, tendon or joint pain or stiffness that remains after the first few minutes of running.

Types of Running

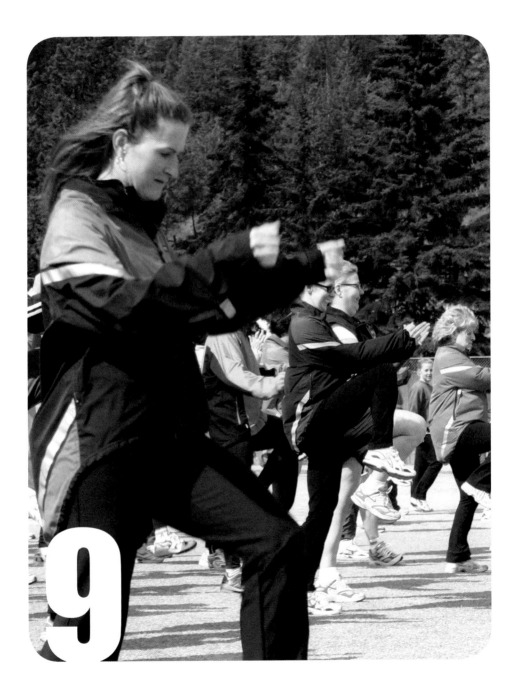

9

Basic running is as simple as putting one foot in front of the other quickly, but there are various kinds of running that can be used for different purposes: speed work, for instance, such as interval training and fartleks, helps a runner run faster; hill work builds strength; long runs build endurance. This chapter looks at the various types of running and how you can incorporate them into your training program.

Types of Training

Long Runs

Long slow distance is the foundation of your entire running. Think of it as long slow distance fun. The consistency and progressive nature of the long slow run provide you with a gentle buildup of endurance strength. This adaptation phase prepares you to be on your legs for an extended period of time.

Tempo Runs

An "up tempo" hard run once per week will improve your coordination and leg turnover rate. Before starting these high-quality speed sessions, run your hills for strength.

Form Drill

Once or twice per week these increases in accelerations will snap your legs and lungs into another gear. These drills are fun sessions, with short, medium and long bursts of speed, followed by as much recovery as you feel necessary. The Swedes have a grand name for this speed play; they call it "fartlek." During these sessions you should constantly check on your running form and focus on "belly breathing."

Social Runs

For most runners, this run is the Wednesday run, or practice run, at your local Running Room. These runs are done at a comfortable "talk test" pace with other runners. The social aspect of the easy runs provides a rest and recovery day and sparks your motivation level. The social run is a great way to expand your circle of friends.

Races

A race can provide a goal. Runners need goals to stay motivated. A group can inspire and motivate each other when training for a common goal or target. Alone, it can be daunting; together we can do it. A race can test your current fitness level or set a new benchmark in your own personal best quest. A race can be in familiar surroundings or in different places. For many, there is an added thrill of running away from home—in a group! A race is also a chance to collect a new T-shirt and some tasty goodies at the finish line. Some even have medals for all finishers. Medals really inspire a runner to continue to run and to collect even more medals! Races provide each runner with their own special bragging rights to share with family and friends.

Easy Runs

These recovery massage-type runs are fun and highly recommended. In all my years of running and coaching I have yet to come across a runner who has been injured by running too slowly. So this easy run is a safe day. Enjoy these injury-free, slow, easy days.

Running Drills

(Teaching a Duck to Dance)
For years, Olympic coaches have been using drills that focus on the muscles and tendons specifically used in running. The exercises develop the full range of motion of the leg muscles, the hamstrings and the quadriceps, along with improving running form and coordination.

Running Drill Rules

+ Be gentle in your whole approach to the drills.

+ Think of the coordination involved, as well as the strength.

+ Keep it fun. This is not work, it is play. Enjoy yourself.

Stretch and warm-up before your practice.

High-knee Drill

This drill will work your feet, ankles, Achilles tendons, calf muscles, abdominal muscles and the driving muscles in your butt. Take it easy, this is high-quality stuff. In addition to all of the muscle groups, you should also be working on your rhythm and coordination.

+ Start with high-knee walking, lifting your knees as high as you can.
+ Keep your posture erect.

- Drive your knees forward to waist height.
- Rise up on your toes.
- Lean slightly forward, but keep your posture erect.
- Think of the lift coming from your abdominal muscles.
- Start with a distance of 25 m and gradually work your way up to about 100 m.
- Think of a slow-motion action.
- Progress to high-knee running.
- Foot strike is quick and light—you are on hot coals!
- Think high knees and fast reflex action—you are prancing.

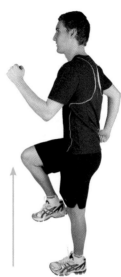

Kick Some Butt

Ah ha, this sounds like just the kind of drill you've be looking for to vent some of that nonrunning stress. Well, I have some good news and some bad news: the good news is that you get to kick some butt; the bad news is that it's your own butt you'll be kicking.

The purpose of this drill is to primarily work on your body position while improving your coordination and flexibility. We have all seen runners who seem to sit back as fatigue sets in during the later stages of a long run. This drill will help you attain a slight forward lean, which improves your form and ultimately your running times by getting that old buddy gravity to do some of the work for you.

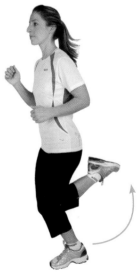

- Look slightly in front of where you are running.
- Keep your arms and hands loose at your sides.
- Get up on the front of your feet.
- Run with your feet kicking back.
- Try to kick high enough to kick your own butt, so to speak.
- Do repeats of 50–75 m.
- Your arms will help to balance you, although it will feel awkward at first.

Yahoo Jump

Most of us can recall this one from our youth. If we had done 20 of these a week, we would have developed all of the running muscle groups well, particularly the hip flexors.

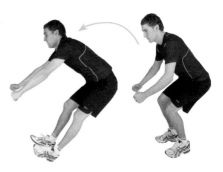

+ Stand with our feet together, flat on the ground.
+ Jump forward, keeping your feet together.
+ Kick both legs forward.
+ Land with your feet together.
+ Swing your arms to assist in the jump.
+ Do a total of about 75–100 m.
+ Holler a loud yahoo! (optional).

Old Goose-step Drill

This is no Mother Goose drill: it looks easy, but once you try it you will discover that it's a great workout for your feet, ankles, quadriceps and hamstrings.

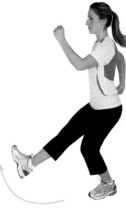

+ Run up on your toes.
+ Kick your legs forward keeping them straight.
+ Keep your knees locked.
+ Your arms should be bent at a 90-degree angle.
+ Keep your steps short and fast.
+ Chase the old goose for only about 50–100 m. Remember you're looking for quality, not quantity.

Pedal-to-the-Metal Bursts

This drill is a fun power acceleration in which you start slowly and then continuously accelerate for 100 m. Try to maintain the form and coordination that you have been practicing in the other drills. Relax, keep your breathing regular and concentrate on a steady acceleration. Even if you start slowly, you will find that you quickly reach your maximum speed. Learn to dig out that extra effort to find the additional speed within yourself—it is a great reward to find the extra speed that has been hiding from you.

Follow-the-Wacky-Leader Fartleks

The running blahs descend on all of us from time to time. They may come from a long period of intense training for a particular goal, or a recent bout of inclement weather can set you off. The best way to rid yourself of the blahs is to get some fun back in your running. I have used this fun drill with my running clubs over the years when things seem to be getting too serious.

First, call out a number as you point to each runner to number everyone in the group—it doesn't matter whether there are just two runners or a large group. Head out on your run, starting with five minutes of easy running to keep the group together. In order, each runner must decide on a fun fartlek or drill that the rest of the group has to participate in. Each drill should be 5 to 10 minutes long. Here are a couple of suggestions to get you started.

Park Bench Jump

Run a loop of about 150 m and jump over a park bench. Hands are permitted.

Beast Hill Workout

My long-time training partner Mike O'Dell started this one when he spotted a killer hill of 150 m with what looked like a grade of 60%. The rules call for only one hill repeat. No crawling is allowed and cheering is compulsory for everyone who reaches the top.

Hill Training

Depending on where you live, hills may be a part of your life every day or they may be something that you've heard of, but not in your part of the world!

Hills are a wonderful way to add some resistance to your training. When you overcome resistance to your training, your muscles get stronger and the intensity of your training increases. Runners have used hills for decades as a way to increase endurance, strength and speed.

Let's talk about how to do the hill sessions. First, and not surprisingly, you should find a hill. The hill should be 400–600 m in length and should have an incline of 6–8%. Prior to starting the hill session, be sure that you have warmed up and are relaxed and fluid. If after your warm-up you still feel fatigued from the previous day, do not do the hill session. This high-quality session should only be done when you are fully ready to work hard.

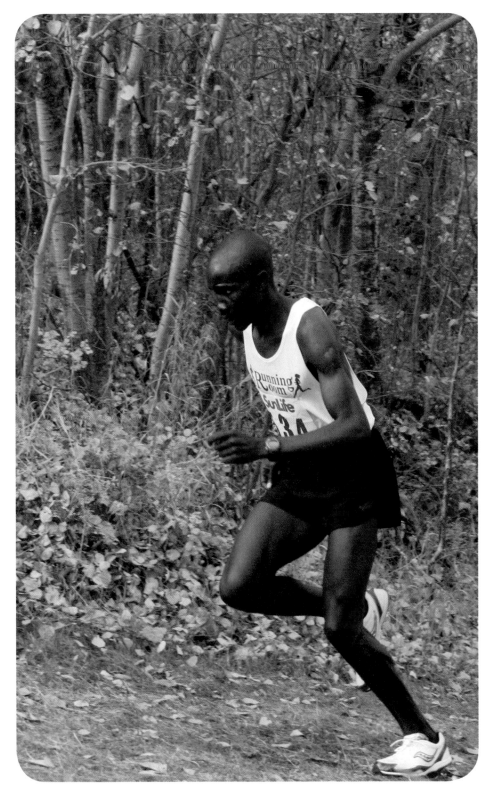

Proper Hill Form

When you are warm and ready, start at the top of the hill and walk down easily. Think of this as part of your warm-up or recovery from the previous hill. When you get to the bottom, don't stop and rest. Resting just gives you time to think about the task at hand and will often get you thinking negatively.

+ Begin your journey up. Try to maintain the same stride frequency as you would on flat ground; shorten it as you adjust to the grade.

+ Don't forget to swing your arms. Although your arms don't actually propel you up the hill, they can be important to maintain proper form and leg speed. Your arms are always in rhythm with your legs. When you find your leg turnover slowing near the top, pump your arms a little faster and your legs will be sure to follow.

+ As you run, be sure to keep your posture erect, rather than leaning too far forward. Try to look parallel to the surface of the hill. In doing this an amazing thing happens: the hill appears to flatten and is not as tough as if you looked up with your eyes while keeping your head down.

+ Concentrate on good form and increase the rhythm of your arms slightly as you near the crest of the hill. Push over the crest.

+ Keep your chest up and out. Keep your breathing relaxed.

+ Think of the power coming from your legs; they are strong and efficient. The key is to maintain the same effort as you go up the hill. Your speed will slow slightly and increase again as you reach the crest of the hill. Keep the same effort at the crest and walk past the top before turning around.

+ Never stop once you have reached the top. Continue a slow jog or a walk. This hill training is pretty intense. By continuing to keep moving, you will enhance your recovery and be ready sooner for your next repeat.

+ Start with four hill repeats and increase by one repeat each successive week, working up to a maximum of 12 repeats. After a hill session, allow at least two days of recovery before you attempt another quality workout.

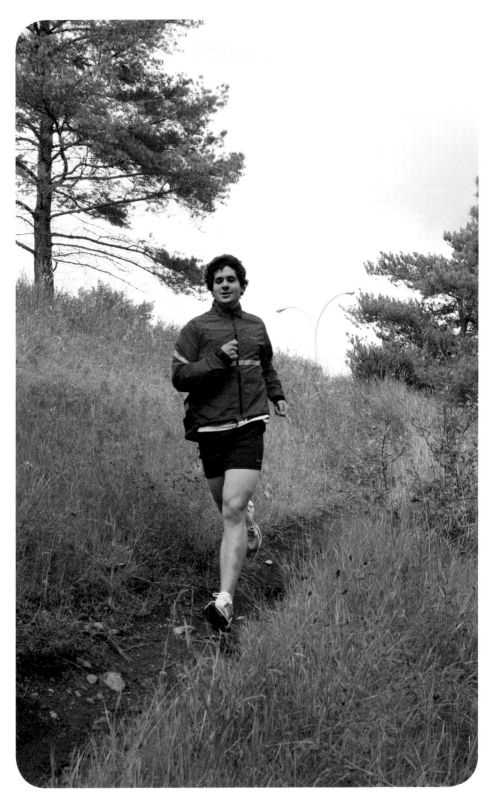

Hill Training Summary

1. Warm-up walk and cooldown walk
2. Erect posture
3. Visualize a flat hill
4. Start with 4 repeats
5. Maximum 12 repeats
6. 2 easy days after workout

Downhill Running

A good number of runners make running downhill difficult and risk injury by leaning back and putting on the brakes as they run down the hill. Here is a tip to improve your running times and reduce the risk of injury; gravity is your training buddy. With a slight lean down the hill, gravity will pick up your pace with no additional effort. Many runners lean back into the hill, but this takes more effort and is slower. Open your stride slightly, lean forward and away you go with your new training buddy. Come race day the experience of the hill sessions pays big dividends as you pass runners not only on the uphills but at the crest and on the downhills as well.

Intensity

For those using their target heart rate, intensity is 80% of maximum heart rate. If you are not using heart rate as your gauge of intensity, then pace yourself so that you are running up the hill as fast as you can without having to stop and rest. Always rest for at least as long as it takes to run up the hill or until your heart rate is below 120 bpm. Rest is part of your training.

Be careful if you are doing the hill session with a group. Remember, it is not a race but a quality, individual workout. Run to the hill and do the warm-up with the group, but the hill is yours alone to conquer at your own speed. Hills are magic stuff if treated with respect and some common sense.

Another ingredient that hills add is character. As you do the hill repeats, mentally, or if it helps, verbally, repeat the words "character, character." On race day when you discover a hill on the course think back to the hill sessions and the word "character." No race course will have 12 repeats in it. Hills build your confidence level and increase your self-esteem, as well as prepare you mentally to be a better athlete.

A once-a-week investment in the "visually flat" hill session will make you a better athlete both mentally and physically.

Speed Training

Nailing on the roof is the last thing we do in our training analogy, which means we work on speed training. This should not take place until six to eight weeks before the event. Speed training should really be thought of as the fine-tuning done in preparation before race day. Even then, if sufficient base and strength training are not completed by this time, speed training may be contraindicated.

What Is the Purpose of Speed Training?

Speed training isn't for everyone. If you are a first-time marathoner or a time goal is not your priority, then continuing to work on your long-term fitness should be the most important aspect of your training.

For those looking for more specific results in the marathon, speed training may become an important phase in preparation for the event. The principle of training specificity states that what a person does in their training will directly affect how they do in their races. Generally this means that if you want to run an 8-minute kilometer in your event, you'd better get your body used to or able to run at that pace in training.

How Hard and How Far?

Pacing is a critical aspect to successful speed training because it involves running a set pace over a specified distance. Short distances are used in speed training because the pace is hard enough that it can only be maintained for a short period of time (three to six minutes). To keep pacing simple, use your race paces for 1 mi., 5 km and 10 km. Each interval should be finished in approximately the same time. If you are burning out or slowing the pace during the last intervals, you probably started too fast. If you are becoming faster throughout the workout, you most likely started off too slowly. The idea is to maintain the desired pace for the entire workout. Try not to become discouraged. Pacing really takes practice.

Rest between intervals is a very important aspect of speed training. A good rule of thumb is to rest for as long as it takes you to run the interval. You can then adjust the rest period depending on your pace or how you feel. During your rest period, try to remain active (walking, slow jogging). Stopping or bending over to rest will delay recovery and promote feelings of nausea or light-headedness. Remember, too much rest can defeat the purpose of the speed work and too little can poop you out before any training can be accomplished.

The nice thing about speed training is that the total distance covered during the workout isn't really the most important aspect. Interval distances at these paces should be no longer than 1500 m and no shorter than 400 m (use the faster paces for the shorter distances and the slower for the longer distances). For most runners, three to five intervals of a moderate length is a good place to start.

The longer the total distance you cover, the longer your intervals should be resulting in fewer repetitions. To progress, add no more than 500–1000 m of speed work per week.

The Speed Training Workout

There are three components of a speed training workout and all three are critical to this type of training's success.

The Three Components of Speed Training

1. Warm-up
2. Speed workout
3. Cooldown

1. Warm-up:

As mentioned earlier, the warm-up is crucial to any workout, but especially so in speed training. Speed training puts a lot of stress on the running muscles as it forces you to run at race pace or faster. Warm-up should consist of at least 10 minutes of light aerobic activity (slower running) followed by 5 minutes of prestretching. A prestretch doesn't require you to hold the stretches for as long a period. In addition, you may want to cut down on the number of stretches you do and really focus on the working muscles of the legs and lower back.

2. The Workout:

Plan, plan, plan. Always know what you are going to do before you get to the track or the start of a run.

3. Cooldown:

Cooldown is more crucial after speed training because you have been working at a much higher intensity. Cooldowns after speed training should always include light aerobic activity (10 minutes of slow running) and stretching.

Nutrition

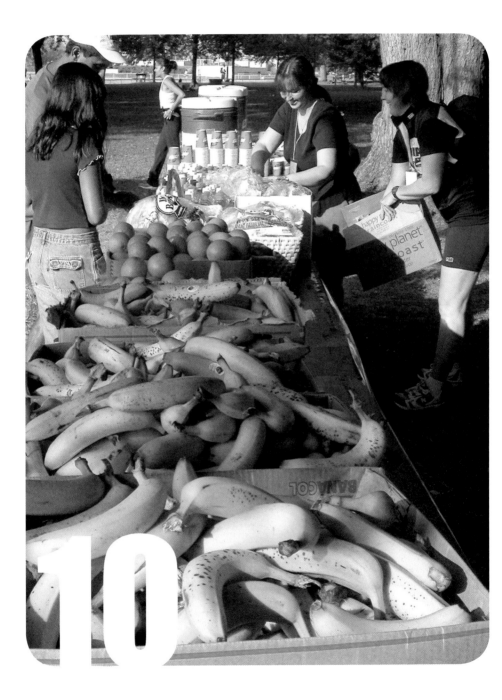

10

Nutrition Overview

There are literally volumes of books dedicated to the topics of nutrition and weight control. A single chapter can only brush the surface of our understanding of nutrition, but the following pages should help provide you with appropriate guidelines to make healthy eating part of an active lifestyle.

A major issue facing most of us is how to make better choices in our daily intake of food and liquids. Think of one glass of water filled with our daily intake of calories and another glass filled with your daily output of calories through exercise and daily living. Simple enough. If you are at the perfect weight and body fat content, then you will strive to have the same amount of water in both glasses. For the vast majority of us trying to lose a few pounds, however, the goal is to have a larger glass for the output than for the input. (In reality, most of us enjoy more input than output.)

Many people become obsessed with the fat and oil contents of their food while neglecting to take note of the total number of calories consumed. Too many calories taken in, even from healthy foods like salads, breads and lean meats, still get converted to fat for storage, which is why exercise is so vital. The most important thing is a balance between the amount of exercise we get and the amount of food we consume. Intelligent choices in our food selections are what can really give us an advantage in weight management. More importantly, we must think of our total well-being rather than just management of our body weight.

The Scale

Do yourself a favor today and give your scale away, preferably to someone you don't like. For the most part, it is only an accurate measure of how much water we have consumed and whether or not we are well hydrated.

Rather than using a scale to chart your progress, take some measurements of your chest, arms, thighs, calves, hips and waist. Mark them down and revisit the measurements every couple of months.

An even simpler way to see our body change is to get a tight pair of pants, one that you can just barely stuff yourself into, and mark them. Those pants will be your benchmark of fitness today and into the future. Once a week, try on the pants to see how they fit.

Alternately, for those of you who are brave and not particularly concerned about modesty, stand naked in front of a mirror. What you see today is the start point. Once a week, make your trip to the full-length mirror. I do suggest that this be done alone; the mirror can be blatantly honest, and this is not the time for critics.

Healthy Eating for the Long Run

Training for a marathon or half marathon can challenge your body beyond what you ever thought possible. The human body undergoes a multitude of very positive physical changes in response to endurance training. Blood volume expands to allow greater amounts of oxygen to reach body cells, muscle mass increases, and the body becomes adept at storing the fuel that will carry it to the end of the race. These changes allow you to finish your event "up-right and smiling." However, significant work is required on your part if you hope to reap these benefits. Consistent training, high-quality eating habits and obtaining adequate amounts of rest are all needed to lay the foundation that will support you during the many miles that lay ahead.

No two marathoners or half marathoners are alike! Despite this, long distance runners often share similar nutrition-related concerns and questions. "What does a good training diet look like?" "Should I be using sport drink?" and "What exactly do you do with gel?" are issues that all marathoners have faced. The good news is that crafting a well-balanced diet, like a really good, long run, is enjoyable and easy to do, provided you keep a few basic principles in mind.

Sports Nutrition Basics

Long distance runners, regardless of their experience or pace, are athletes in the truest sense of the word. Frequent, longer duration training sessions increase nutrient requirements. Responding to these heightened needs will help you maximize your training and strengthen your performance on race day.

Calories Count

Endurance training profoundly affects metabolism or the way the body uses energy (calories). Training for a marathon or half marathon involves hours of prolonged activity. The stress imposed by this kind of training dramatically increases a runner's need for energy. If this need is not met through a high-quality diet, chronic fatigue, rapid weight loss and a decrease in physical performance can occur, making consistent training next to impossible.

Balance, variety and moderation are the keys to a sound training diet. This means that no one food or food group is over or under emphasized. In practical terms, a healthy training diet:

+ Provides abundant amounts of whole grain products, vegetables and fruit
+ Contains moderate amounts of protein and fat
+ Limits (not eliminates) less nutritious foods, such as margarine, butter, higher-fat snack foods, sweets, alcohol and caffeinated beverages.

When you eat is almost as important as what you eat. A regular, consistent eating pattern is essential in terms of helping endurance athletes meet their calorie needs. Most marathoners and half marathoners need to eat at least three meals and three snacks each day to match the energy that they expend during training. Infrequent eating, skipping meals and chronic weight loss dieting can make getting enough calories very difficult. Avoiding these practices will enhance performance and allow you to make the most of your training runs.

Carbohydrates: Training Fuel

Carbohydrate is an essential nutrient that serves as the body's prime source of fuel during physical activity. In addition, carbohydrate is essential for utilizing or "burning" fat as a source of energy. Without adequate amounts of carbohydrate your body will be unable to draw on your fat stores to fuel your run.

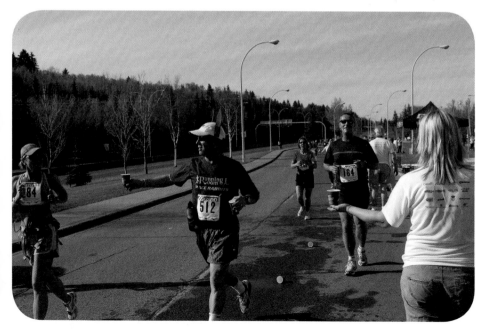

In foods, carbohydrates are found in two forms: simple carbohydrates (sugars) and complex carbohydrates (starches). In the body, both forms are digested or broken down to give glucose, the sugar that fuels all of our cells. During activity, glucose circulating in our blood can be withdrawn for use as an immediate source of fuel. Endurance athletes can also store glucose in their muscles and liver in a complex form called glycogen. Glycogen functions much like a backup or reserve fuel tank on a truck or motorcycle. During prolonged activity, the body can dip into its glycogen "tank" or stores for an added source of glucose.

Carbohydrate intake can make or break a long distance runner. When carbohydrate intake is marginal, glycogen is not stored in the amounts needed to support runs that last for more than an hour. As a result, endurance drops dramatically in runners who do not take in enough carbohydrate. This phenomenon, which sport nutritionists call "hitting the wall," can end even the best-trained athlete's dreams of glory. Depleting your glycogen stores has the same effect as a car running out of gas—things come to a halt. You cannot rebuild your glycogen stores during a long run or training session. Recognizing this, it's critically important that you take in enough carbohydrate on a daily basis. At least 55–65% of the energy (calories) in a distance runner's diet should come from this nutrient. Translated into food, this is a diet that contains approximately:

5 to 12 servings of grain products, where one serving equals:
+ 1 slice of bread
+ 30 g of cold cereal
+ 175 ml (¾ cup) hot cereal
+ ½ bagel, pita, or bun
+ 125 ml (½ cup) cooked pasta or rice

Plus 5 to 10 servings of vegetables and fruit, where one serving equals:
+ 1 medium-sized vegetable or fruit
+ 125 ml (½ cup) fresh, frozen, or canned vegetables or fruit
+ 250 ml (1 cup) salad
+ 125 ml (½ cup) vegetable or fruit juice

Marathoners and half marathoners should aim for the middle to upper ends of these serving ranges in order to meet their heightened needs for carbohydrate.

Fluid Intake

Fluids: Wetter is Better!
Water, like carbohydrate, is a critical nutrient for long distance runners to focus

on. Unfortunately, water intake is often overlooked, a practice which can have disastrous results.

Water is essential for:
+ Regulating body temperature
+ Transporting glucose and other nutrients to cells
+ Removing waste products.

All of these processes suffer when water intake is inadequate and dehydration can result. Dehydration or lack of body water is a very real concern that all runners need to be aware of. Left unchecked, dehydration curbs endurance and overall physical performance. In extreme cases, dehydration can be deadly.

Fluid Myths

Many myths exist about water and other fluids. For example, runners often mistakenly believe that you only need to drink when you are thirsty. This is not true.

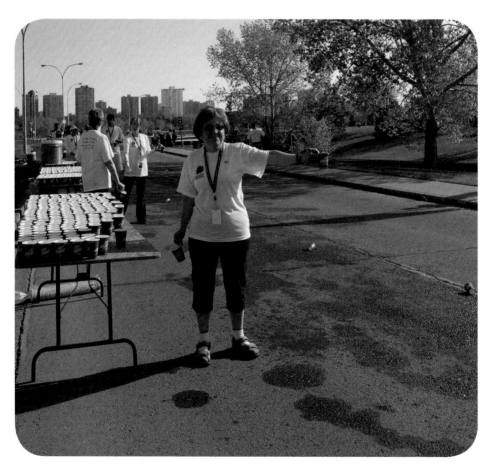

In fact, by the time you become thirsty you are usually already dehydrated. Many people also believe that you can treat dehydration while continuing to run. Again, this is more myth than fact. Treating dehydration involves taking in substantial amounts of fluid (e.g., 1 L or more) over a relatively short period of time. Most runners could not consume this much fluid and continue to run in comfort.

How Much Is Enough?

Endurance running dramatically increases your need for water and other fluids. You may have heard that you should take in 8 cups (2 L) of fluid each day for good health. However, what many people do not realize is that this recommendation describes the minimum amount of fluid required by an inactive person. It does not account for prolonged activity and is far too low to meet the needs of marathon and half marathon runners.

Significant amounts of body water can be lost during the course of a long run. Sweat losses of 500 ml (2 cups) of body water per hour are not unusual. These losses must be replaced or physical performance will drop off.

More is better when it comes to taking in enough fluids. Healthy, active people are unlikely to "over do it" with fluids, and concerns about "water overload" are largely unfounded. If you are not a "big drinker" you may need to focus on this aspect of nutrition for a while in order to change your behavior. Keep the following guidelines in mind to make sure that you are getting enough fluid:

- Drink regularly when you are not active—sip 125 ml (½ cup) to 250 ml (1 cup) per waking hour of your day.
- Center some of your fluid intake around your runs or other activities.
- Drink 500 ml (2 cups) of fluid in the two-hour period before exercise.
- Take time out to drink 150 ml (²/₃ cup) to 300 ml (1¹/₃ cups) of fluid every 20 minutes during exercise.

What Counts as Fluid?

In general, all decaffeinated, nonalcoholic beverages contribute to your daily fluid intake. This includes water, sparkling water, caffeine-free teas and coffee, fluid replacement sport drinks, juices and milk.

Some liquids can actually promote dehydration. Use regular coffee and teas, caffeinated soft drinks and alcoholic beverages in moderation to avoid this effect.

Do I Need to Use Sport Drinks?

Sport drinks or fluid/electrolyte replacement beverages help to "top up" blood glucose levels. This, in turn, helps to preserve or "spare" your glycogen stores and promote endurance. Sport drinks also replace minerals like potassium and sodium that are lost during exercise. Research indicates that during prolonged activity (i.e. more than one hour of activity) these products may improve performance. Not all runners can tolerate sport drinks. Recognizing this, it is important to experiment with sport drinks during training to assess their impact on your individual performance. Never, ever try a sport drink on race day if you have not already tested it during training. And keep the following tips in mind when experimenting with these products:

+ Choose a commercially prepared sport drink. Commercially prepared fluid replacement drinks contain carbohydrates, sodium and other minerals in amounts that are well absorbed and most likely to be tolerated. Steer clear of recipes for homemade sport drinks, which can be difficult to formulate to the specifications needed to maximize performance.

+ Following the manufacturer's directions when preparing sport drinks from a powdered mix. Add the exact amount of water specified on the label to prepare a drink that provides appropriate amounts of carbohydrates and minerals.

+ Drink small amounts at regular intervals. Consuming large volumes of sport drink in a relatively short period of time can promote bloating and abdominal cramping.

+ Keep it cool. Cool, rather than ice cold, fluids are easier to drink in the amounts needed to keep you well hydrated.

How Can I Tell If I'm Getting Enough Fluid?

There are a number of simple things you can do to assess your fluid intake:

1. Check out your urine! Well-hydrated people produce urine in relatively large amounts and they urinate frequently. Examining the color of your urine can also give you an indication of your fluid status. If you are taking in enough fluid, your urine will be pale colored, similar to dilute lemonade.

2. Weigh in before and after exercising. If you've lost an appreciable amount of weight during a workout it's not body fat. Instead, what you are seeing

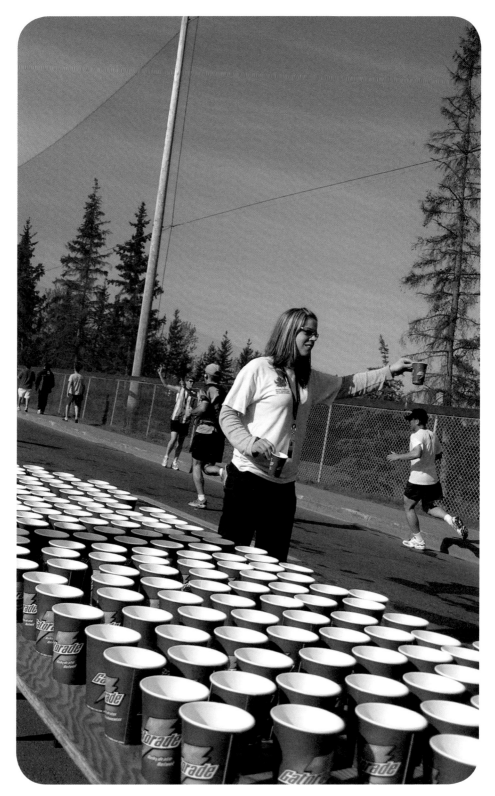

is fluid loss. Remember that a 0.5 kg (1 lb.) weight loss is roughly equal to 500 ml (2 cups) of water that have been lost and need replacing.

3. Know the symptoms of dehydration. Dehydration is a continuum of physical symptoms that are quite subtle at first but progress in their intensity as more and more water leaves the body. Common signs of dehydration include thirst, headache, fatigue, irritability, chills and nausea. If you experience any of these symptoms during a run you need to stop and rehydrate.

Caffeine

Here we defer to the experts! When it comes to nutrition or sports medicine, the Running Room is associated with many professionals who provide us with a wealth of knowledge that is current and accurate. Susan Glen and Heidi Bates are regular contributors to the Running Room training programs and web site on all issues related to nutrition. You will see both names popping up throughout this chapter, and we thank them for their contribution.

Caffeine and Running
By Susan Glen, MSc Nutrition

As soon as we started selling Power Gels out of the Kinsmen Running Room location (and we sell a lot, since we're located in a fitness facility) our customers asked why there was caffeine added to the strawberry-banana flavor. This led to many in-store discussions about caffeine and running.

Many runners make a cup of coffee a part of their prerun/prerace routine. But what effect does caffeine really have on performance?

There are several ways caffeine may improve performance in endurance events. Caffeine stimulates the central nervous system which facilitates neuromuscular function by improving muscle contraction/reaction time. This effect on the CNS may also lead to a decreased perception of fatigue.

Another potentially beneficial effect of caffeine for runners is an increased concentration of free fatty acids in the blood and increased uptake and utilization of these fatty acids by muscle tissue. This, in turn, spares the muscles' limited supply of glycogen.

The importance of this effect is illustrated by the term "hitting the wall," which is the point at which a person's glycogen stores have been completely depleted. All of this makes caffeine sound like it's the ultimate aid for the long distance runner. However, there is a downside to the use of caffeine.

10 Nutrition

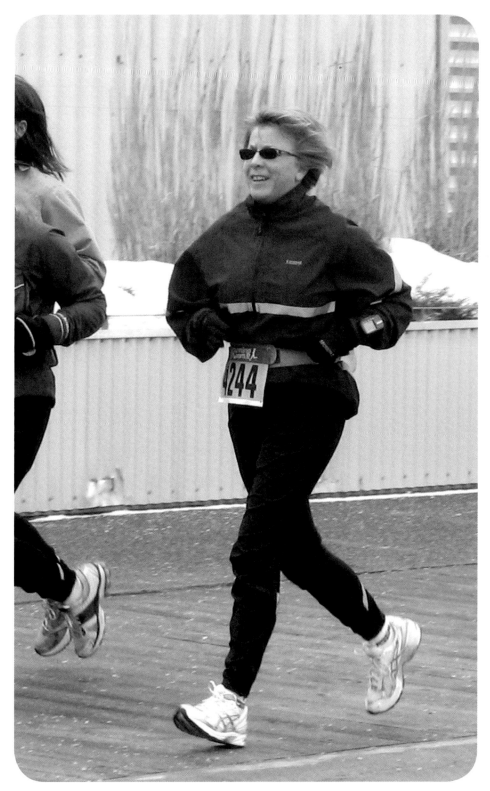

The first and best-known negative effect is that caffeine is a potent diuretic. Staying well hydrated is one of the keys to quality runs in training and competition. Therefore, ensure that you increase your fluid intake if you are going to take caffeine prior to working out. Caffeine also increases the secretion of acid into the stomach which can lead to cramps and stomach pain—definitely two things you don't need in the middle of a long run.

Before you decide whether or not caffeine is for you, there are a few other factors to consider. One is that tolerance is easily built up. Therefore, the effect that caffeine may have on your performance will be limited if you are a regular coffee, cola or tea drinker. So give yourself two or three caffeine free days before trying it out in your program. As well, like all other changes to your running program, try it out first in training and not in competition. If you do decide to use caffeine, the optimum dose for positive effects is 2–3 mg/kg of body weight. (There are about 80 mg in a cup of brewed coffee and 40 mg in a can of Coke.) The effects of caffeine peak around 30 minutes after ingestion and continue for two to three hours.

Caffeine or not? Armed with the facts, you can decide what's best for you!

Losing Weight

Weight Management

More than one runner has entered a marathon or half marathon training program hoping to lose significant amounts of weight. Given the amount of training that is involved in marathon running, this sounds like it should be a relatively simple goal to achieve. However, what runners often do not realize is that weight loss requires dietary changes that can hamper performance and make their dream of completing a marathon or half marathon more challenging.

Weight loss is directly related to energy (calorie) intake. To lose weight you need to take in fewer calories each day than you are using through normal metabolism and daily activities. Unfortunately, cutting calories during periods of intense training can impair performance by reducing glycogen stores, altering immune function and slowing muscle recovery. With this in mind, you may be better off trying to trim down during your personal off-season, when training is moderate and rest is plentiful. If this is not possible, it's important to temper your goals and aim for very slow and gradual weight loss over a longer period of time.

Eating on the Run

Pre-Run Eating

"What should I eat before a run?" is a common question and one that can haunt you if you have incorrect information. Eating at the wrong time or choosing the wrong kind of foods can produce symptoms like nausea, vomiting and diarrhea, experiences that rarely make for a fun run!

Eating before activity, or pre-event eating as sport nutritionists refer it to, serves some very important purposes. A sound pre-event meal or snack can:

+ enhance endurance
+ prevent hunger and dehydration
+ promote mental alertness.

Different people tolerate eating before activity differently, and experimentation is important for finding the exact combination of foods that works best for you. While some runners can happily down a breakfast of pancakes, sausages and coffee before a run, others may feel nauseous after eating only a granola bar and a glass of juice. Use your longer training runs to try out different foods and food combinations.

Timing is critical in terms of pre-event eating. Foods need time to be digested in order to serve as a source of energy. Recognizing this, it's important to allow two to four hours between a moderately sized meal and the start of a workout. Smaller snacks or liquid "meals" can be consumed a little closer to the start of a run, perhaps as late as one hour before you hit the road.

For runners who enjoy training in the morning, a bedtime snack is critical. A nutritious snack, eaten just before bed, helps to keep blood glucose levels stable. This approach, coupled with a very light snack in the hour prior to a run, may help you sneak in a bit more sleep before you train.

Some foods offer greater benefits than others as pre-event meal choices. Foods rich in complex carbohydrates, such as breads, pasta, cereals or grains, are broken down quickly to provide the body with a source of glucose and are ideal choices before exercise. Fluids help to hydrate the body and should be part of all pre-event meals.

Some foods are not suitable for inclusion in a pre-event meal. Many people have difficulty tolerating the following kinds of foods, which should be eaten with caution before activity:

+ High sugar foods: honey, regular soft drinks, syrups, candy and table sugars. These foods can cause abdominal cramping and diarrhea.
+ High fiber foods: bran cereals and muffins, legumes (e.g. beans, peas, lentils) and raw vegetables. High fiber foods can produce bloating, gas and diarrhea.
+ High fat or high protein foods: butter, margarine, salad dressings, peanut butter, hamburger, hot dogs, etc. Fat and protein take longer to digest than carbohydrate and are not a good source of quick fuel during exercise.

Examples:

Pre-Event Meals and Snacks

Breakfast
250 ml (1 cup) Rice Krispies
250 ml (1 cup) skim milk
1 banana
250–500 ml (1–2 cups) plain, cool water

Snack
1 large cinnamon-raisin bagel
250 ml (1 cup) orange juice
250 ml (1 cup) low fat yogurt
125 ml (½ cup) strawberries

The Golden Rule of Pre-Event Eating

Conquering the challenge of the marathon or half marathon distance is a thrill few runners ever forget. To make the most of this experience stick to eating foods that you have tried many times in training and that you know you tolerate well. The excitement of racing, when coupled with a food you can't tolerate, may place you in the awkward position of searching for a restroom (or bush) on the run. Never, ever eat something on race day that you haven't already tested several times during training.

By Susan Glen, MSc Nutrition

For people running their first marathon, planning what to eat on the days leading up to the race and on race day can be almost more difficult than running the 42 km. Below I have outlined some guidelines for prerace eating.

One Week To Go

This is the time when you most dramatically taper your training (and probably go a little crazy in the meantime). Because you are decreasing your exercise time you don't need to increase your intake to prepare for the race. By maintaining your calories you will provide your body with the extra fuel it needs to prepare for the race. To optimize your glycogen stores in your muscles you may need to increase your carbohydrate intake slightly over this period. Aim for 65–70% of your calories to come from carbohydrates during this period. This intake of carbohydrates combined with the decrease in muscle glycogen utilization (from tapering) will ensure your glycogen stores are peaked for the race. It is important to remember that storing glycogen in your muscles requires water. For each gram of glycogen stored, 2–3 g of water must also be stored in your muscles. This brings us to the next important nutrition goal for the week prior to your marathon. HYDRATE, HYDRATE, HYDRATE! During the pre-race week aim to take in 2–3 L of water a day and limit your intake of caffeine and alcohol, which can increase fluid losses. This will ensure your fluid levels are topped off for the race (to limit dehydration) and will give your body the fluid it needs to store glycogen in your muscles.

The Day Before

Don't eat any unusual foods the day before a race; stick with what you know. The last thing you need is to find out you don't agree with Aunt Margaret's borscht or the new restaurant down the street. After breakfast try to limit your intake of fiber. This is especially important for people who experience problems with cramps or diarrhea during long runs. By decreasing your fiber intake the day before you will decrease the amount of residue your intestines are dealing with. (It is important to make sure you have adequate fiber two days before to prevent constipation when you decrease your fiber). Plain pasta, white bagels and white rice usually work well for people who need to control their fiber intake the day before a race. As redundant as it sounds, remember to keep drinking water. Your water bottle should never leave your side the day before a marathon.

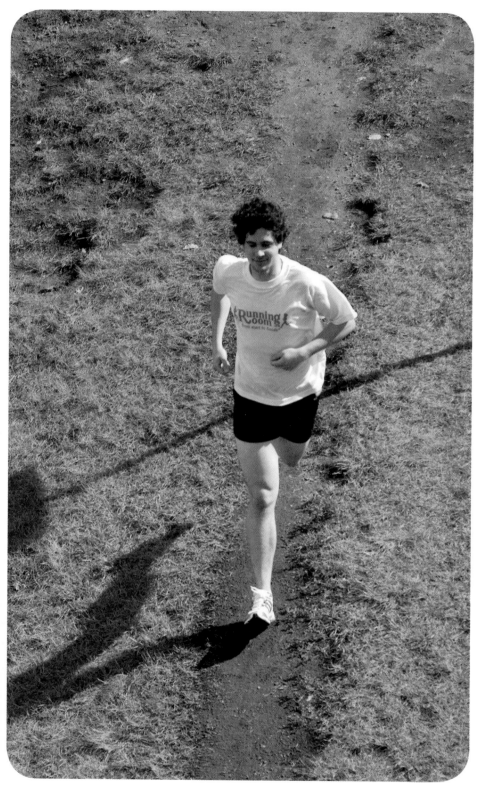

There is no need to eat a large meal the night before your race. The last thing you want to happen is to wake up still feeling full from supper. Eat a normal-sized, carbohydrate-rich meal no less than 12 hours before start time (e.g., if your race starts at 7 a.m. you should be finished supper by 7 p.m. the night before).

It's Race Day

What you eat the morning of the marathon will have little effect on your race. The most important thing to remember is that whatever it is, you should have tried it at least once in training. If you are sure that a yogurt smoothie is the right premarathon breakfast for you, make yourself one before some of your long runs and see how well you do. Knowing that you are eating something familiar that has gotten you through some of those 18-mi. training runs will help give you confidence for the race. Most people find that a small meal (200 to 400 calories) works best, but the key is finding out what works for you.

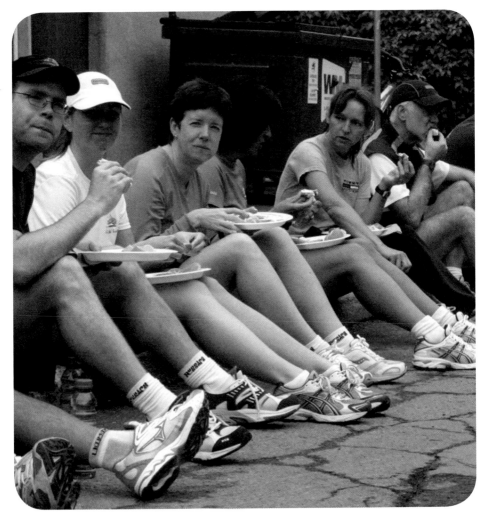

During the Race

As with everything on race day, you should be prepared well in advance. Make a plan for what you intend to eat and drink during the marathon and try it out in training. By taking in carbohydrates during the race you will help spare your muscle glycogen reserves and avoid "hitting the wall" (the same applies to your long training runs). Aim to take in 0.5–1.0 g of carbohydrate per kilogram of your body weight each hour. This can be in any form: fluid, solid, gel or a combination of all three. The trick is to find out what works for you. To avoid dehydration you should take in 0.5–1 cup of water or diluted sports drink every 15 minutes, starting 5 minutes into your run. Don't wait until you're thirsty. The key to nutrition before and during a marathon is preparation. By making a plan and trying it out in training you can be sure that come race day you will be ready to run and keep on running.

Weight Loss

What Works for Weight Loss?

To look at the plethora of magazine articles, diet books and web sites, you might think that there isn't anything that works as far as long-term weight management is concerned. In fact, just the opposite is true. Registered dietitians and nutrition researchers have a very clear picture of the approaches that best support weight loss, as well as those that don't:

+ Begin by rethinking your focus. View weight loss as one, small part of a larger plan to "retrain" your overall lifestyle. Focus on developing healthy eating habits rather than dieting restrictively to drop a few pounds quickly. Remind yourself that learning new habits is difficult, and expect to experience periods of frustration along the way.

+ Be realistic. Aim for a goal weight that is ideal for you. This may not be the same as your "ideal" weight from a chart or your lowest adult weight. Instead, a realistic goal weight is one that you can maintain without resorting to constant dieting or extreme exercise programs. It is a weight that allows you to fully enjoy the activities of daily life and that gives you a sense of well-being.

+ Keep moving! Exercise plays a critical role in weight loss and long-term weight maintenance. Traditional weight loss diets frequently ignore the important link between exercise and weight maintenance. Without regular exercise, dieters tend to lose some muscle tissue along with any body fat that is lost. Loss of muscle tissue tends to slow metabolism (the rate that you

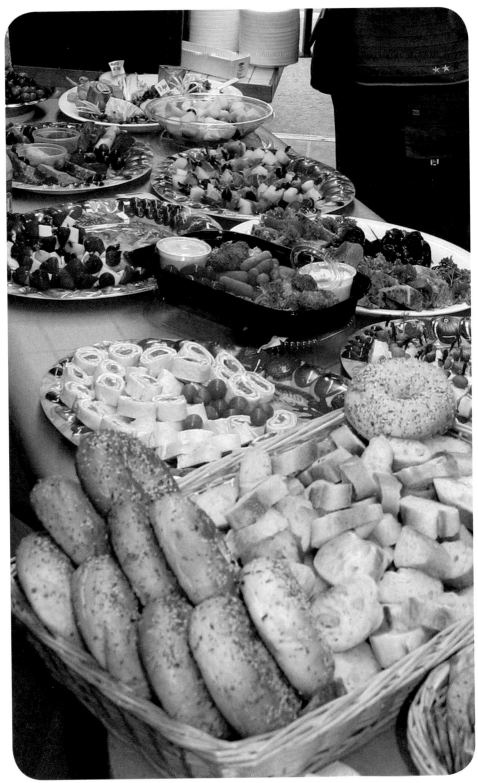

burn calories). As a result, inactive dieters are much more likely to regain any weight that they have lost when they abandon their diet and return to a less restrictive way of eating. Regular exercise can help to prevent this situation from occurring.

+ Be wary of fad diets. Fad diets are everywhere, and despite their compelling marketing these kinds of eating plans rarely lead to long-term weight loss. Most cannot verify the miraculous results that they promise and some are potentially quite harmful. In general, unsound weight loss plans:

  + Promise rapid or dramatic results.
  + Restrict one or more foods or food groups.
  + Promote so-called "miracle" products, supplements or food choices.
  + Encourage bizarre eating patterns or food combinations.
  + Suggest that their approach is painless and easy.

+ Focus on eating for health instead of dieting. Traditional weight loss diets are often nutritionally imbalanced, overly restrictive and woefully unsuccessful. As a result, most people cannot stick with this kind of eating pattern long-term, and achieving a healthy weight becomes impossible. Aim for a nutrient-rich eating style, based on Canada's Food Guide to Healthy Eating, that is low enough in calories to promote gradual, healthy weight loss.

+ Opt for small changes instead of a complete lifestyle "renovation." Changing behavior takes work, and building new eating habits or creating an active lifestyle are no exceptions. However, you can make things much easier if you phase in change slowly over time. Research shows that people adapt best to small changes rather than complete lifestyle "renovations." Recognizing this, don't aim to change your eating habits overnight. Focus on revamping one meal or one food choice at a time, letting yourself become comfortable with your new approach before adding anything new.

Nutrients During the Run

Eating during a run is a strategy designed to keep blood sugar or glucose levels high and promote endurance. Research shows that athletes who consume carbohydrate-rich foods or beverages during prolonged activity benefit from enhanced performance.

A wide variety of foods and drinks are available to provide long distance runners with the carbohydrates needed to keep blood glucose levels within the normal range. Sport drinks, gels or "gu," energy bars and even dried fruits are all items that you can use to "top up" your carbohydrate stores during a run.

Like the ideal pre-event meal, the definition of a perfect "on the run" snack varies from runner to runner. Keep the following points in mind as you look for foods to eat during activity:

Portability is important. Ideal on the run food choices are non-perishable, lightweight and easily contained.

Taste matters! Most runners will need to take in between 30 g and 60 g of carbohydrate per hour to keep blood glucose levels in the normal range during activity. Translated into food or beverage choices this equals:

- 1 to 2 packages of sport gel
- 1 sport bar
- 500 ml (2 cups) of sport drink
- 60–80 ml (¼–^{3}/8 cup) raisins

Unless you enjoy the taste, taking in the recommended amounts of these foods or beverages will be a challenge.

Experiment. The ability to tolerate sport gels, bars and drinks is highly individual. While some runners swear by these products, others are unable to tolerate even small amounts. Discover what works best for you by experimenting with a variety of carbohydrate-rich snacks during your long training runs.

Recovery Eating

Marathon running is intensive, and after a long run or race the body needs to be refueled. Eating well after exercise can help to speed your recovery and allow you to train at a consistently high level.

Keep the carbs coming! The body is primed to replace its glycogen stores following a long or rigorous bout of exercise. Make the most of this situation by choosing carbohydrate-rich foods and drinks immediately after finishing a workout. Continue to snack on foods like bagels, muffins, cereal and milk, fruits and fruit juices for several hours to fully restore muscle glycogen.

Keep up the fluids! Continuing to take in plenty of fluids after exercise helps to combat dehydration by replacing water that was lost from your body during exercise.

Hyponatremia and Running

Recent media reports have made the issue of fluids and hydration very confusing, which is too bad because it is actually a very straightforward issue. The American College of Sport Medicine (ACSM) says this about hydration, a statement that I completely endorse:

Hyponatremia is a dangerous condition that may arise when athletes consume too much water or sports drinks, diluting or disrupting the body's sodium levels. ACSM experts in sports medicine and exercise science point out that while hyponatremia is a serious concern, excessive fluid consumption resulting in hyponatremia is unlikely to occur in most athletes, and hydration is important for all active people. Water and sports drinks, when consumed as recommended, are not dangerous to athletes. And while hyponatremia has gotten more attention lately, far more athletes are affected by dehydration.

A good example of this comes from the experience at the 2004 Boston Marathon. According to The Boston Globe, "The main tent, which contained approximately 240 cots, was mostly full of dehydrated runners complaining of nausea, diarrhea and vomiting." Hospital officials reported a single case of hyponatremia in this year's marathon, involving a runner who was released after treatment.

With all of this in mind, it is truly unfortunate that the media and some individuals in the sport community have positioned overhydration and hyponatremia as larger concerns than dehydration—the evidence paints quite a different picture if you really look at things.

The American College of Sport Medicine stands by its current stand on fluids and hydration:

+ It is recommended that individuals drink about 500 ml (about 17 oz.) of fluid about two hours before exercise to promote adequate hydration and allow time for excretion of excess ingested water.

+ During exercise, athletes should start drinking early and at regular intervals in an attempt to consume fluids at a rate sufficient to replace all the water lost through sweating (i.e., body weight loss), or consume the maximal amount that can be tolerated.

+ It is recommended that ingested fluids be cooler than ambient temperature (between 15° and 22°C).

- Fluids should be readily available and served in containers that allow adequate volumes to be ingested with ease and with minimal interruption of exercise.

- Addition of proper amounts of carbohydrates and/or electrolytes to a fluid replacement solution is recommended for exercise events of duration greater than one hour since it does not significantly impair water delivery to the body and may enhance performance.

- During exercise lasting less than one hour, there is little evidence of physiological or physical performance differences between consuming a carbohydrate-electrolyte drink and plain water.

- During intense exercise lasting longer than one hour, it is recommended that carbohydrates be ingested at a rate of 30–60 g/h to maintain oxidation of carbohydrates and delay fatigue. This rate of carbohydrate intake can be achieved without compromising fluid delivery by drinking 600–1200 ml/h of solutions containing 4–8% carbohydrates (the standard for most commercially produced sport drinks mixed to the manufacturers' specifications).

- Inclusion of sodium (0.5–0.7 g/L of water) in the rehydration solution ingested during exercise lasting longer than one hour is recommended since it may be advantageous in enhancing palatability, promoting fluid retention and possibly preventing hyponatremia in certain individuals who drink excessive quantities of fluid.

The full guidelines can be found at: http://www.acsm-msse.org/pt/pt-core/template-journal/msse/media/0196.htm

Heidi M. Bates, BSc, R.D.
Nutrition Consultant
Tri-Nutrition Consulting

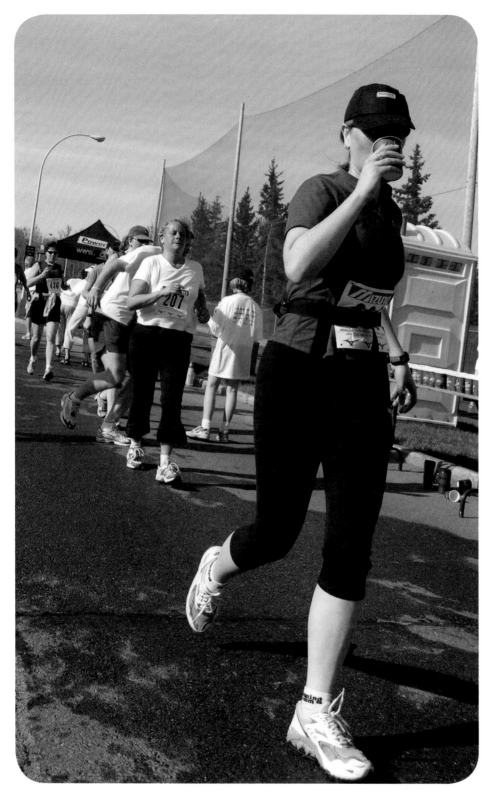

Strength Training

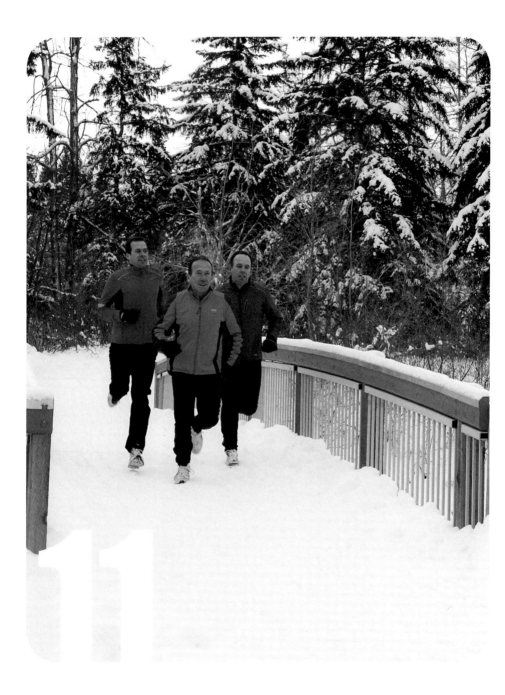

Body Weight Strength Exercises

While stretching helps reduce the risk of injury by keeping muscles and fibrous tissue from becoming rigid and inflexible, strengthening helps to prevent injury by keeping weak muscles from being overpowered by stronger ones. The three basic opposing muscle groups for training include:

+ Abdominal vs. lower back
+ Quadriceps vs. hamstrings
+ Anterior shin muscle (front of leg, below knee) vs. calf/Achilles.

Also important is the iliotibial band, as this band is vital in stabilizing the lower leg during running. It is the most commonly inflamed structure on the outside of the knee, and in runners it is a frequent cause of pain and soreness at the outer hip.

The hamstring is vulnerable to strains if it is overpowered by the quadriceps' strength. The hamstring therefore demands both stretching and strengthening in a total conditioning program. While your quadriceps are often strong already, they can also benefit from further strengthening to help prevent many of the overuse problems that involve the kneecap.

Strengthening exercises should be done after running, rather than before. For maximum benefit it is recommended that you follow this routine three to four times per week.

Foot Exercises

Why train the foot? Well, the longitudinal rib and the cross rib of the foot take a great deal of punishment during running, particularly during the landing and push-off phases. The ligaments and the aponeurosis plantaris that directly support the two ribs are passive tissues that cannot be trained; instead, the muscles of the foot can and must be trained in order to reduce the risk of injury. Your feet do a great deal of work for you during running, so give them some special attention each day and watch your strength improve over time.

Start with this simple exercise: drop a towel on the floor, stand with one foot on the towel and one off, and try to pick up the towel with your toes. After several weeks, proceed to this next exercise, which will strengthen your foot muscles, toe joints, ankles and knees; stand in a bucket filled with sand or rice and squeeze the sand or rice with your toes for 10 minutes.

Ankle Exercises

Your ankle acts as a powerful lever during running. Over time, runners develop powerful running-specific muscles, but they sometimes neglect the development of improved coordination. Spend some time on these two drills and not only will they help improve your base running but they may help prevent a turned ankle on one of your runs.

The Flamingo

Start by balancing on one leg for 30 seconds without touching down with the other leg. When this balance becomes easy, try it with your eyes closed. (figure 7-a) You will notice it's much harder to hold a balanced position without visual cues. After mastering the blind flamingo, try bending your raised leg slightly at the knee and then do some toe raises. (figure 7-b, figure 7-c)

Over the years I have spent a fair amount of time in airport lineups, and I have found the flamingo to be the ideal exercise—not only do you get some interesting looks, but you must be careful not to lose your space in the line while your eyes are closed. (By the way, while the flamingo does require the one-legged stand, the pink tights are optional.)

Balance Kicks

This drill can be done on a flat surface, or to increase the complexity try it on a rebounder. Stand on one leg, kick your other leg back, balance and hold for 20 to 30 seconds. (figure 8-a) Switch legs and repeat. Repeat the exercise with kicks out to the side and in front of you. (figure 8-b, figure 8-c) These positions will seem awkward when you first try them, but over time, as your balance improves, they will become more fluid—you may even think of signing up with the Dallas Cowboys cheerleading squad.

Push-ups

Yes, I am sorry to break the news to you, but your old phys-ed teacher was right; push-ups are good for you. Push-ups work on all the upper body muscle groups, improving your running form and posture. We all know how to do them; it's getting around to doing them that's a problem. This single exercise could replace a lot of time in the weight room if only we didn't find it so boring. Check off a daily 25 or so. Be sure to keep your back straight. (figure 9-a, figure 9-b)

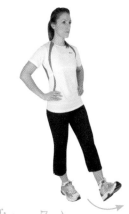
(figure 7-a)

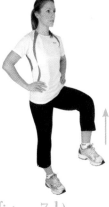
(figure 7-b)

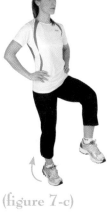
(figure 7-c)

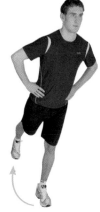
(figure 8-a)

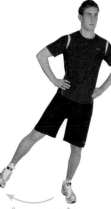
(figure 8-b)

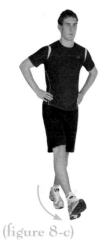
(figure 8-c)

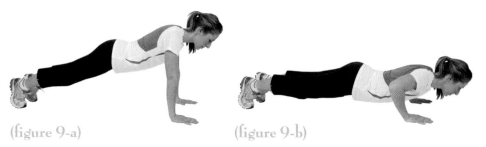

(figure 9-a)

(figure 9-b)

Sit-ups (the right way)

We have all seen the many infomercials on the benefits of the latest abdominal equipment on the market. Well, save yourself a few bucks; do these sit-ups as part of your daily routine and those abs of steel will be yours! The great benefit of this sit-up is it works all the abdominal muscles from the rib cage through to the groin area. You, too, could have that infomercial "six-pack belly."

Lie flat on your back with your knees bent and your feet flat on the floor. Be sure to do an abdominal tuck to flatten the small of your back against the floor. (figure 10-a) Now extend your arms to put your hands on your thighs and then curl up your upper body, sliding your fingertips up to your knees. Keep the small of your back on the floor. (figure 10-b) Hold for a count of 10 and then lower yourself back to the floor. Start with about 25 repetitions and build from there.

Step-ups

Find a sturdy bench you can step on that isn't too high (your knee shouldn't bend tighter than 90 degrees when your foot is on the bench). Step up onto the bench and stand up straight before you step down. Alternate your feet each time. This drill works the upper leg muscles and hip flexors. (figure 11-a, figure 11-b)

Calf Raises

Stand on the edge of a step with your heels hanging over so that your toes carry your weight. (figure 12-a) Slowly raise and lower yourself. (figure 12-b) Start with both feet and then try one foot at a time. You can add a light weight after a few weeks of single-leg raises. This drill improves the strength and flexibility of the lower leg muscle group.

Benefits of Strength Training

- Helps reduce the risk of injury.
- Prepares your muscles for faster running.
- Makes you stronger on hills.
- Enhances the rehabilitation of skeletal and muscular injuries.

A Belly Full of Strength

Achieving your personal goals may revolve around improving your core strength. So stop ignoring your weak pelvis and turn your attention to some core abdominal and pelvic strength.

Runners get plenty of leg development through running. Many runners incor-

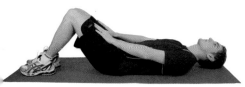

figure 10-a

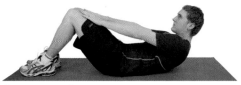

figure 10-b

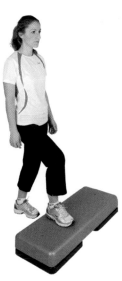

figure 11-a

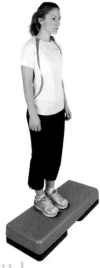

figure 11-b

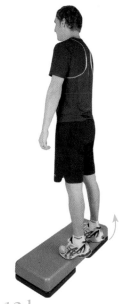

figure 12-a

figure 12-b

porate hill training, intervals for leg strength and some resistance weight training for the upper body. The muscles in your pelvis are continually stressed by running. Yet, many runners totally ignore the abdominal and psoas muscles*.

The pelvis is the platform of your body. During running it absorbs shock and transfers the weight of your torso and upper body to the legs. The stronger the platform, the better it absorbs the shock of each foot strike. Our body absorbs three to four times our weight on each foot strike, so maintaining strong pelvic muscles will reduce the risk of injuries.

The abdominal muscles provide stability to the body, and the psoas creates the impulse of energy that initiates leg movement. Abdominal muscles, the washboard muscles in our stomach area, are easy to identify and see. The psoas you cannot see. This long muscle works through the pelvis and inserts on the inside of the top of your thighbone. It is the primary initiator of your running movement. To prevent muscle imbalances and all sorts of injuries, both the abdominal and psoas muscles need to be strengthened.

Relax and enjoy this circuit routine. Start by laying flat on your back with your knees up and together. Your feet should be flat on the floor, about a foot from your butt.

*Muscle, psoas: Muscles of the lower back (the loin). There are two psoas muscles on each side of the back. The larger of the two is called the psoas major and the smaller the psoas minor. The word "psoas" is Greek for loins, the muscles of the lower back.

The Crunch

Place a towel between your knees and squeeze, contracting the inner thigh muscles. (figure 13-a) Curl your upper back to your thigh muscles while doing a pelvic tilt; keep your lower back tight to the floor. (figure 13-b) Hold this for 5 to 10 seconds. Return to the starting position, take a breath and relax and then repeat a total of 10 times to a count of 5 to 10. This crunch will work the abdominal, the psoas and the adductor muscles of the inner thigh.

The Hipster

Sit upright perpendicular to the floor. Use your arms for support, lean back and place your hands palms down on the floor shoulder width apart. (figure 14-a) Keep your knees together, extend your legs straight out and bring your knees back towards your chest. (figure 14-b) The heels are kept 6 in. off the ground throughout the routine. Repeat 20 times with a smooth and steady action. This builds strength in the psoas, hip flexors and lower abdominal.

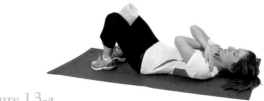

figure 13-a

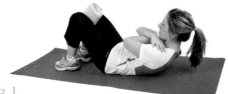

figure 13-b

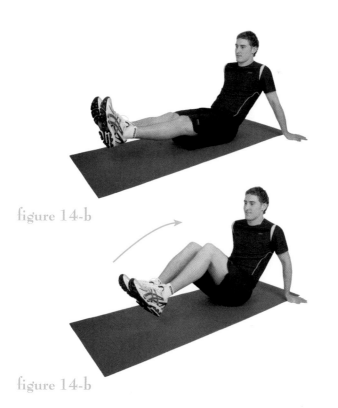

figure 14-b

figure 14-b

The Crossed Leg Crunch

Rest your right ankle on your left knee. (figure 15-a) Now curl your left shoulder up towards the inside of your right knee. (figure 15-b) Hold the crunch for 5 to 10 seconds, repeating 10 times. Now cross your legs the other way and repeat on the opposite side for 10 repetitions. This routine will strengthen your oblique stomach muscles and help prevent upper body rotation while running.

Knee slider

Place the palms of your hands on your thighs. (figure 16-a) Slowly slide your hands towards your knees and lift your upper back. Contract your abdominals and keep your lower back tight on the floor. (figure 16-b) Curl hold for a count of 5 to 10 and repeat 10 times. This strengthens your upper abdominals. Do this circuit training three times per week and watch your running times improve!

Quadriceps

Terminal Extensions

Sit down, bend one leg and extend the other. Place a rolled towel under the knee of the extended leg. Lean back on your elbows. (figure 17-a) Straighten the extended leg and lift 2 in. above the towel. (figure 17-b) Hold for three seconds. Complete 10 repetitions; then repeat with the other leg.

Hamstrings

Hip Extensions

Lie on your stomach with legs extended. Raise one leg 6 in., keeping your knee straight. Hold for three seconds. Keep hip muscles relaxed. Complete 10 repetitions; then repeat with the other leg. (figure 18-a)

Tibialis Anterior

Ankle up-and-down

Sit down with your legs extended and together. Place a loop of Thera-Band around your feet. Bend one knee and pull that foot towards your head. Hold for three seconds. Complete 10 repetitions; then repeat with the other leg. This exercise helps prevent shin splints. (figure 19-a)

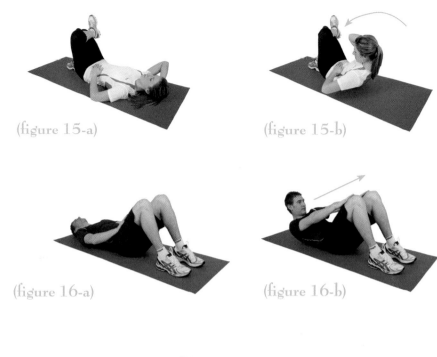

(figure 15-a)　　　　　(figure 15-b)

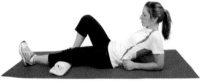　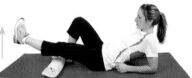

(figure 16-a)　　　　　(figure 16-b)

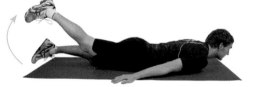

(figure 17-a)　　　　　(figure 17-b)

(figure 18-a)

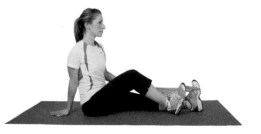

(figure 19-a)

Post Tibialis

Ankle Eversion

Sit down with your legs extended and together. Place a Thera-Band loop around your feet and hold. (figure 20-a) Point your toes down and out. (figure 20-b)

Peroneals

Ankle Inversion

Repeat previous with your legs crossed. (figure 21-a, 21-b)

Weight Training

Give Your Running a Lift:

A smart weight training program can be a big benefit to just about every runner.

Weight Training for Runners:

It is important that your weight program be tailored specifically for your running requirements—you want to develop muscular endurance and strength to enhance your running.

Work with weights that are no more than 70% of the maximum you can lift. Work on doing 12 repetitions of each, with no more than one minute rest between each set. Do three sets of each 12 repetitions. To maintain flexibility, be sure to concentrate on performing a full range of motion; your movements should be smooth, fluid and controlled. Once you have accomplished three sets of 12 repeats you can increase the weight.

Prior to lifting, do 10 minutes on the stationary bike to warm up. After your routine do another 10 minutes cooldown.

Perform your strength exercises two or three times per week, using the hard-easy system—load and rest, load and rest—will make you stronger, faster and more energized.

+ Improving your posture and your body mechanics—good form leads to speedier, more efficient running.

+ Helping prevent or overcome injuries—strong muscles withstand stress better than weak ones.

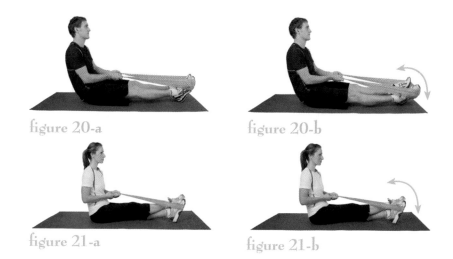

figure 20-a   figure 20-b

figure 21-a   figure 21-b

How to Make Weight Training Work for You:

As a runner, you'll want to develop greater muscular endurance in your legs, arms, lower back and abdomen. Muscular endurance is the ability of a muscle or group of muscles to perform repeated contractions against a light load for an extended period of time. Training for muscular endurance will allow you to improve in strength without gaining the muscular bulk of a body builder.

To reach this goal, work out with weights that are fairly light—no more than 60–70% of the maximum weight you can lift—and work on doing more repetitions:

+ 3 sets of between 12 and 20 repetitions.

+ Abdominal exercises should be done in sets of
  30 to 50 repetitions.

Begin your program with a couple of weeks of lighter weights so you can practice good form. Start with fewer repetitions and gradually work your way up to 12 to 20 over several sessions. If you begin to struggle before the set is ended, the weight is too heavy. If you do not feel a slight "burn" in the last few repetitions, the weight is too light. The object is for you to maintain the rhythm and range of movement throughout the set even though you know that you are having to work hard towards the end of the set. When 3 sets of 20 are becoming easy, it is time to increase the weight or resistance. If you do move up, be sure to start off with fewer repetitions and go through the same process again.

Weight Exercises

Balance the muscle groups. Most human actions cause muscles (or muscle groups) to work in pairs, one moving the limb in one direction and the other moving the limb back to the starting position. This implies a certain balance between the muscles that does the action (the agonist) and the muscle that returns the limb to the starting position (the antagonist).

Progress by the weaker leg. You have a stronger and a weaker side. Basically everyone does. When you are doing an exercise with both legs, one is working harder than the other, which simply tends to accentuate the difference in strength that you started with.

Runners and walkers doing exercises for leg strength should make sure to avoid this strength difference. The cyclical nature of our activities involving thousands of muscular contractions of each leg in each walk or run means that any significant strength difference between the two legs will surely come back to affect us sooner or later.

By all means, start doing leg exercises with both legs, just to get comfortable with the action. But after a few sessions, you may wish to consider doing what some athletes do to equalize their strength. Reduce the weight and do the exercise with one leg at a time. You will quickly find which leg is stronger. Concentrate on the weak one; bring it up to the strength of the stronger one before you start working the strong leg again. At least do more sets with the weak one. Your session may initially take a little longer, but the time to achieve balance in your leg muscles is a very worthwhile investment indeed.

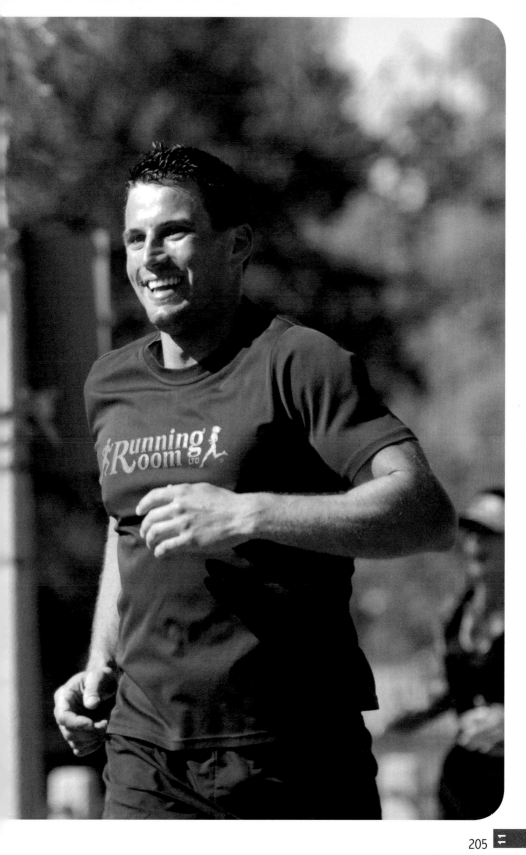

Squat:

The squat is very effective in working the quadriceps, hamstring and gluteal muscles. There are three main variations. Done properly, none of the variations is unsafe. For aerobic sports, the "quarter squat" is perfectly adequate for our needs. In a quarter squat, the knees are bent to 90 degrees only. (In a half squat, the knees are bent a little more so that the thighs are parallel to the ground. In a full squat, the knees are bent even more so that the buttocks are closer to the ground.)

1. Use a squat rack or at the very least two spotters to load the bar onto your shoulders. Modern squat racks are designed to control the weight if you can't.
2. Stick your chest out and your shoulders back. This opens a "platform" on each shoulder where the bar can comfortably rest. (figure 22-a) In this position the bar needs only to be steadied by your hands. If you find yourself grasping the bar tightly with "white knuckles," find a more comfortable position before you begin the exercise. In this comfortable position, a pad or towel around the bar is generally not necessary, but feel free to use one if it makes a difference for you. Do not load the bar onto the vertebrae in your neck.
3. The squat motion feels exactly like sitting down on a chair. Your feet are shoulder width apart. If you are at all unsure of your balance, feel free to put a chair underneath you so that you can literally sit down if necessary. (figure 22-b)
4. If you would still like to feel more stable, try putting each heel on a weight disk before you begin the exercise. Keep your weight on your heels.
5. Lower the weight slowly; raise it a little more quickly.

Leg Press Leg Extensions:

Like the squat, the Leg Press is an exercise directly related to walking and running. You are pushing against a resistance with your feet, exactly like you do when you walk or run. Leg Press machines come in various forms. Generally, you sit and push pedals away from you with your legs, starting from a bent position until they are extended. (figure 23-a, figure 23-b) Some even have you lying down and pushing the weight upwards, providing additional support for the back.

For runners and walkers, a particularly effective form of the exercise is the Reverse Leg Press, which is possible only on some leg press machines. In the Reverse Leg Press, you are able to stand with your back to the pedals and support yourself by holding onto a pole behind the seat. You can then put a foot into one of the pedals and push the weight away from you in a motion similar to the push of a classic cross-country skiing action.

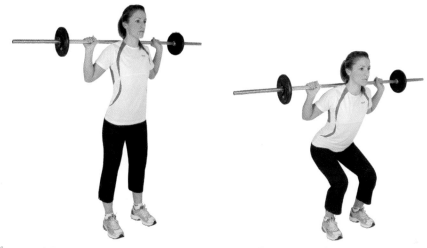

figure 22-a   figure 22-b

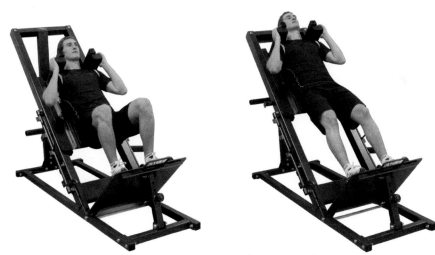

figure 23-a   figure 23-b

Leg (Hamstring Curl):

If you are doing squats or leg presses, you are working the muscles in the front of your thigh (the quadriceps). To maintain the balance between muscles, you need also to work the muscles in the back of the leg (hamstrings). This is done with the Leg Curl or Hamstring Curl. The traditional hamstring curl is done lying on the front on a bench. The feet fit under pads at the end of a bench allowing you to lift the weight simply by bending the knees. (figure 24-a, figure 24-b) More advanced benches are raised in the middle or adjustable for length. This reduces the awkwardness some people feel on a flat bench. You may even find equipment that allows you to sit upright, curling the legs underneath you. This has the advantage of isolating the hamstring muscle, removing the back muscles that tend to creep into the exercise when you are lying down.

Calf Press:

Lift the bar to your shoulders as in the squat exercise, keeping your back straight and your head up. (figure 25-a) Raise your heels off the floor as far as possible, and then lower them back to the floor. (figure 25-b) Works the calf muscles (gastrocnemius and soleus).

Dumbbell Fly:

Lie on your back on a bench with a dumbbell in each hand and your arms extended directly over your chest. (figure 26-a) Slowly lower the dumbbells directly out to the sides until your arms are parallel with the floor. (figure 26-b) Then bring your arms back slowly to the starting position, keeping your arms extended as you do.

Dumbbell Side-raises:

Stand erect with your arms at your sides and a dumbbell in each hand. (figure 27-a) Raise the dumbbells upward from your sides, keeping your arms fully extended, until your hands are slightly above shoulder level. (figure 27-b) Works deltoids, trapezius.

Arm Curl:

Stand with your back straight, your head up and your feet slightly spread. Grasp the bar in an underhand grip (palms up) with arms fully extended. (figure 28-a) Then slowly curl the bar up to your chest. (figure 28-b) Hold for a count of two, and lower it to the starting position. Be careful to lower the bar slowly rather than let it drop from its own weight. Keep the bar under control at all times. Works the biceps.

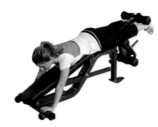
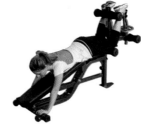

figure 24-a   figure 24-b

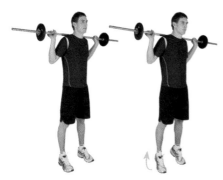
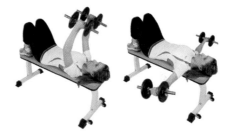

figure 25-a   figure 25-b   figure 26-a   figure 26-b

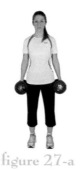
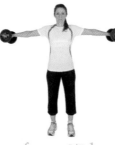

figure 27-a   figure 27-b

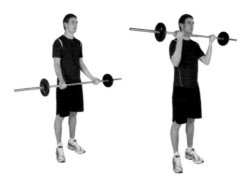

figure 28-a   figure 28-b

Bench Press:

Lie on your back on a bench or the floor with your back flat against the surface and the bar over your chest. (figure 29-a) Then slowly press the bar straight up until your arms are fully extended, and then lower it slowly to the starting position. (figure 29-b)

Bent Row:

Focuses on pectorals. Bend over at the waist, keeping your back as flat as possible and your head up. (figure 30-a) Grasp the bar in a widely spaced overhand grip and raise it slowly to your chest. (figure 30-b) Lower it slowly to the floor and repeat. Bend your knees if necessary. Works back (latissimus dorsi).

Press Behind the Neck:

Stand erect with the bar resting on your shoulder. (figure 31-a) Press the bar directly up over your head and lower it slowly to the starting position. (figure 31-b) Works posterior aspect of deltoid (shoulder).

Upright Row:

Stand with your back straight and your head up. Hold the bar in an overhand grip with arms fully extended. Keep your hands about 6 in. apart. (figure 32-a) Slowly raise the bar along the front of your body until your hands are under your chin. (figure 32-b) Lower it slowly to the starting position and repeat. Works shoulder and neck.

Triceps Extension:

Stand erect with the bar pressed straight overhead. Your hands should be about 8 in. apart. Then lower the bar slowly behind your head by bending your elbows. (figure 33-a) Slowly raise the bar to the starting position and repeat. Works triceps. (figure 33-b)

Weight exercises shown here train major muscle groups and when used together, develop a good general muscle tone. If you are not sure how to do an exercise, ask a qualified professional or instructor to show you how.

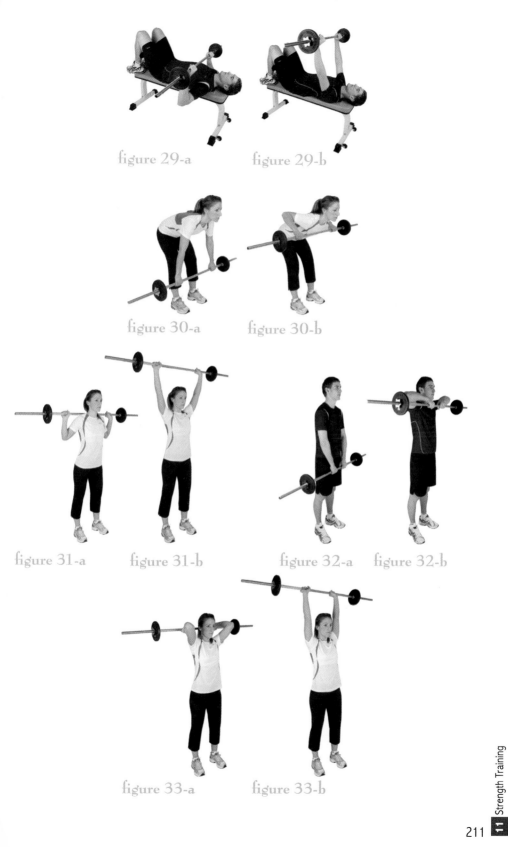

figure 29-a   figure 29-b

figure 30-a   figure 30-b

figure 31-a   figure 31-b   figure 32-a   figure 32-b

figure 33-a   figure 33-b

Cross Training &
Core Strengthening

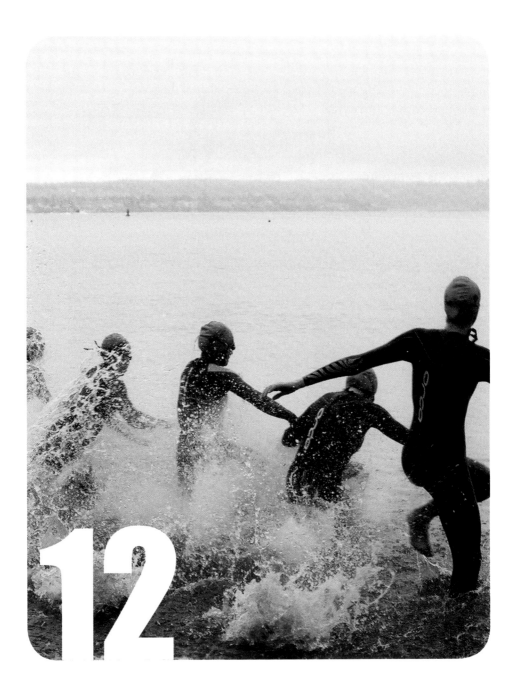

12

Introduction

What Is It and Why Do It?

Simply put, cross-training is using one or more sports to enhance your overall fitness. So by adding sports like swimming or cross-country skiing to your running schedule, you'll be building overall strength that can't help but improve your performance.

Does Cross-Training Work?

It sure does! Cross-training strengthens your whole body, not just your legs, and it lets you maintain a high level of fitness without straining or injuring sport-specific muscles and joints. Besides that, cross-training adds welcome variety to your workouts—a variety that keeps you going month after month.

What Can Cross-Training Do For You?

1. Enhance the quality of your training so you get maximum results in minimum time.
2. Reduce your risk of injury.
3. Add mental variety to your workout schedule.
4. Help you stay fit during recovery from an injury.
5. Strengthen individual muscles as well as your overall body strength.
6. Promote smooth action between muscle groups.
7. Improve endurance levels.

Overview

How It Works

Some skeptics might ask, "How will swimming help improve my running?" It is really very easy to explain, but first you need to know a bit about the adaptations to training. Generally, through exercise training we teach our bodies to become more efficient at breathing and delivering oxygen to the muscles, and our muscles become stronger. We can divide the adaptations to training into two categories:

Cardiovascular:
Heart, Lungs, Blood

Muscular:
Muscles used for exercise

All aerobic exercise of sufficient intensity and duration will promote adaptations in both categories. What will change from activity to activity is the location of muscular adaptations. Running requires the use of the legs. Swimming, on the other hand, requires mostly the arms. In these two sports the muscular adaptations to the training will be, for the most part, in completely different muscle groups. But both swimming and running are super aerobic activities. They will both promote adaptations in the cardiovascular system.

Back to our question. How will swimming improve my running?

Swimming will improve the efficiency of the cardiovascular system, which is also a requirement of running. These adaptations in the heart, lungs and blood will carry over from sport to sport. While the muscular adaptations don't carry over, the benefit is that you will be promoting whole body fitness, which in the long run is healthier than just focusing on the strength and efficiency of one body part.

- The best cross-training regimen will use a wide variety of activities.
- Swimming and running are the best examples because they utilize very different muscle groups. Find activities that will stress different muscle groups.

- Avoid activities that are too similar because the predominant muscle groups may not receive adequate rest, resulting in fatigue or injury.

- Try combining weight-bearing and non-weight-bearing activities. For example, swimming and running, cycling and running, or rowing and running. This gives the joints a chance to rest and repair from the constant forces experienced during weight-bearing activity.

Resistance Training

Cross-training works best when more than one aerobic activity are combined throughout the week. Weight or resistance training gives cross-training a bit of a twist. Resistance training promotes whole body improvements in strength. The adaptations to strength training are very different from aerobic training. So don't expect vast improvements in your running performance with this type of training. Try not to be confused—the benefits of moderate resistance training a couple of times per week are vast. Having stronger muscles, tendons and balanced joints will help decrease your chance of injury and will also help you tone up the spots that your aerobic activities might miss.

Benefits

+ Enhance the quality of your training so you can receive maximum results in minimum time.
+ Reduce your risk of injury.
+ Add mental variety to your workout schedule.
+ Help you stay fit even when injured or sore.
+ Strengthen individual muscles as well as overall strength.
+ Promote smooth action between muscle groups.

Three Great Aerobic Sports

1. Cycling:

Whether you have a sleek road-racing bike or a sturdy all-terrain model, cycling can

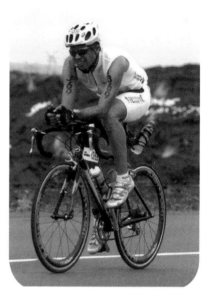

+ Increase muscle balance between quadriceps and hamstrings
+ Increase flexibility in hips and knees
+ Increase ability to run up hills
+ Increase leg speed
+ Increase cardiovascular endurance.

But if you haven't been on a bike since grade school, you may find your first outing taxing, especially on your hands, buttocks and shoulder, neck and leg muscles. The most sensible and enjoyable start to a cycling program is a slow one.

For the most comfort on a long ride, get a bike that fits you. Your muscles, joints and cardiovascular system will thank you.

If you run five or six days a week, begin by substituting bike rides on one or two of those days. At first, you should ride only 10–15 km (6 –9 mi.). Soon, you'll find yourself able to ride 25–30 km (15.5–19 mi.) in a little over an hour on a flat course.

For fitness purposes, 4 km (2.5 mi.) of cycling is roughly equivalent to 1 km (0.6 mi.) of running.

2. Swimming:

Swimming is the sport that cushions your muscles and still gives you a great workout. By adding a swim to your weekly workout schedule, you can boost your aerobic fitness, upper-body strength and muscular endurance.

If you're not already an experienced swimmer, your first strokes in the pool may be difficult. Your best approach, then, is to wet your feet gradually.

A good first goal might be just to swim one lap of a 25 m pool. Eventually, you'll want to swim 1 km (40 laps in a 25 m pool) without stopping. Time isn't a factor in the beginning, but you should work steadily to increase your speed. Use the freestyle stroke since it will give you the best overall workout.

One kilometer of swimming gives you about the same workout as 5 km of running.

3. Cross-Country Skiing:

Cross-country skiing does more than just replace the pounding and jarring of running with a kick and glide that's gentle on your legs. It provides an unparalleled cardiovascular workout. That's because it works the large muscles of your arms, torso and back as well as your leg muscles.
But, as with any other new activity, it's best to start cross-country skiing slowly, then build your mileage as you become more accomplished.

For the easiest start, head to a Nordic centre that sets tracks on its trails. The tracks will keep you moving along in a straight line so you can concentrate on your form without worrying about the terrain.

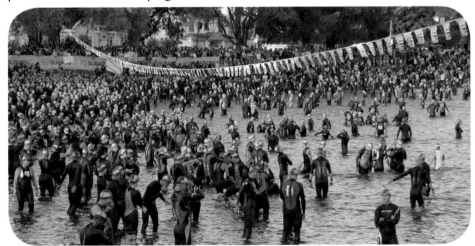

Even for the beginner, cross-country skiing does require special equipment—skis, boots, bindings, poles and light but warm clothing. Initially, rent the equipment just to make certain you like the sport. Once you're sure, consult a seasoned skier and inquire at several Nordic shops to get skis, poles and bindings that match your size and ability.

Water Running

Today's athletes are looking for ways to train more intelligently and give the body a chance to recover between quality workouts. Water running is a great alternative to running and one that is the closest in emulating running. It gives the athlete the same release that they receive from dry land running without the impact.

Many athletes have discovered the benefits of water running as a result of implementing it during an injury. People are able to water run when an injury keeps them from running or cycling. Most have then followed up by incorporating it into their regular workouts as a cross-training exercise. It is a great way to work on form, and you can get a quality workout without the pounding of the road. Many athletes achieve improved recovery by running in the water. Water running will help maintain range of motion, flexibility and cardiovascular fitness.

Many people use water running as an alternative medium for training. Be sure to check with your doctor, as many injuries will still allow you to water run.
You should get to a pool that is deep enough that the water is over your head. Some runners train without a flotation device, but you can better concentrate on

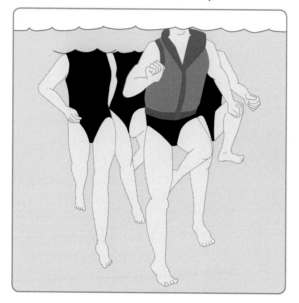

your form if you wear one. The Running Room recommends the Aqua Jogger. A flotation device will assist in the primary concern: the maintenance of good posture.

The flotation device should keep you above water, at about neck level. You must maintain an upright position as you begin your normal running motion. The most common error is to lean too far forward, so concentrate on keeping an upright position, with your shoulders back. As you run, bring your knees up high and tuck your heels under your buttocks. Keep your arms synchronized with your legs and focus on driving your elbows back and pointing your toes forward as you run. This sprinter's form will enable you to improve the range of motion as you run. You will find that you become more fluid in your form at the hip joint. The knees and ankles will become stronger and more supple. Most people who have used water running have reported improvement in their form and performance on the roads.

You can do both long and slow workouts in the water, as well as high-intensity workouts. A great way to recover from a long run is to do a 45-minute water run. You will find that water running is somewhat deceptive in that you do not feel the workout at first. Water running will leave you fatigued but not sore. The Running Room recommends that the first workouts start with about 30 to 45 minutes, depending upon your current level of conditioning. For long runs you can work up to two hours in length.

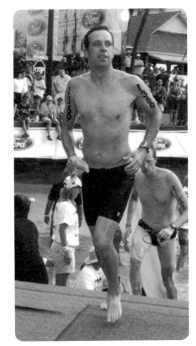

Whether you are using the water running as an alternative to running owing to injury or as a cross-training workout to supplement your workouts, most people have found that water running can become an integral part of their total running program.

Water Running Tips
1. Use a flotation device
2. Upright position
3. High knees
4. Tuck heels under buttocks
5. Drive elbows back
6. Point toes
7. Think sprinters form
8. Concentrate on form
9. Relax
10. Power

High-Intensity Workout

Start with four intervals of 15-second hard workouts with 15 seconds of rest between the hard efforts. Next start a ladder by doing four hard intervals of 30 seconds with a 20-second recovery, then 45 seconds with a 30-second recovery, then 60 seconds with a 30-second recovery. Finish going off back down the ladder—4 x 45, 4 x 30 and 4 x 15.

Do a 10-minute warm-up and a 10-minute cooldown.

This is about a 45-minute session with 16 minutes of anaerobic work.

This is much longer than we would have you do on dry land, so the bonus is a high-quality workout with a low level of injury risk, plus some alternative training to keep it fun.

Good Water Running Form

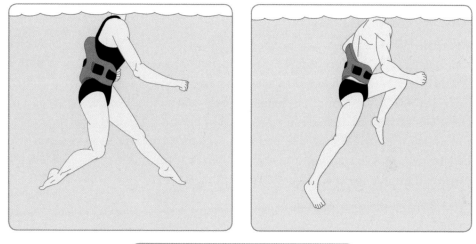

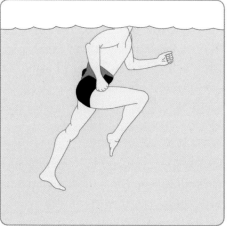

Building Core Strength

Cross training works best when more than one aerobic activity is combined throughout the week with core strength training using weights or some other form of strength exercise. This is a form of cross training that will really complement your aerobic work.

Running success is a combination of your cardiovascular system (heart, lungs and blood) and your muscles. The energy you are producing is transferred to the ground by your muscles. This transfer moves you forward. The stronger your muscles are, the more effective your running form.

Runners do not have to spend the amount of time in the gym that participants in power/speed events often do. Moderate core strength training twice a week will have a significant effect on your aerobic activity. Your muscles will be stronger; so will your connective tissues, resulting in more stable and balanced joints. This applies regardless of gender and it applies to adults of all ages.

As an aerobic athlete, you may not be familiar with core strength exercise, weight room equipment and procedures. The weight room in a modern fitness center is a bright, airy place filled with safe, interesting equipment. It is also staffed by trainers who are more than happy to help you with a program designed to complement your chosen aerobic activity. Do not be intimidated by the fitness room—with a little knowledge and some practice you will soon discover the benefits of strength training. You will feel better, stand taller, experience less injuries and be able to walk longer and faster.

Core Exercises on the Ball

Exercise ball workouts have become very popular over the last few years. They are a great way to lose weight and get in shape and are inexpensive. You do not need to go to a gym because the exercise ball is convenient and easy to use at home. A primary benefit of exercising with an exercise ball is that the body responds to the instability of the ball to remain balanced, engaging many more muscles to do so. These exercises on the ball help strengthen core muscles. They also improve balance and overall coordination. Those muscles become stronger over time to keep balance.

We will demonstrate a few great exercise ball techniques that will soon become a core part of your fitness program. Most of these moves are not advanced exercises that require previous experience with an exercise ball, so enjoy this great training technique.

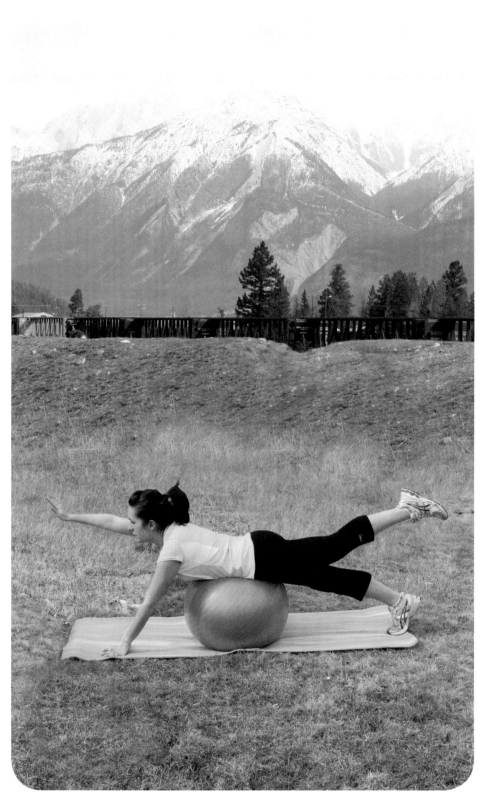

Ten Simple Exercises

Before you begin the workout, warm up with five minutes of walking or stretching that gets your heart pumping.

1. Inner-Thigh Crunch

Targets: inner thighs and abdominals

Lie on your back with your knees bent at 90 degrees and your shins parallel to the floor. Place the ball between your knees and squeeze your legs together to hold it there. If you have lower-back pain, place your hands under the small of your back for support. (figure 34-a)

Keeping your lower back on the floor, inhale and lift your heels (with your knees still bent) toward the ceiling. Exhale and lower your feet and legs back to the starting position. (figure 34-b)

Repeat 10 times.

2. Bridge

Targets: back of thighs, buttocks and abdominals

Lie on your back with your legs extended, feet hip width apart, and calves and ankles resting on the ball. (figure 35-a)

Exhale, engage your abdominal muscles, and lift your butt toward the ceiling, taking care not to arch your back. Hold for two to five seconds, and then slowly lower yourself back to the starting position. (figure 35-b)

Make this move more difficult by moving the ball closer to your ankles or easier by resting it under your knees. Try for 10 repetitions.

Once you've mastered this move, add a kick. With your butt lifted, shift your weight to your right leg and raise your left leg 90 degrees, keeping your leg straight. Focus on squeezing the thigh and butt muscles in your right leg.

Repeat on the other side for a total of 10 repetitions.

3. Push-Up

Targets: chest, triceps, abdominals, shoulders and back

Lie on the ball on your stomach. Carefully walk your hands forward on the floor until the ball is centered on your thighs. Extend your legs and hold your body in a straight line. (figure 36-a)

Inhale, bend your elbows and lower your chest to the floor. (figure 36-b)

Exhale and push back up to the plank position. Keep your back flat. If this is too difficult, perform the move while resting on your knees.

Repeat as many times as you can, eventually working up to 10 repetitions.

The Benefits of Using an Exercise Ball

As you will learn later in this chapter, strength training boosts your metabolism by building lean muscle mass. With an exercise ball and a little space, you can build muscle and increase your metabolism with a full-body workout. You will enjoy the following benefits:

+ improved balance
+ better coordination
+ increased flexibility
+ enhanced muscle tone
+ stronger core

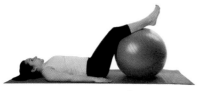

figure 34-a

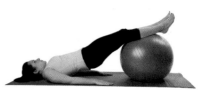

figure 34-b

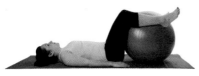

figure 35-a

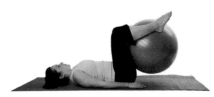

figure 35-b

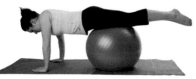

figure 36-a

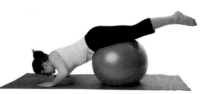

figure 36-b

12 Cross Training and Core Strengthening

4. Standing Ball Squeeze

Targets: abdominals, hips, lower back and inner thighs

Stand upright with your hands on a wall or chair for balance. Place the ball between your legs. (figure 37-a)

Kneel forward in a squatting position so your knees hug the ball. Let go of the wall (or chair) and hold your body in a stable stance. This move challenges almost all of your muscles as they work to keep you balanced and steady. (figure 37-b)

Hold the position as long as you can, with a goal of 30 seconds.

This exercise is more difficult with a big ball and easier with a smaller one. This move works your entire body, but you'll feel it most in your inner thighs.

5. Back Extension

Targets: back and shoulders

Facing away from a wall, kneel with the ball in front of you and place your hands behind your head with your elbows bent. Lean forward onto the ball, holding your feet against the wall for stability. Your chest should rest across the top of the ball. (figure 38-a)

Exhale and lift your chest up, stopping when your back is extended in a straight line. Squeeze your shoulder blades together and hold your back tight. Inhale and slowly lower back to the starting position. (figure 38-b)

Repeat 10 times.

Bump up the difficulty by extending your arms straight in a Superman position while you perform the exercise.

6. Hamstring Curl

Targets: abdominals and back of thighs

Lie on your back with your knees bent and your heels resting on the ball. (figure 39-a)

Lift your butt, inhale, and use your feet to push the ball away from you until your legs are straight. (figure 39-b)

Exhale and pull the ball back to the starting position. After 10 repetitions, exhale, tuck your abdominals, and roll back down onto your back.

Once this move becomes easy, take it up a notch by performing the move one leg at a time. In the starting position, shift your weight to your right leg and lift your left leg off the ball. Do the exercise as before, moving the ball with your right leg

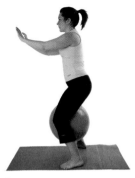

figure 37-a

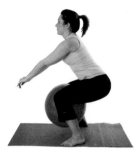

figure 37-b

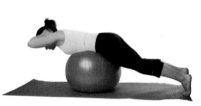

figure 38-a

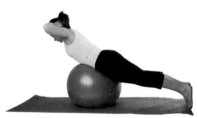

figure 38-b

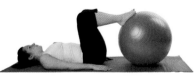

figure 39-a

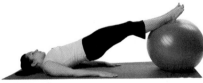

figure 39-b

while your left leg hovers above the ball.
After 10 repetitions, switch legs.

7. Ball Rotation (figure 40-a, b)

Targets: abdominals and backs of thighs and shoulders
Lie with the ball under your shoulders and lower back. Extend your arms straight up over your chest, with the palms together. Hold your body in a straight line from hips to knees. Tightening your glutes and abs, slowly twist your body to the left, sweeping your arms parallel to the floor, then back up, repeating on the other side. Try not to collapse the body or roll too far, but really use your abs. Repeat 10 times.

8. Ball Twist (figure 41-a, b)

Targets: abdominals, inner thighs and shoulders
Get into a pushup position with the feet on either side of the ball (turning your ankles so that you are hugging the ball). Hold your body in a straight line with your abs pulled in, hips straight and hands directly under your shoulders. Slowly twist the ball to the right while trying to keep your shoulders level, then to the left. Don't sag in the middle. Repeat 10 times.

9. Opposite Limb Extension (figure 42-a, b)

Targets: lower back, buttocks and hamstrings
Lie with your stomach on the ball and stabilize yourself with your toes and hands. While looking down at the floor, extend your left arm and your right leg simultaneously, hold for two seconds, and return to the starting position. Repeat with the opposite arm and leg combination. Repeat 10 times.

10. The Beetle (figure 43-a, b)

Targets: abdominals, lower back, buttocks, hamstrings and shoulders
Lie down on a matt with the legs and arms straight up. Place the ball between the feet and hands while squeezing to keep the ball in place. Lower your left arm and your right leg simultaneously towards the floor. Keep the knees bent and limit how far you lower the arms and legs. Do not touch the floor. Bring your arm and leg back up, returning to the starting position. Repeat and with the opposite arm and leg combination. Repeat 10 times.

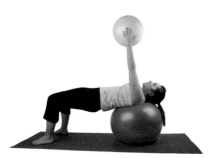

figure 40-a

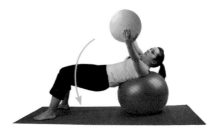

figure 40-b

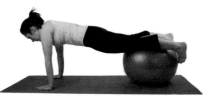

figure 41-a

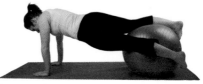

figure 41-b

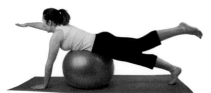

figure 42-a

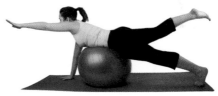

figure 42-b

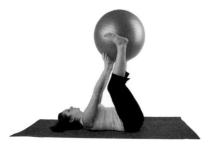

figure 43-a

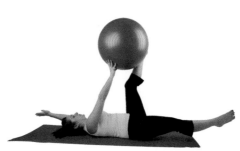

figure 43-b

12 Cross Training and Core Strengthening

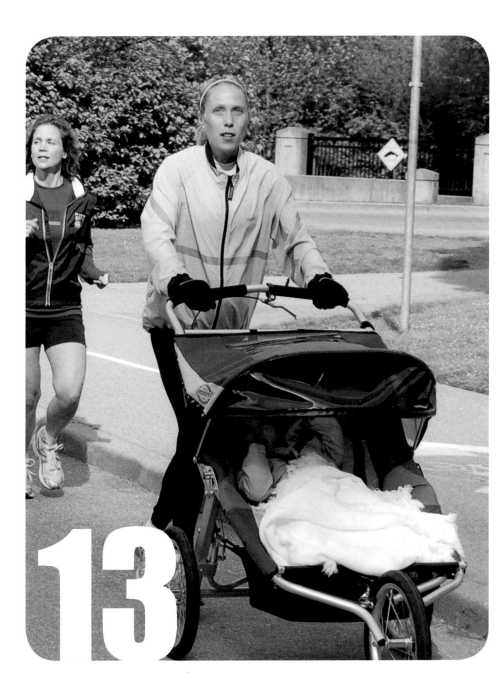

13

Special Health Concerns for Female Athletes

Women often have questions about exercise related to the menstrual cycle and reproduction. By knowing the answers and learning how to avoid the pitfalls, women can benefit from a full exercise program.

For both men and women, regular exercise offers weight loss, reduced levels of harmful cholesterol, fewer sick days and an improved self-image. Those who exercise have less low backache, headache, anxiety, depression and fatigue. Weight-bearing exercises build and maintain strong bones in both sexes. The points to note about exercise concern the physical differences between men and women:

+ Menstrual symptoms, including a group called molimina (appetite changes, breast tenderness, fluid retention and mood changes) are eased.
+ Stronger bones developed with weight-bearing exercise may help prevent osteoporosis that often occurs after menopause.
+ Women tend to have smaller hearts and less lung capacity. Their muscles are smaller and they have more body fat. Despite this, women can still achieve a lower heart rate and blood pressure, loss of body fat and increased strength by doing aerobic exercise.

Iron Pumping

Iron—Pumping Power for Active Women

Iron is an essential nutrient that is critical for overall good health. Unfortunately, many women do not get enough iron in their diets and as a result anemia, or low blood iron levels, is a common concern, particularly for active women.

Iron is a key component of hemoglobin, the factor in our blood that carries oxygen to body cells. If you do not take in adequate amounts of iron, your body will not be able to make hemoglobin in the amounts that are needed to load your cells with oxygen. As a result, the body becomes unable to fuel itself during rest and activity. Symptoms such as relentless fatigue, listlessness, irritability and difficulty concentrating are common in women suffering from iron shortages or deficiencies.

Physiology puts women at greater risk for iron deficiencies than men. Women aged 13 to 49 years rank at the top of the list when it comes to iron requirements. Menstruation causes this significant need for iron. Iron is lost on a monthly basis in menstrual flow. If these losses are not replaced, iron deficiency can easily occur.

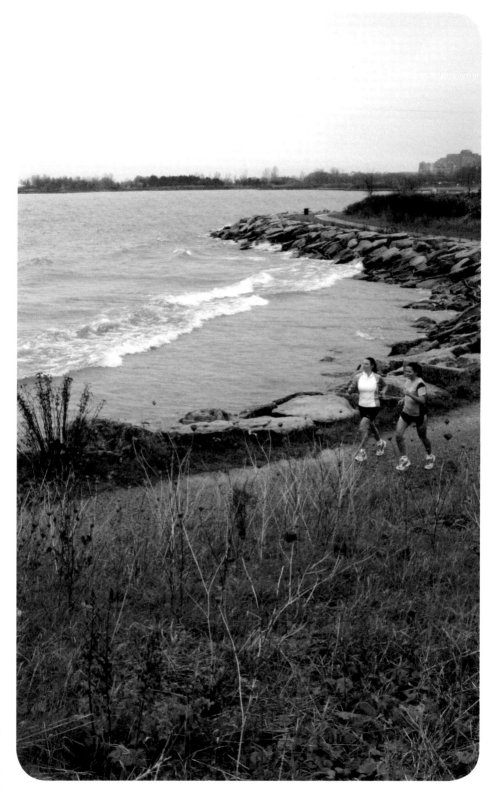

Activity, especially intense activity, can further increase iron requirements in women. Iron is lost in sweat that is generated during exercise. In addition, physical activity can cause red blood cells and muscle tissue to breakdown, which, in turn, causes iron to be lost from the body in significant amounts. These losses need to be replaced or iron shortages can occur.

Iron Intake

Iron-Rich Eating

Healthy eating can help you obtain all of the iron you need to stay healthy. Choosing a wide-variety of iron-containing foods is the key to meeting your needs.

Iron in foods is found in two forms: heme iron and non-heme iron. Heme iron—found in red meats, fish and poultry—is readily absorbed and used by the body. All other foods—including eggs, vegetables, fruits and whole grain products—contain the non-heme form of iron. This form is not absorbed as well as heme iron.

Increasing Your Iron Intake

Use the following strategies to make sure that you are getting enough iron:

1. Forget chronic dieting and low-calorie eating plans. At any given time 70% of women are dieting to manage their weight. This obsession with low-calorie eating can make it difficult, if not impossible, to obtain all of the iron needed for optimum health. Many low-calorie diets simply do not provide enough iron-rich foods to meet a woman's needs. Opt for a well-balanced, healthy diet plus regular exercise like running if weight management is a concern.

2. Include sources of heme iron in your diet on a regular basis (e.g., three to four times per week). Foods rich in heme iron include red meats, fish and poultry. Contrary to some media reports, red meats can be a nutritious part of a woman's diet. It is not necessary to exclude red meats from the diet in the name of good health.

3. Have some vitamin C with each source of non-heme iron. Vitamin C helps the body to use non-heme iron more effectively. Foods rich in vitamin C include citrus fruits and juices, tomatoes, broccoli and bell peppers. This strategy is particularly important for vegetarians, who may not choose any sources of heme iron.

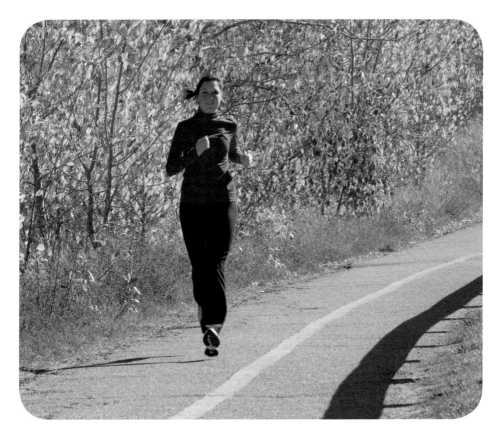

4. Cook in cast iron pots and pans. Some of the iron from this type of cook-ware will be transferred to the foods that you eat.

5. Be on the lookout for any signs of iron deficiency. If you constantly feel tired or listless see your doctor. A simple blood test can let you know if you are short of iron.

References:

1. National Eating Disorder Information Centre Web Site. www.nedic.on.ca

Eating Healthy

Bone Up with Healthy Eating

Healthy eating provides the building blocks for healthy bones and is critical for preventing osteoporosis. Two nutrients, calcium and vitamin D, are essential for bone health at all stages of life. Unfortunately, research shows that many women do not get enough of these nutrients.

Calcium is an essential nutrient that our bodies need on a daily basis in order to maintain optimum health. Ninety-nine percent of the calcium in our bodies is stored in our bones. The remaining one percent is found in blood and is used to regulate heartbeat and blood pressure, clot blood and contract our muscles. If we do not get enough calcium in our diets, the body "tops up" blood calcium levels by withdrawing calcium from our bones in much the same way we withdraw money from a savings account. Over time, too many "withdrawals" can lead to bone breakdown. Taking in enough calcium can prevent this problem from occurring.

The national health recommendation for women aged 19 to 49 years is to take in 1000 mg of calcium each day. This translates into three to four servings of calcium-rich foods each day. Examples of calcium-rich foods include:

Food	Portion Size	Calcium Content
Milk (whole, 2%, 1%, skim or chocolate)	250 ml (1 cup)	300 mg
Yogurt (plain or flavored)	175 ml (¾ cup)	250 mg
Calcium-fortified beverages (e.g. soy, rice)	250 ml (1 cup)	300 mg
Firm cheese (e.g. cheddar, Swiss—regular or low fat)	1 cube	250 mg
Processed cheese slices	2 slices	250 mg
Salmon (canned with bones)	1 can	250 mg
Sardines (canned with bones)	1 can	250 mg

Supplements Are Important

Calcium Supplements

It is important to think "food first" whenever possible in order to meet your nutrient needs. Our bodies are designed to extract nutrients from whole foods in a way that is often not duplicated by supplements. In addition, whole foods contribute to your overall nutritional health by providing multiple nutrients in a single serving.

Seek the advice of your physician, registered dietitian or pharmacist if you are considering calcium supplementation. A wide variety of supplements in varying dosages and prices are available. A knowledgeable health care provider can help you choose the supplement that best meets your individual needs.

Vitamin D

Vitamin D is calcium's partner in bone health. Without adequate amounts of vitamin D, the body cannot effectively use the calcium it gets from food. As with calcium, many North Americans do not get enough vitamin D.

As children we often learn that our bodies can make all the vitamin D that we need from sunlight. This is only partially true. In fact, research shows that between October and March in North America we do not make substantial amounts of vitamin D from sunlight, owing to low exposure and variations in the angles of the sun's rays. Sunscreens can also interfere with this process, and the growing trend towards regular use of sunscreens means that sunlight is not a reliable source of vitamin D for many people.

Food sources of vitamin D are essential for meeting women's needs. Good sources of vitamin D include fortified milk, fortified soy beverage and fatty fish like salmon. Choose one to two servings of these foods on a daily basis to obtain all of the vitamin D that you need.

Osteoporosis is a health concern that no woman wants to deal with. Recognize that you can do much to prevent this serious condition. Be active and eat well—your bones will grow to thank you.

Running Builds Bones

Women's Running: Building Bones to Run on

Over the past decade, osteoporosis prevention has become an issue of key concern for women. Osteoporosis is a chronic condition where, over time, bones become very weak and very brittle, and break very easily. According to the Osteoporosis Society, one in four women will be affected by this condition, which is often severely debilitating.

Lifestyle plays a profound role in building strong bones. Active living and healthy eating both help to lower a woman's risk for osteoporosis.

Running Builds Better Bones

Consistent physical activity helps to stimulate bone growth and development. As a result, women who are active on a regular basis tend to have stronger bones and a greatly reduced risk for osteoporosis. While all forms of physical activity help to promote bone health, weight-bearing activities—activities where the weight of your body is supported by your bones—are especially important. These kinds of activities, which include running and walking, place mild stress on our bones and encourage the body to build bones that can withstand the test of time.

Hormonal Changes

Effect on Menstrual Cycle

For some women, especially those with little body fat, too much exercise can reduce the levels of hormones (estrogen and progesterone) that control menstruation. The results may range from normal periods with no egg produced to infrequent and light periods (oligomenorrhea) to no periods at all (amenorrhea). For girls near puberty, the onset of periods may be delayed by intense training. Changes in the menstrual cycle can have an effect on fertility, although this usually only occurs with excessive training.

Effect on Bones

Estrogen and progesterone help bone growth. If hormone levels are low for a long time, such as during too much exercise, calcium will be lost from the bones. This loss is similar to that which occurs after menopause. It may result in broken bones, especially the spine and hips. More often, however, bone growth is improved with exercise.

Reversing the Effects

The reason for exercise-related hormone changes are complex and not well understood. What is known is that these changes can be reversed with small reductions in training or small weight gains. Certainly women who have irregular periods, no matter what the cause, should see a doctor. Women who have a history of irregular periods could have their bone density measured to determine if there has been any associated bone loss.

Iron Levels

Active women must maintain proper iron levels in the body. Iron is found in hemoglobin, which is in the red blood cells carrying oxygen from the lungs to the tissues. Iron is also an important part of many body proteins and cell components. Women who menstruate risk having low iron because of the regular loss of blood (and therefore iron) that occurs each month. Very active women have an added risk because their bodies absorb less iron. They also lose iron with sweat and have a breakdown of red blood cells in some of the tissues.

Red meat provides the best source of iron. Any red meat and the dark meat of poultry provide a form of iron called heme iron, which is more easily used than the iron found in vegetables and grains. It is most effective when combined with vegetable proteins. For example, split-pea soup with ham, or chicken soup with lentils are high-iron combinations. Vitamin C, plentiful in fruits, will also increase iron absorption.

Some people who restrict meat from their diets are also counting calories. These people may cut back on other food groups which supply iron. One way to increase iron, especially if calories are being limited, is to choose breads, cereals and pasta with "enriched" or "fortified" on the label.

The single or combined effect of loss of iron through menstruation, exercise and diet restrictions may cause iron deficiency. The symptoms of low iron include tir-

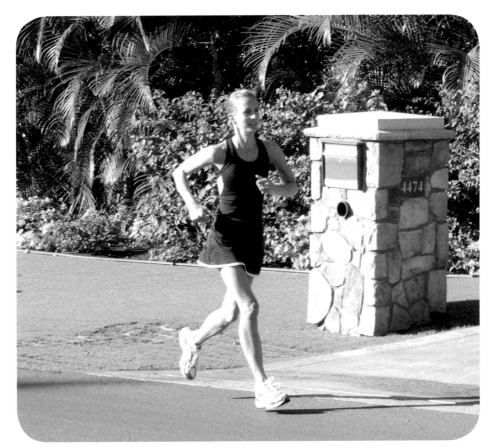

ing easily and poor performance. If iron stores become too low, anemia will result and the added symptoms of this include paleness, greater fatigue and shortness of breath.

All women should eat a diet with enough iron (see table). It is also important that they have hemoglobin levels checked on a regular basis by a doctor. For those at risk of low iron, the body's iron stores should be measured.

Increasing Iron Intake

To be sure you are taking in enough in your food, try the following:

At each meal, eat foods that are high in vitamin C. Vitamin C helps the body use iron. Drink orange juice with an iron enriched cereal, or combine pasta with broccoli, tomatoes and green peppers.

Sources of Iron	Amount	Iron (mg)
(contain heme iron)		
Pork chop	3.5 oz	4.0
Lean ground beef	3.5 oz	3.4
Lamb (leg)	3.0 oz	2.1
Turkey (dark)	3.0 oz	1.9
Chicken	3.0 oz	1.0
Tuna	3.0 oz	1.0
(contain non-heme iron)		
Dried apricots	12	6.0
Dates	9	5.0
Baked beans	1/2 c	3.0
Kidney beans	1/2 c	3.0
Raisins	1/2 c	2.0
Spinach	1/2 c	2.0
Green beans	1/2 c	1.0
Enriched pasta	1/2 c	1.0

Risk of Injury

A question often asked about women in sports is whether they are at higher risk of injury than men. This concern, without basis in fact, kept women from taking part in many sports until recently. For example, women were not allowed to compete in the marathon at the Olympics until 1984.

The body's response to exercise is the same for both sexes. Each sport puts demands on the body and carries its own risk of injuries. Women are at no greater risk of those injuries than men and should be allowed to take part in any sport. If a training program is suited to the level of fitness, women are no more likely than men to suffer injury. Any sports injury should be treated promptly by a doctor.

Exercise During Pregnancy

One concern to women in sport is exercise during pregnancy. For this special case, pregnant women should discuss the exercise program with a doctor.

Conclusion

Exercise is a key to good health for everyone. Women should take part in regular exercise and sport, not only for their health but also for the pure pleasure of participation.

Amenorrhea

This is a term used to describe the cessation of a woman's menstrual periods after she has been menstruating on a consistent basis. It occurs mostly among women under 30 years of age, but can affect any women through the age of menopause. Amenorrhea can be harmful to the body, particularly the bones and reproductive systems, if it is allowed to continue for a substantial length of time, usually more than one year. Its effects are reversible, if treated.

A menstrual cycle is called a "regular period" if the interval between periods is in the range of 25 to 30 days. If the frequency of periods is greater than or less than this interval, then the periods are considered to be irregular. In this case, the woman may not be ovulating, but the body continues to have periods as reactions to the same hormonal changes that occur among those with regular periods. This condition is generally only a problem if the woman is trying to conceive.

Harmful Effects

In addition to the problems associated with infertility that occur with both irregular periods and amenorrhea, the other harmful effect is that of decreased bone mass, leading to an increased risk for osteoporosis. The amounts of estrogen associated with decreased menstruation also makes these women more susceptible to bone fractures and skeletal injuries. The hormonal imbalances have also been associated with slightly higher risk of uterus and breast cancer.

Low Body Weight Theory

Athletic amenorrhea was originally believed to be due to a low amount of body fat, together with mileage training. This theory has not held up to scrutiny by many researchers, and although there remains an association between these factors and menstrual dysfunction, the relationship is not causal. Thus, some women with low body fat continue to have regular periods, and some running very high mileage also continue to menstruate regularly. Some researchers have suggested that perceived stress, or mental stress, also has an important effect. The intensity of training and/or competition may also contribute to amenorrhea, as some women only lose their periods during times of high stress (either mental or physical). The bottom line may be that every woman's body, personality and experience is so different that one can't predict the effects on menstrual function. An important point to remember is that a gradual adaptation to training can reduce both the physical and mental stresses on a person, thereby diminishing a woman's chance of disrupting her cycle.

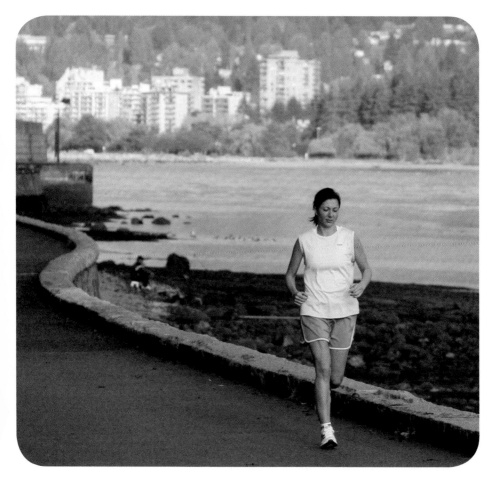

What Can Be Done

Almost all problems associated with amenorrhea are reversible once menstruation begins again. A reduction in training is usually sufficient to bring about normal menses. Calcium supplements and other hormonal medications (such as birth control pills) can also be prescribed by a doctor. Eating a diet that is rich in calcium-containing foods, such as dairy products, leafy green vegetables, seafood, etc., is also helpful.

In the end, it is extremely important that women stay in tune with their bodies through any training program and be aware of the serious side effects related to irregular or complete cessation of menses. They should watch for disturbances in the menstrual cycle as warning signs that something is wrong. Factors that are associated with amenorrhea (in no particular order) are:

1. Rapid weight loss/low body fat
2. High-intensity training and/or volume
3. Failure to adapt fully to training
4. The mental perception of training
5. Internalized (self-applied) pressure to perform
6. The desire to meet high (external) expectations
7. Higher than normal or sudden changes in total life stress

Once identified, measures can be taken to eliminate obvious factors in order to restore a woman back to healthy menstrual functioning.
*(adapted from Peak Running Performance, 1992; 2(3): 5-8)

Exercises and Pregnancy

Fit Mom

Introduction

The aim of this section is to provide a basic guide for exercise during pregnancy for the active woman. It is not intended to be a complete manual. It does not set out a full range of exercises in detail but simply provides examples to facilitate the planning of a suitable exercise regimen while pregnant. Planning and implementation of your exercise regimen while pregnant should be under strict supervision of your doctor.

Little is known about the effects of a mother's exercise on the fetus. Care must be taken when fitness begins with pregnancy because both exercise and preg-

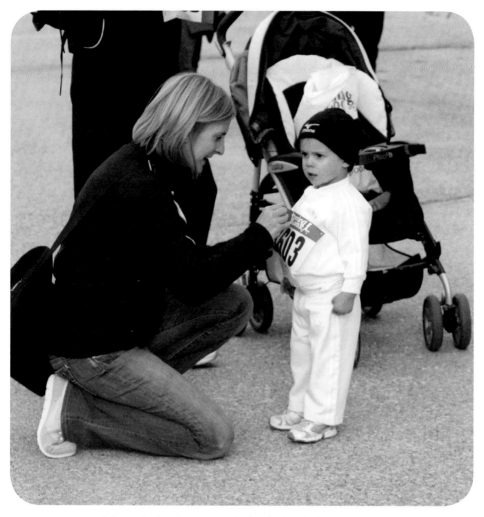

nancy are stressful on the body, particularly the back, hips, knees and other joints and muscles. In most cases, a reasonable, noncompetitive exercise program based on current level of fitness may be the beginning of lifelong fitness. If you are already active, you can probably continue to do so, modifying it as the pregnancy advances, monitoring how you feel and what your doctor recommends. A woman, especially during pregnancy, has to make sure she has good pelvic floor and abdominal muscle support before even jogging. Consult your doctor prior to starting.

Benefits

The benefits of maintaining your exercise program throughout your pregnancy are not well documented. That should not detract from your own perceptions of your program. The advantages to exercise training in general become advantageous to the pregnant woman also. The most commonly reported benefits are:

1. Maintained aerobic capacity
2. Increased insulin sensitivity
3. Improved muscular strength
4. Decreased pain perception
5. Positive well-being
6. Self acceptance

Exercise training not only increases aerobic capacity but also influences the insulin sensitivity in the muscles. Increased insulin sensitivity increases the body's capacity to mobilize and oxidize fat and decreases the rate of glycogen depletion in the muscles during exercise.

A few scientific investigations have reported that women who maintained their fitness level while pregnant had elevated levels of B-endorphin during labor and delivery, thus pain perception was reduced in women who exercised throughout their pregnancy. These adaptations to exercise training may assist in preparing women for the physical and psychological stress of labor. Improved muscular strength may be especially beneficial in preventing back pain, may help in feeling agile and may facilitate carrying added weight and dealing with the change in centre of gravity.

The physiological and anatomical changes in a woman's body during pregnancy are perceived to inhibit exercise. The anatomical changes occurring, such as laxity in the joints and ligaments, together with increased weight and the continuing shift in the centre of gravity, may mean that pregnant women are more susceptible to injury. The extent of the body's adjustment depends on many factors, both external and internal. Individual factors such as age, body weight and health status are significant, as well as the type of exercise undertaken and the environment in which it is performed.

Be sure to discuss your individual changes and requirements with your physician.

Psychological Benefits of Exercise During Pregnancy

Psychological and emotional well-being are one of the greatest advantages to exercise. For the pregnant woman, this can be the greatest benefit to maintaining a fitness regimen during pregnancy. Your motives for being active in the past may have been primarily conscious or unconscious. Fitness may have given you

1. Measurable achievement (essential for your self-esteem)
2. Externalization and diversion of conflicts (the shifting of attention from internal conflicts to external challenges)
3. Enhanced sense of mastery (a sense of satisfaction by engaging in something you know is beneficial to you)
4. Physical exercise as hard work (the feeling of accomplishment after completing a hard workout)
5. Expression of aggression (pent-up aggression and hostility can be discharged through physical activity)
6. Opportunity for social interaction (interaction with people similar interest and motivations)

Being physically active during pregnancy should not be done out of fear (of looking pregnant, gaining weight, losing endurance) but with enjoyment. This will contribute to your sense of well-being and self-confidence and give you greater emotional and physical resilience. A word of caution, this is a good time to dispel that old saying, "No pain, no gain." Think "No pain, more brain" instead. Keep your level of intensity well within your limits.

There is no question that the improved stamina, resilience, physical well-being and greater self-reliance will prepare a woman to the real challenges, both physical and emotional, inherent in pregnancy, childbirth and beyond.

Tips for Maintaining a Safe Exercise Environment

Ask yourself these questions:
1. Is the area appropriate for the activity?
2. Is the area relatively safe and free from latent defects and danger?
3. Is the area free from rapid and changing environmental conditions?
4. Is the area relatively safe from criminal activity?
5. Is the area populated?
6. Is the area close to emergency facilities?
7. Is the area close to shelter and assistance?

Risks

Guidelines for exercise during pregnancy vary from woman to woman. Whether she is a highly trained athlete or has been participating in a fitness program for only a short time, the risks a pregnant woman faces and the precautions she should take are similar. All are to follow the strict advice of their physicians. Safety for both the mother and the fetus should be the primary concern. The following list shows a few of the risks for those undertaking physical exercise during pregnancy:

Maternal Risks

1. Increased risk of musculoskeletal injuries
2. Cardiovascular complications
   a. Supine hypotension
   b. Aortocaval syndrome, arrhythmias
   c. Heart failure
3. Spontaneous abortion
4. Premature labor
5. Hypoglycemia

Fetal Risks

1. Fetal distress
2. Intrauterine growth retardation
3. Fetal malformations
4. Prematurity

Neonatal Risks

1. Decreased adipose tissue
2. Hyperthermia

Although some of the listed risks may be theoretical, caution should be exercised to prevent potential complications. If you experience any of the following symptoms, stop exercising and contact your doctor immediately:

- Pain
- Bleeding
- Dizziness
- Back pain
- Palpitations

- Tachycardia (abnormal, rapid heartbeat)
- Pubic pain (or any cramping)
- Shortness of breath
- Faintness
- Difficulty walking

Guidelines for Exercise During Pregnancy

The American College of Obstetricians and Gynecologists (ACOG) has developed these guidelines for exercise during pregnancy. In general, these guidelines are based on a consideration of the physiological changes that take place at this time. Your physician should be made aware that you are undertaking a fitness program and will advise you of any limitations, contraindications, alarming signs and special concerns.

1. Regular exercise (at least three times per week) is preferable to intermittent activity. Competitive activities should be discouraged.

2. Vigorous exercise should not be performed in hot, humid weather or during a period of febrile illness.

3. Ballistic movements (jerky, bouncing motions) should be avoided. Exercise should be done on an absorbent surface to reduce shock and provide sure footing.

4. Deep flexion or extension of joints should be avoided because of connective tissue laxity. Activities that require jumping, jarring motions or rapid changes in direction should be avoided because of joint instability.

5. Vigorous exercise should be preceded by a five-minute period of muscle warm-up, which can be accomplished by slow walking or stationary cycling at a low resistance.

6. Vigorous exercise should be followed by a period of gradually declining activity that includes gentle stationary stretching. Because the connective tissue laxity increases the risk of joint injury, stretches should not be taken to the point of maximum resistance.

7. Heart rate should be measured at times of peak activity. Target heart rates and limits established in consultation with the physician should not be exceeded.

8. Care should be taken to rise gradually from the floor to avoid orthostatic hypotension. Some form of activity with the legs should be continued for a brief period.

9. Liquids should be taken liberally before and after exercise to prevent dehydration. If necessary, activity should be interrupted to replenish fluids.

10. Women who have led sedentary lifestyles should begin with physical activity of very low intensity and advance activity levels very slowly.

11. Activity should be stopped and the physician consulted if any unusual symptoms appear.

Developing an Exercise Prescription During Pregnancy

The goal of exercise during pregnancy should be to maintain the highest level of fitness consistent with maximum safety. Given this constraint, it is not possible to maintain optimal cardiovascular fitness nor to maintain strength training levels achieved in the nonpregnant state. No single exercise program will meet the needs of all women. The ideal exercise program will involve a variety of activities, such as walking, swimming, cycling and modified forms of aerobics and dance.

Your Heart Rate as a Measure of Intensity

For any activity, your heart rate is the best indicator of how hard you are working. In the past you may have used a target heart rate zone for which all your training would be in the limit of that zone. By using your heart rate in this way you ensured that your training was hard enough to evoke a training effect and not so hard that fatigue would accumulate over a few training days.

During pregnancy your heart rate will be one of the most valuable tools in assessing your body's response to your fitness program. It is important to note that the added stress of pregnancy is reflected by changes in heart rate both at rest and exercise.

Your heart rate response to a given intensity of submaximal exercise increases progressively during pregnancy, as does your resting heart rate. This change has important implications if you routinely use heart rate as a means of prescribing the intensity of your exercise routine.

Guidelines

Under unsupervised conditions, the intensity of the exercise should be reduced by approximately 25%, maximum maternal heart rate should not exceed 140 bpm and the period of strenuous exercise should not exceed 15 to 20 minutes, interspersed with low-intensity exercise and rest periods. Moderating activity in this way may significantly reduce the incidence for the previously listed risks.

Creating an Individualized Program

Whether you continue to participate in the same activities or take on a different routine, adjustments will have to be made in terms of intensity, frequency and duration of exercise.

There are many proposed but not proven benefits of exercise for pregnant women. These include a shorter labor and delivery, prevention of varicose veins, thrombosis and leg cramps and improved mental outlook. Exercise appears to help some women cope with the pain of labor. When proper exercises are used there may be some benefit in pregnancy, such as maintaining proper posture and preventing lower back pain, and after birth in facilitating recovery. Some of the stretching routines may have to be modified to prevent injuries.

Pregnant women who participate in exercise programs should be examined periodically to assess the effect of their exercise program on the developing fetus. They may have their programs readjusted to their level of tolerance or discontinued if necessary.

Moderation and individualization should be advised, and there is no reason not to modify such activities if they are too difficult to perform as originally prescribed. For example, the sit up from the semirecumbent position is a good exercise for the abdomen, but as the abdomen starts to protrude, perhaps a sit-back, where the mother begins in the upright position and slowly lies down into the semirecumbent position would be more appropriate.

Supine exercises should not be performed in pregnancy under any circumstances. This precaution is to avoid the high incidence of orthostatic hypotension and aortocaval compression syndrome. It is very important to remember that there is already major stress on the lower back in pregnancy because of the extra weight in the stomach area, so all the exercises that required the mother to be on her back need to be done in the semirecumbent position or preferably sitting position with the legs bent and the knees up.

Consistency is the most important part of any exercise program; if the individual is not willing to exercise regularly, she would probably be better to significantly reduce the intensity of her exercise program. By doing so, she will prevent injuries associated with sporadic exercise.

Pregnancy is the ideal time for behavior modification.

Warm-Up and Cooldown

Each activity should begin with a 10 to 15 minute warm-up period and end with a 10 to 15 minute cooldown. During exercise, maternal heart rate should not exceed 140 bpm. The cardiorespiratory changes, as well as changes in the ligaments and joints, require that special care be taken to exercise safely.

Recreational Sports Activities

It is not known if a pregnant woman has greater risk of strains and sprains than the general population. It should be noted that there is an orthopedic risk associated with some of these activities, and continuation of the activities through pregnancy may increase in risk.

Pregnant women should avoid all activities in which there is body contact to reduce the risk of injury to the abdomen and reduce the intensity of other games, such as racket sports and some field games, to reduce the risk of injuries to the extremities.

Running

This is an activity that should not be initiated after pregnancy has begun. For those who wish to continue their running program throughout their pregnancy, certain precautions should be taken during the first trimester if certain common complications occur, e.g., nausea, vomiting or poor weight gain.

Ketosis and hypoglycemia are more likely to occur during prolonged strenuous exercise in pregnancy.

Because of the nausea, vomiting and general feeling of fatigue or lethargy prevalent in pregnant women, many will not be able to run long distances.

Recommendations

During the first trimester, the recreational athlete should reduce mileage to no more than 3 km (2 mi.) per day. (This is to reduce the risk of hyperthermia and dehydration.) Because pregnant women are running to maintain fitness rather than training for competition, the shorter distances should suffice. If women want to exceed these recommendations, this activity should be coordinated with their physician to allow closer follow-up.

During the second and third trimesters, increased body weight may make running more difficult. Other factors, such as lower limb edema, varicose veins and joint laxity, may also effect performance.
Because of joint laxity, women need to be especially alert to their running path.

Walking

Walking is always an alternative to running. Especially as the pregnancy progresses, running may become uncomfortable.

A walking program could consist of a 6–10 km walk depending on the terrain and the temperature. This activity is a more than reasonable alternative to running. The same precautions should be taken in preventing dehydration and hyperthermia.

Guidelines for Walking and Running

1. Do not begin a running program while pregnant.
2. Reduce mileage to a maximum of 3 km per day.
3. If temperature and humidity is high (temp = 39°C or higher) do not exercise.
4. Wear running shoes with proper support.

Guidelines for Avoiding Hyperthermia

There are a number of precautions active women can take to avoid hyperthermia while exercising during pregnancy. If high thermal loads cannot be avoided:

1. Acclimatize gradually to the ambient temperature
2. Avoid the worst of the heat by exercising early in the morning or in an air-conditioned facility
3. Wear appropriate clothing that will permit free evaporation of sweat
4. Drink plenty of fluid
5. Do not exercise when ill
6. Use the buddy system to monitor heat distress.

Fitness Class During Pregnancy

Benefits

1. Work out in a group
2. Maintain cardiovascular endurance
3. Maintain muscular endurance and strength

Because aerobics is a weight-bearing activity, the same concerns that are associated with running should be considered by the mother (heat stress, potential joint and ligament injuries, unrecognized fetal distress). As the pregnancy progresses, some movements in these classes will have to be modified to suit the changes occurring during the pregnancy.

Guidelines

1. Specific exercises that should be avoided include over-extension and exer-

cises performed on the back (supine position).

2. Avoid hard surfaces when exercising. Limit repetition movements to 10.
3. Warm up and cooldown gradually.
4. Modify your intensity of exercise (switch from high to low impact, reduce the number of steps under platform).
5. Avoid highly competitive classes.

Bicycling During Pregnancy

Cycling is a non-weight-bearing activity. The risks of musculoskeletal injury are far less than with weight-bearing activities, such as running and aerobics.

Bicycling is not without risk, particularly stationary cycling. The ability of the body to dissipate heat is compromised by the lack of circulating air. As well, cycling may put undue stress on the lower back if riding in the more aerodynamic position, such as on a road bike. These risks can be reduced by:

1. Cycling on a stationary cycle with a fan
2. Using a more upright position
3. Strengthening the abdominal wall
4. Where available, trying the newer recumbent bikes (sitting in a reclined position while pedaling). A Tri-road bike is a preferable choice. Pregnant women find them particularly comfortable.

Guidelines

1. The program can be started during pregnancy.
2. A stationary cycle is preferable to standard cycling owing to weight and balance changes (especially after the seventh month).
3. Cycling may cause lower back stress.
4. Cycling should be avoided out of doors during high temperatures and high pollution levels.

Weight Training During Pregnancy

If weight machines are used more frequently than free weights, the risk of damage to the baby from dropping weights is decreased. Free weights can still be used, but the need for a "spotting" partner becomes of increasing importance.

Care is needed in developing weight-training programs for the pregnant woman. These programs can easily cause injury to the spine or discs because of the relaxation of the joints and ligaments.

Any program that works the entire body, promoting toning and flexibility, can be recommended within moderate limits.

One potential problem is the transient hypertension caused by the Valsalva maneuver. Proper breathing techniques (exhaling during a lift) will keep this from happening.

The Valsalva maneuver*, due to improper breathing, may cause:
1. Orthostatic hypotension
2. Decreased perfusion of the uterus.

*Valsalva maneuver: A maneuver in which a person tries to exhale forcibly with a closed glottis (the windpipe) so that no air exits through the mouth or nose as, for example, in strenuous coughing, straining during a bowel movement, or lifting a heavy weight. The Valsalva maneuver impedes the return of venous blood to the heart.

Low weights and moderate repetitions should make a sufficient program to maintain flexibility while toning the muscles. While engaging in a weight-training program during pregnancy ensure that you:
1. Decrease weight as the pregnancy progresses.
2. Do not exercise in the supine position.

Guidelines

1. Training with weights can be cautiously continued throughout pregnancy.
2. Heavy resistance on weight machines should be avoided.
3. The use of heavy free weights should be avoided.
4. Proper breathing is necessary to avoid the Valsalva maneuver.

Water Running and Aquasize During Pregnancy

Running in the water is such an efficient exercise that many injured athletes have jumped out of the pool and run personal best times after not having run on land for up to a month. Running in the water allows you to follow the same action as running on land, using water as the resistance, but without the forces of impact on the bones and soft tissues of the legs. For most, sessions of running in the pool will improve range of motion, help with flexibility and maintain the cardiovascular system.

What about during pregnancy? Water running is a great way to relieve the stresses of normal running. The cool water surroundings help keep core temperature at normal levels, and the difference in cardiovascular benefits are minimal. What does change, however, is the technique used for running in the water. Normally, water running is done in deep water. With the help of a floatation device, either a life jacket or buoyant waist belt, you are able to remain above the surface and remain in the upright position. While pregnant, a floatation device may not be comfortable, so workouts will have to take place in shoulder deep water. In this situation you stride through the water. Swing your arms naturally against the water to provide an upper body workout. For variety, stride sideways, backward and forward. You may even want to try some aerobic dance steps.

Deep water workouts and water exercise are most fun when done in groups. Check with your local community pool or Running Room for the closest water exercise program.

When deep water running, you should be trying to simulate your running action as much as possible. Don't lean too far forward. Bring your shoulders back and you knees up high, tucking them under your buttocks. Your arms should move in time with your legs. Begin with 15 to 30 minutes in the pool, depending on your fitness level.

Nutrition During Pregnancy

Information provided by Capital Health, AB

You and Your Baby

Pregnancy is a special nine months in which your body undergoes dramatic changes. The foods you eat provide nutrients for the growth and development of your baby and your own body tissues. By eating properly you are more likely to have a healthy pregnancy and baby.

Weight Gain

You may be worried about whether you are eating enough for your baby. The easiest way to check this is to look at your weight gain. Generally, women gain 9–16 kg (20–35 lb.). Women who are underweight before pregnancy should try to be in the upper end of this range, and those who are overweight may gain towards the lower end. Your doctor may recommend a goal for you.

During the first three months of pregnancy you will gain little, probably 1–2 kg (2–4 lb.). Most weight is put on during the last six months, at a rate of 0.4–0.5 kg (¾–1 lb.) per week.

If you were to gain 11 kg (24 lb.) during your pregnancy, the weight would be distributed among many components. As you would suspect, the fetus, the placenta that feeds it and the amniotic fluid that surrounds and cushions it are the largest part—5 kg (10½ lb.). The increases in maternal blood and energy stores (such as fat) to support the fetus are the next largest at 2 kg (4 lb.) each. Your breasts and uterus together increase by about 1.3 kg (3 lb.). Finally, there is a 1 kg (2½ lb.) increase in tissue fluids.

Your gain should be slow and steady. A sharp weight gain owing to water retention at about the 20th week is called preclampsia. This is a complication of pregnancy whose cause is unknown. It is marked by high blood pressure and protein loss in the urine. Any sudden increase in weight should be reported to your doctor.

Choose Quality

Your appetite may increase slightly in the first three months of your pregnancy, and even more in the last six months. But eating for you and your growing baby doesn't mean eating twice as much as before.

Actually, the daily increased energy need is very small. You'll need 100 calories more per day in the first three months and an extra 300 calories per day for the rest of your pregnancy. One hundred calories is one medium banana, 200 mL (¾ cup) plain yogurt, 30 g (1 oz.) cheese, six soda crackers or one glass of juice.

+ If you are using metric,1 calorie = 4.184 kJ (kilojoule)

Because your need for nutrients also increases, the extra energy is best obtained through foods high in essential nutrients. Throughout your pregnancy, you need to concentrate on quality foods. Check your diet, use Canada's Food Guide to help you evaluate your choices for quality as well as quantity.

What about junk food? What do you do when you are trying to eat well, but you really want a jelly donut or a package of potato chips? Firstly, see if you can substitute. Can you satisfy your craving for chips with whole grain crackers? Will a bagel make you forget the donut? How about a whole wheat bagel?
If you can't trade, eat it (but try for a small serving). The nutritional quality of your diet will not be ruined by eating a less-than-perfect food. And an occasional treat may keep your craving from becoming an obsession.
Try to keep it all in perspective. Yes, you need to eat well, but you need to have pleasure from your food. You can have both.

Special Nutrient Needs

As you would expect, your need for nutrients increases during pregnancy. The following ones are especially important in the development of your baby:

1. Protein: for growth of all cells, including bones, muscles and blood vessels.

2. Iron and Folic Acid: because your body has more blood, carrying nutrients to your baby.

3. Calcium and Vitamin D: to make strong bones and teeth.

4. Vitamin C: for healthy skin and gums and strong blood vessel walls.

Eating Upsets

Morning sickness can occur at any time of the day. The reasons for the nausea and vomiting, which is common in the first trimester, aren't well understood. Diet-related suggestions include:

+ Eat dry foods, such as crackers, dry toast or cereal, just before getting out of bed in the morning.
+ Eat small quantities of food frequently, for example, six to eight times per day. Try to include a small amount of food containing protein, such as meat, fish, eggs and cheese, at these meals.
+ Drink fluids about half an hour after meals, or have your beverages between meals, rather than with them.
+ Limit the amount of fat and fatty foods eaten.
+ Limit your consumption of coffee, tea and alcohol.
+ Avoid food odors by eating cold foods or those at room temperature.

Additional suggestions for women with nausea include:
+ Avoid tight waistbands and underwear.
+ Have minimal emotional stress with maximum emotional support
+ Get plenty of rest.
+ Use stress reduction techniques, e.g., breathing exercises, yoga.
+ Have fresh air in the bedroom while resting and in the kitchen while cooking.

Heartburn, bloating, indigestion and belching are most common in the second and third trimesters as the growing baby crowds the stomach. To assist with these discomforts:

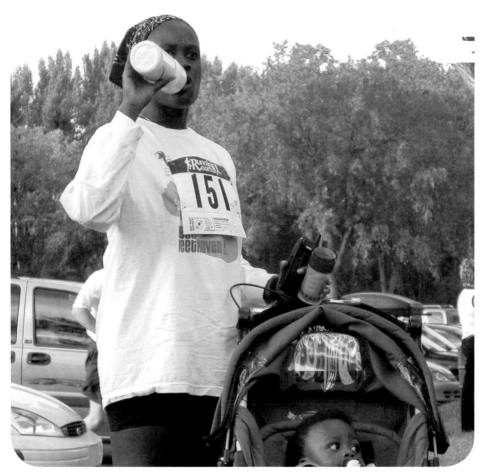

- Eat smaller quantities of food frequently and eat slowly
- Avoid highly spiced foods, fatty or fried foods, and any foods that bother you—not all foods affect everyone the same way
- Avoid coffee, tea and alcohol
- Drink fluids between meals rather than with meals
- Avoid bending or lying down for one to two hours after eating (if you wish to lie down, prop up your head).

Antacids interfere with the absorption of important minerals, such as calcium and iron. Baking soda has a high amount of sodium and is not recommended.

Constipation

Constipation is a frequent complaint in the second half of pregnancy. At this time your digestive system slows down to increase the absorption of nutrients from food, and the growing fetus presses on the digestive tract. Iron supplements may increase constipation. To ease constipation:

- Include plenty of fluids in your diet, at least 1.5–2 L (6–8 cups) per day of water, milk, juice and soup (prune juice may help).
- Use high-fiber foods in your meals: raw and dried fruits; vegetables; bran and other whole grain cereals and breads; nuts and seeds; cooked and dried peas, beans and lentils
- Remember that irregular eating times may contribute to constipation
- Avoid coffee and tea, which are constipating to some.

As Well...

- Have some moderate exercise every day—take a walk.
- Avoid taking laxatives or mineral oil. These products can decrease the absorption of nutrients from your food. If you require a laxative, consult your doctor or pharmacist.
- Although a regular, unrushed toilet time may require some schedule reorganization, it helps prevent constipation, as does an immediate response to the need for a bowel movement.

Spacing Pregnancies

From a nutrition standpoint, there should be a least 24 months from the end of one pregnancy to the start of another. This time is required to allow you body to completely recover from pregnancy and lactation, and to rebuild body nutrient supplies.

In practice, this is not always possible. Discuss this with your doctor.
Some health units have community health nutritionists, and all have community health nurses who can answer your questions during pregnancy. Contact your local health unit for further information.

Goal Setting During Pregnancy

Goal setting to create a fitness plan during pregnancy must be based on your feelings, your doctor's advice and your individual conditioning.

A. Prenatal Conditioning
What did I do for fitness before I got pregnant?

Please write down your answer. Include number of times per week and length of time for each session.

_____

_____
_____
_____
_____
_____
_____
_____

Your prenatal fitness level will help you to develop goals that are realistic during pregnancy.

B. Goal Setting During Pregnancy
What is my fitness plan during pregnancy?

1. Long-term Goal

_____
_____
_____
_____
_____
_____

Keep a logbook.

2. Short-term Goals
First Trimester

Doctor's Advice

_____
_____
_____

My Goals

_____

Modify

_____

Doctor's Advice

_____
_____
_____

My Goals

_____
_____
_____

Modify

_____
_____

Third Trimester (the extra weight and gravity will have an effect)

Doctor's Advice

_____
_____
_____

My Goals

_____
_____
_____

Modify

_____
_____

Babies very rarely come on the predicted date.
We've gone past our due date!

Modify

_____
_____
_____
_____

C. Post Natal Goal Setting

At this time your entire life is going through many changes. Your body is going through changes and your lifestyle is changing. Do not become discouraged if you feel your long-term fitness goal is not being met. Everything must be modified.

D. Finally I get to do something

1. Start slow.

2. Establish new short-term and long-term goals.

3. Decide best days and best times to work out.

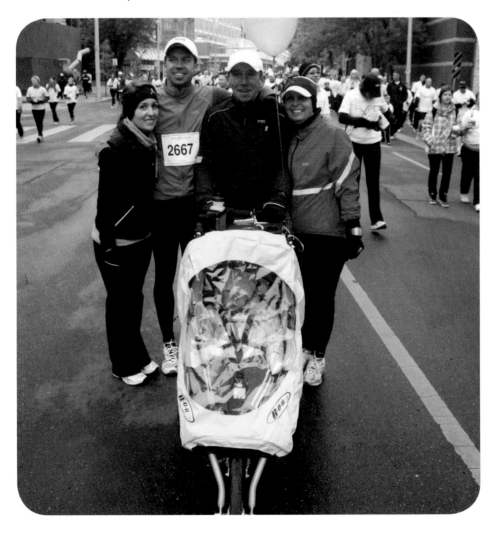

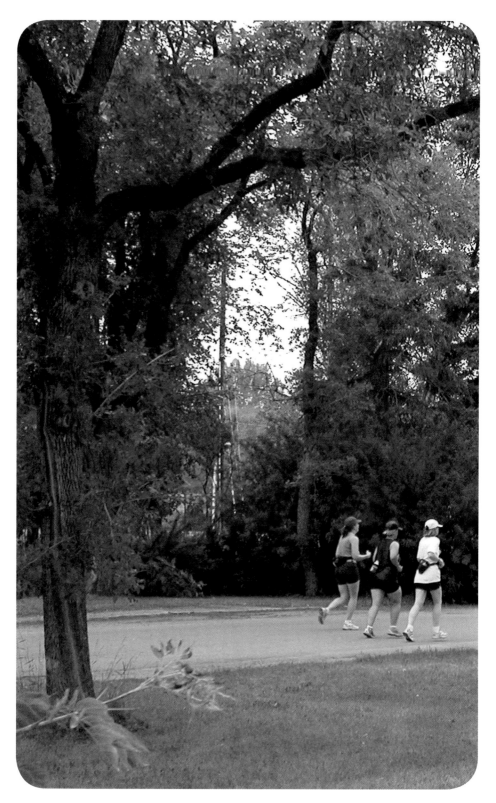

1st Trimester

Weekday	Walking	Running
Monday	Rest	Rest
Tuesday	20–30 min	30–45 min
Wednesday	Rest	Rest
Thursday	20–30 min	30–45 min
Friday	Rest	Rest
Saturday	35–45 min	30–40 min
Sunday	20–30 min	60 min (walk 1 min/run 4–10 min)

2nd Trimester

Weekday	Walking	Running
Monday	Rest	Rest
Tuesday	20–45 min	30–45 min (walk 1 min/run 4–10 min)
Wednesday	Rest	Rest
Thursday	20–45 min	30–45 min (walk 1 min/run 4–10 min)
Friday	Rest	Rest
Saturday	45–60 min	40–60 min (walk 1 min/run 4–10 min)
Sunday	20–45 min	20–45 min (walk 1 min/run 4–10 min)

3rd Trimester

Weekday	Walking	Running
Monday	Rest	Rest
Tuesday	20–30 min	30–45 min (walk 1 min/run 1–10 min)
Wednesday	Rest	Rest
Thursday	20–30 min	20–30 min (walk 1 min/run 1–10 min)
Friday	Rest	Rest
Saturday	35–45 min	30–45 min (walk 1 min/run 1–10 min)
Sunday	Rest	Rest

Injuries

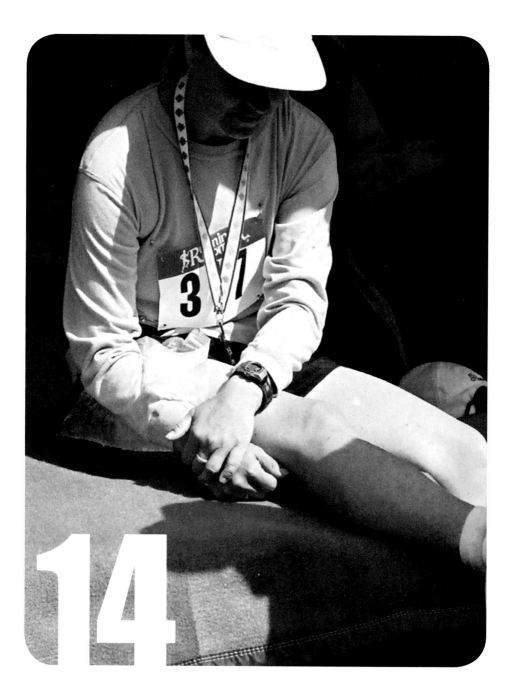

14

Running Injuries

Most runners are highly motivated and extremely devoted to their sport. They think that if they don't get their run in they won't feel quite right. While they are in pursuit of those miles, many forget to listen to their bodies.

Avoiding injury is not impossible if you pay attention to your training techniques and don't try to do too much, too soon. The best way to prevent most athletic injuries is to maintain good muscle strength and flexibility.

Most running injuries are from overuse, so tune in to your body and listen to what it's telling you. If you're cranky or more impatient than usual, you may need a few days of rest. Other signs of fatigue are a susceptibility to colds or flu, difficulty falling asleep, an inability to sleep well, a higher than usual resting pulse rate or more than the usual aches and pains in the limbs. The one running maxim you should never forget is "any pain, no brain."

> Common Causes of Injury
> + Too many miles, too quickly
> + Running in improper or worn-out shoes
> + Insufficient rest, such as running too hard on "easy" days
> + Lack of a good mileage base
> + Forcing a run when you're tired
> + Pushing too hard during intervals and tempo runs
> + Too much speed training or too many hills

Biomechanics

Running form and shoe selection are two big factors that can lead to running injuries. We covered shoes earlier in the book; now we are focusing on how the foot works and how that relates to the rest of our body.

For some, running injuries are either minor or nonexistent; for others, it seems like we're constantly battling one nagging pain after another. As with everything, the key to recovering from injury is to always remember that any injury has a cause (wrong shoes, sudden change in training volume or intensity, etc.) and until that cause is corrected, treatment (rest, drugs, etc.) will not be effective.

Here are some very straightforward lessons on the importance of biomechanics. Remember to keep these suggestions in mind:

1. Lead with your hips.
2. Keep your body tall, with your head up, and avoid leaning forward.
3. Strike down with your heel and roll off your toes in a flowing motion.
4. Don't clench. Clenching (hands, arms, eyes) transfers stress to other parts of the body and makes running in comfort difficult.
5. Avoid swinging your arms excessively, lifting your knees upward, etc. These types of movements waste energy and make running a challenge.

Common Questions about Injury

Question:

I feel like I'm in a losing battle to my running injuries. Everyone I talk to seems to have a different opinion about what I should do. I'm not sure who to listen to.

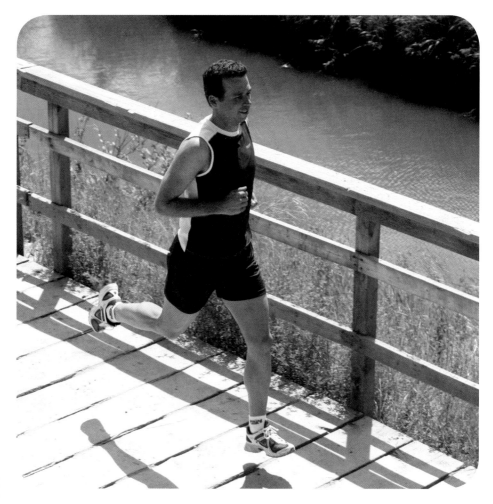

Answer:

You're not in a unique predicament. When it comes to injuries, it seems like everyone is an expert. Your best choice is to seek out a medical professional who treats runners (sports physician, physiotherapist, chiropractor, etc.) and have them assess your condition. If you find the cause of your injuries, healthy running won't be far behind.

Checklist for Running Through Injury

Run

1. If there is no pain walking or going up or down stairs.
2. If the pain or stiffness is only present at the start of the run.
3. If the pain does not worsen as you keep running day after day.
4. If stretching or icing before your run keeps the pain under control.
5. If the benefits of running exceed the negative effects and you are not creating chronic problems that will affect your activities of daily living.

Don't Run

1. If there is substantial swelling or bruising.
2. If the pain is intense and gradually worsening as you run.
3. If the pain after the run is disabling.
4. If you have an upper respiratory problem that is concentrated in your chest.
5. If you have to drastically alter your running form in order to run.

If the Pain Starts at the Start of the Run but Disappears

1. Continue to run, but spend more time stretching in your warm-up.
2. Start your run at a slower pace.
3. Warm up with walking, cycling or other low-impact aerobic activity.
4. Consider running later in the day if you have been running in the morning.

If the Pain Starts Partway into Your Run

1. You can continue as long as the pain does not continue to worsen.
2. If the pain is intense when it starts, stop and stretch or walk and try to resume running.
3. Try to stop running before the normal onset of your pain if you know it won't go away until you stop (i.e. IT band syndrome).
4. Do part of your workout running and cross-train for the rest.

1. Cut your workout distance in half until the problem is brought under the control
2. Make sure you stretch and ice after you run, even before the pain or stiffness starts.

1. Start with at least 50% of your usual training volume.
2. Increase your volume by 10% per week if all goes well.
3. Take rest days and do some cross-training.
4. Don't race until you are ready.

Runner's Stitch

Question:

I took a break from running over the winter and as I tried to get back into it this spring, I began getting a stitch in my right side, in the same place at the same time each run. I've found that if I stop and stretch during this time, it works itself out but returns again. I've tried breathing differently, holding my arm above my head when I feel it coming on, massaging the area that hurts and nothing seems to be working. Any suggestions?

Answer:

You are doing some of the things that will usually help alleviate what's commonly called "runner's stitch." The truth of the matter is, sports medicine professionals are not in agreement about the cause of this discomfort. One of the things I have found in working with runners is to have them start off very slowly and gradu-

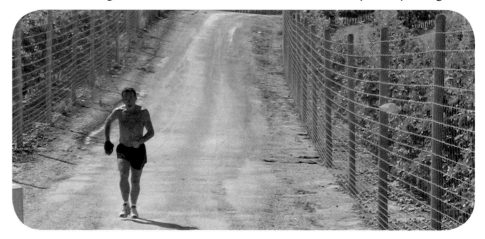

ally build up the intensity of their run. Many have found that the sudden start to a run and their labored breathing in the first 10 minutes is the source of the discomfort. Another thing to concentrate on is "belly breathing." Concentrate on breathing deeply in your diaphragm rather than high in your chest. Pursing your lips as you breathe out also helps in fully exhaling and relaxing the diaphragm. Try to really focus on staying as calm as possible and keep your breathing relaxed and controlled. All of us have a tendency to start our runs with too much intensity, rather than working at a gradual build up in intensity.

Chafing

Question:

When I do a long run, I get very sore nipples (I am male, 47 years old). On my last run, they got sore and at about 18 km they started to bleed. They are still sore two days later. Is this unusual? How do I prevent it from happening?

Answer:

Your discomfort is very common among runners as they increase their mileage. The chafing is caused by salt in your perspiration. At longer distances, we sweat longer and often you will notice this sweat and salt on your face, etc. The salt can cause chafing in the nipple area, under the arms, between the thighs and for women along the bra line.

A lubricant like Bodyglide will help. Wearing CoolMax material rather than cotton can be beneficial. Cotton retains sweat and salt, whereas CoolMax transports the sweat to the outer layer where it can evaporate.

For severe cases or for nipples that are currently chafed, use a liquid product like Second Skin, which is a liquid bandage. These products cover the injured area with a thin, breathable coating that allows the area to heal and protects from further injuries. NipGuard or bandages are best to prevent nipple chafing.

Speed Related Injuries

For many runners, listening to their bodies is the best way to avoid injuries. During periods of stress, our body sends us signals and we learn the difference between residual soreness after a good run and the tight pulling sensation indicating an injury has occurred or is about to occur. Our technique, footing and intensity combined with the surface we are running on contribute to the maintenance of muscular, cartilage and bone injuries.

Injury Prevention Tips

1. Watch for early signs of overtraining, pay close attention to fast running, down hill running, curved or uneven surfaces.

2. Days of high intensity should be followed by low-intensity days. This hard/ easy system is applied to both the days of the week and month of training. Much like we have hard/ easy days, after a period of 4 weeks of increased intensity, we need a cut back of one week to moderate intensity.

3. You will note in my recommendations for speed we have you running at about 85–95% of your maximum heart rate. Running at 100% carries with it a great risk of injury. Speed training sessions spark your running performance but be cautious not to overdue it.

4. Build warm-up and cooldown portions into all high-intensity workouts. High-intensity workouts include hills, speed sessions, tempo and fartlek runs.

5. Warming up prior to your run acclimatizes your body to the rigors of the run by increasing the blood flow to your working muscles. Your warm-up should be at about 40–50% of your maximum heart rate.

6. A cooldown of at least 10 minutes helps flush out lactic acid from your muscles, slowly lowers your heart rate to its resting state and restores your body's resting equilibrium.

7. Having flexible muscles and tendons is crucial to injury prevention and to running your best times. A stretch should never hurt; be gentle. Work on your flexibility and range of movement.

8. Be patient in your training; improvement in performance comes with time. Injury interrupts one of the key aspects of your program—frequency.

9. With any severe pain, seek medical attention.

10. Keep your training challenging and enjoyable by pushing beyond your current comfort level. You will discover an improved performance and stay injury free, if you balance the high-intensity sessions with rest.

Overuse vs. Traumatic Injuries

Definition

There are two types of injuries that an athlete may encounter: one caused by an acute trauma, the other resulting from overuse.

The Traumatic Injury

The traumatic injury is violent and sudden, such as sprains, lacerations, torn ligaments, pulled muscles or broken bones caused by a fall. These types of injury usually require immediate professional treatment. If the injury causes immediate pain, swelling, inability to use the injured body part or severe pain that does not subside in 30 to 40 minutes, the injury should be examined by a professional. If the athlete hears or feels a crack, tear or pop and the pain persists, help should be sought.

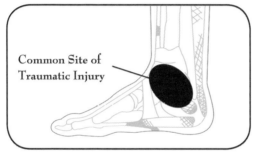

Common Site of Traumatic Injury

The Overuse Injury

Overuse injuries are more common and develop over a long period of time from mild or low-grade, repeated stress. Overtraining results in overuse injuries. Sometimes this type of injury can be associated with anatomical variation, such as flat or high arches or an abnormally sized or positioned kneecap. The knees (e.g., Iliotibial Band Syndrome, Runner's Knee) and Achilles tendon (e.g., Tendonitis) are most adversely affected by overtraining.

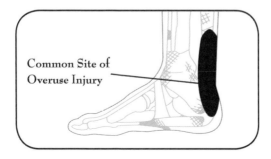

Common Site of Overuse Injury

Causes of Overuse Injuries

+ Anatomical variations, such as high arches, can create biomechanical problems that may lead to an overuse injury

+ More than half of all running injuries are due to training errors. Each run stresses the body. Daily high-intensity training does not allow the body adequate time to adjust and recover. An imbalance of hard and easy workouts can also contribute to injury.

Self-Care for Overuse Injuries

+ Reduce distance and intensity for 7 to 10 days. Never run through pain. Evaluate your training habits.

+ If the pain is severe at the beginning of and during activity, the activity should be stopped completely. If the pain is present at the beginning of activity but lessens and does not return until a few hours later, then the level of activity should be reduced. Other aerobic activities should be considered to maintain cardiovascular fitness.

+ Reduce inflammation by icing the area after activity and by taking aspirin or ibuprofen throughout the day. Encourage healing with a whirlpool, massage or ice and heat therapy.

Prevention of Overuse Injuries

+ Follow the guidelines for self-care.
+ Understand the effects of long-term exercise programs on bones, joints and muscles.
+ Undertake a conditioning program that includes stretching, strengtheningexercises and cross-training.
+ Select the proper shoes and socks.

Running Injuries Summary

Injury Prevention
1. Run every other day.
2. Don't increase mileage more than 10% per week.
3. Never sprint (run all out).
4. Ease into longer or faster running.
5. Don't run a long run and a race on the same weekend.

6. Run the long ones extra slow.
7. Never run fast at the end of a run—cool down slowly.
8. Don't overstretch or perform the wrong stretches.
9. Monitor shoe midsole wear.
10. Stay on stable surfaces.
11. Don't overstride (especially when going uphill, downhill or when tired).
12. Be sensitive to your "weak links."
13. When in doubt, don't run for two to three days.
14. If it doesn't go away, see a physician.

When is it an injury?

1. Swelling.
2. Loss of function.
3. Pain stays for a week.
4. Pain gets worse.

Treatment

1. Don't stretch the injured area.
2. Ice massage.
3. Inflammation? Use compression.
4. Talk to a doctor about anti-inflammatories if swelling persists.

Stay Active

1. Choose alternative exercise which doesn't aggravate injury.
2. The more your alternative exercise simulates running, the less fitness you will lose during recovery.
3. Talk to a physician about massage.

How to Avoid Repeated Injuries

Just as the pain in your knee starts to get better, your hip starts to ache, then your ankle, then back to your knee, and so on. Repeated injuries don't necessarily strike the same place twice, but just like any single injury, they will prevent you from achieving your goals.

A cycle of injuries usually occurs because parts of your body compensate for others, creating a biomechanical syndrome. Think of the body as a moving chain. If a joint or muscle complex is not stable, is damaged or weak, or has scar tissue that alters normal function, then stress will be placed on an adjoining structure in the moving chain. This stress may be the force of gravity, the force of impact, the forces that create stability or the forces that create smooth, coordinated movement. These additional forces may then cause the adjoining structure to be injured—and so the cycle has begun.

A cycle of injuries indicates that you haven't fully healed. If you are favoring one injury, you may develop another somewhere else. One way to stop the cycle is to substitute running with another aerobic sport that focuses the biomechanical stress away from the affected injury site. Cycling, swimming and rowing are usually good substitutions for running.

If you suffer from a cycle of injuries, you may need to find the weak link in your locomotor system—the foot, the ankle, the knee or something else. Treat the weak link with proper support and rehabilitation exercises. If you have a known imbalance, such as flat feet, weak quadriceps muscles, leg length discrepancy, etc., or a history of previous injury, work on eliminating that weakness first.
Always use appropriate shoes to stabilize and cushion. Listen to your body and follow a training program best suited for you and only you. Make your sports medicine doctor, physiotherapist and nutritionist part of your training team.

Basic Care of Injuries

The pain associated with overuse injuries is usually not severe. It is often ignored by athletes, and it is more difficult to determine whether or not an overuse injury needs professional attention. If the pain persists for more than 10 to 14 days after you follow basic self-care treatments, such as decreasing the level of activity, applying ice, taking aspirin or ibuprofen and stretching, you should seek professional help.

Definition

R Rest:
Stop any aggravating activity that could make the injury worse.

I Ice:
The quicker the ice is applied after the injury, the more effective the treatment.

C Compression:
Usually applied using a stretch elastic bandage (tensor type), wrapping towards the heart.

E Elevation:

During and after application of ice, the injured body part should be elevated above the level of the heart.

Suggested Regime for R.I.C.E.

+ Do an initial assessment of the injured structure.
+ Within 5 to 10 minutes following injury, apply ice massage or an ice pack directly to the injured area.
+ An ice pack should be wrapped firmly in place with a wide elastic wrap (be sure to check that circulation isn't impaired).
+ The injured body part should then be elevated well above the level of the heart.
+ Leave the ice pack in place for 15 to 20 minutes.
+ After removing the pack, apply an elastic wrap for compression and continue to elevate the body part.
+ Ice should be applied every hour for as many hours as possible during the first 48 hours.
+ Use compression at all times, except when sleeping.
+ Elevation should continue as often as is practical during this time.

Why Ice?

When you injure yourself, you damage tissue at the site of the injury. Blood vessels inside the tissue break and bleed.

The cold from ice achieves two positive effects. First, cold contracts, so the broken blood vessels close quickly and the bleeding stops. This is also why we do not put heat on an acute injury. Heat expands!

But blood is also a healing agent. We don't want it spilling into places where it's not supposed to be, but we do need it to flow normally through the tiny blood vessels still intact in the tissue. Cold brings blood to a cold area in order to warm it—this is why your cheeks and go red in the winter. The use of ice triggers this protective mechanism. At the same time that the broken blood vessels are being sealed off, the healthy ones are filling with blood. You will notice the redness in the area you are icing after only a few minutes. Good blood flows starts the healing processes almost immediately. But we can only trick the body for so long. This is because another line of defense is triggered in cases of extreme cold. After trying to warm an area without success, the body's blood supply abandons an area of surface cold and concentrates on the protection of the vital parts of the body. (This is what happens in the winter when people suffer frostbite.)

So we do not keep the ice on for too long. Fifteen minutes per hour is plenty. But, for the first 48 hours after an injury, the more hours you can manage with 15 minutes of icing, the better.

How to Ice

1. Your ice pack must allow insulation between the source of cold and the skin. Without this insulation, the skin can freeze and you have a case of self-inflicted frostbite. Plastic bags do not allow this insulation. Water from the melting ice does! You can apply ice directly onto your skin with no problem, as long as you keep it moving. You can wrap ice cubes in a wet towel or face cloth. But ice in a dry plastic bag on the skin will freeze your skin quite quickly. Many athletes keep Styrofoam cups of ice handy in the freezer. They are comfortable to handle and easily peeled back to expose more ice as they melt. They also provide a convenient sized ice surface. In general, an ice massage applied directly onto the skin, but with circular strokes moving over the affected area, is very effective therapy indeed. Rubbing the injury with a handful of ice works best for most injuries.

2. You will feel three stages during your icing. First, of course, your skin feels cold. Second, the injury may actually ache a little, especially if you apply gentle pressure. (The gentle pressure is better than just "patting" the area.) The third stage will occur after about 10 minutes. The ice will act as a mild anesthetic. Close your eyes and have another person very gently tap the place you have iced. You will not be able to feel the tapping.

3. Numbness is the stage you want to reach. For a couple of minutes, you can remove the ice and gently put the injured area through as much range of motion as it can do without pain. While the injury is still acute, ice is what you need. This generally lasts 48 hours and maybe longer. If a slight movement reproduces the sharp pain of the original injury, your injury is still acute. When you feel that the sharp pain has been replaced by a duller ache and a distinct restriction of normal movement, you may move to the next stage in your recovery. If you have visited a therapist, follow the advice you are given. If you are treating the injury yourself, put it through a gentle range of motion and begin as much activity as you can do without causing pain. Pain is absolutely your body's warning signal. Pain indicates that you are causing further damage and delaying your eventual return.

Achilles Tendonitis

Definition

Achilles tendonitis, one of the more common and difficult injuries to treat in athletes, involves inflammation, degeneration or rupture of the Achilles tendon. The Achilles tendon is located at the back of the heel and inserts into the rear portion of the heel bone. It is surrounded by a vascular sheath that provides the tendon fibers with their blood supply.

Symptoms

The symptoms of this injury tend to come in stages or degrees of severity.

Stage 1

The athlete will experience a burning or prickly pain in the Achilles tendon about 1–3 in. above the heel bone. This is the result of inflammation of the vascular sheath and may simply be due to shoe counter irritation.

Stage 2

The Achilles tendon actually begins to deteriorate (tendonitis) and the pain becomes a shooting or piercing sensation that occurs during activity, especially when changing direction or running uphill.

Stage 3

The collagen protein fibers in the Achilles tendon weaken to a point that the tendon will snap or rupture and there will be a great deal of swelling. The main cause of tendon damage is sudden overstretching of tendon fibers. The Achilles tendon must be properly preconditioned to withstand sudden stretches and the strain of body weight during activity. If a chronic tendonitis is ignored and the tendon ruptures, the cells that repair the tendon cannot work quickly enough to heal the damage done by the over enthusiastic athlete.

Causes of Injury

1. The positioning of the tendon in the calf makes it susceptible to running injuries.
2. Overpronation strains the soleus tendon.
3. Oversupination or high arches strains the gastroc-nemius fibers in the calf muscle. Both cause injury high up in the Achilles tendon.
4. Constant rubbing of the back of the shoe against the tendon.
5. Improper shoe selection.

6. Improper warm-up.
7. Direct trauma.
8. A sudden dramatic increase in activity or intensity of activity.
9. Heel bone deformity.
10. A high-mileage, long-term running program that does not incorporate enough rest.

Short-term Treatment

+ Decrease mileage and intensity for 7 to 10 days; never run through pain.
+ Avoid hills during recovery.
+ Ice treatment after running.
+ Flexibility program concentrating on the soleus and gastrocnemius, including stretching and heel lifts.
+ Aspirin or ibuprofen to reduce inflammation.
+ Orthotic devices or proper shoe selection.

Gastrocnemius

Soleus

Achilles Tendon

Common Site of
Achilles Tendonitis

Heel Bone

If the injury persists for more than two weeks, it is recommended that the athlete see a physician.

Long-term Treatment

+ Continuous flexibility program.
+ Orthotic devices.
+ Professional treatment by a physician may be required.

For overall prevention of injury, all athletes should be aware of shoe deterioration and purchase shoes designed to correct any stride problems, such as over-pronation or oversupination.

Iliotibial Band Syndrome

Definition

Iliotibial band syndrome is one of the leading causes of lateral knee pain in runners. The iliotibial band is a superficial thickening of tissue on the outside of the thigh, extending from the outside of the pelvis, over the hip and knee, and inserting just below the knee. The band is crucial to stabilizing the knee during running, moving from behind the femur to the front of it during the gait cycle. The continual rubbing of the band over the bone, combined with the repeated flexion and extension of the knee during running may cause the area to become inflamed or the band itself may become irritated.

Symptoms

The symptoms range from a stinging sensation just above the knee joint on the outside of the knee or along the entire length of the iliotibial band to swelling or thickening of the tissue at the point where the band moves over the femur. The pain may not occur immediately, but it will worsen during activity when the foot strikes the ground if you overstride or run downhill, and it may persist afterward. A single workout of excessive distance or a rapid increase in weekly distance can aggravate the condition.

Causes of Injury

- Iliotibial band syndrome is the result of both poor training habits and anatomical abnormalities.
- Running on a banked surface, such as the shoulder of a road or an indoor track, causes the downhill leg to bend slightly inward and causes extreme stretching of the band against the femur.
- Inadequate warm-up or cooldown.
- Running excessive distances or increasing mileage too quickly can aggravate or cause injury.
- Anatomical abnormalities, such as bowlegs or tightness about the iliotibial band.

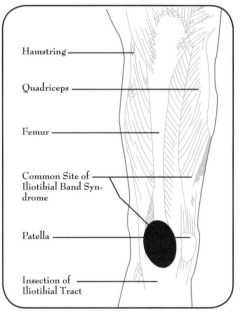

Hamstring

Quadriceps

Femur

Common Site of Iliotibial Band Syndrome

Patella

Insection of Iliotibial Tract

Short-term Treatment

To treat functional problems resulting from poor training:
- Decrease distance.
- Ice knee after activity.
- Alternate running direction on a pitched surface.
- Use a lateral sole wedge to lessen pressure on the knee.
- Stretch to tolerance.

Long-term Treatment

To treat structural abnormalities, such as a natural tightness in the band:

- Stretch, especially before working out, to make the band more flexible and less susceptible to injury.
- In extreme cases, surgery to relieve tightness in the band.
- Both structural and functional problems need to be considered when treating iliotibial band syndrome.

Plantar Fasciitis

Definition

Plantar fasciitis is a persistent pain located on the plantar aspect (bottom) of the heel and the medial aspect (inside) of the foot. The plantar fascia is a fibrous, tendon-like structure that extends the entire length of the bottom of the foot, beginning at the heel bone and extending to the base of the toes. During excessive activity, the plantar fascia can become irritated and inflamed and may even tear if the area is subjected to repetitive stress. Heel contact during the gait cycle exposes a specific area to this stress. This area is known as the medial plantar aspect of the heel, where the plantar fascia attaches to the heel bone. The pain resulting from this injury is most noticeable in the morning when the first few steps are taken and subsides with prolonged walking. Likewise, during athletic activity the pain will occur in the beginning of the exercise routine and subsides as activity continues.

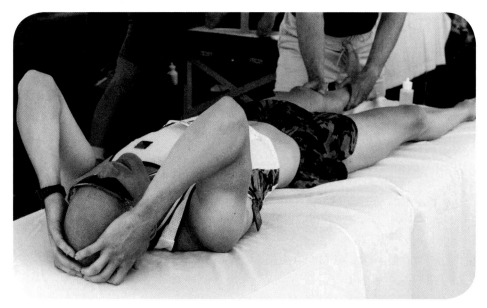

Causes of Injury

- Plantar fasciitis is more common in athletes who have a high-arch, rigid type of foot or a flat, pronated foot. In motion, the plantar fascia experiences continuous stress and excessive pulling, which results in inflammation and pain.
- A high-arch foot has a tight band-like plantar fascia that is rigid during the gait cycle.
- The plantar fascia is stretched by excessive motion in the pronated foot.
- Improper shoe selection can be a cause of the injury; foot and gait type must be considered.
- Stiff-soled shoes can cause stretching of the plantar fascia.
- Overworn shoes allow the foot to pronate more extensively and can result in an injury to the plantar fascia.
- The most common cause is a sudden increase in the amount or intensity of activity within a short period of time.

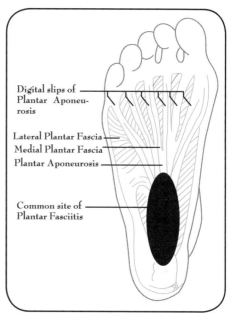

Digital slips of Plantar Aponeurosis

Lateral Plantar Fascia
Medial Plantar Fascia
Plantar Aponeurosis

Common site of Plantar Fasciitis

Short-term Treatment

In determining the proper treatment for plantar fasciitis it is important that the athlete knows and eliminates the causative factors of the injury. A complete medical history analysis, pedal examination, gait analysis and X-rays to check for a heel spur are recommended.

- Ice application and strapping.
- Complete rest or a reduction in the intensity of exercise.
- Physical therapy involving whirlpool and ultrasound.
- Anti-inflammatory medication, such as pills or cortisone injections, to alleviate severe pain in acute cases. These are considered only as a last resort in chronic cases only.

Long-term Treatment

In cases that are persistent, orthotic devices help correct biomechanical problems and alleviate stress and strain on the plantar fascia.

- High arches require softer orthotic devices for shock absorption.
- Flattened arches require a more rigid orthotic to control pronation.
- Plantar fascia and calf muscle stretching exercises to prevent recurrence.

Most patients respond to these forms of treatment; only a very small percentage of patients require surgery.

Stress Fractures

Definition

Stress fractures are tiny, incomplete breaks or cracks in a normal bone caused by repeated trauma or pounding. One of the most misdiagnosed of athletic injuries, stress fractures can happen after a short period of stress, but more commonly after a longer period of continued trauma. When the bone cells cannot rebuild as fast as the repetitive trauma damages them and the bone can take no more stress, the crack occurs. Stress fractures can occur in both the upper and lower body, but they are most common in the foot.

Symptoms

The pain related to a stress fracture begins gradually and intensifies with continued activity. Pain is not always present as an early warning or it is often ignored

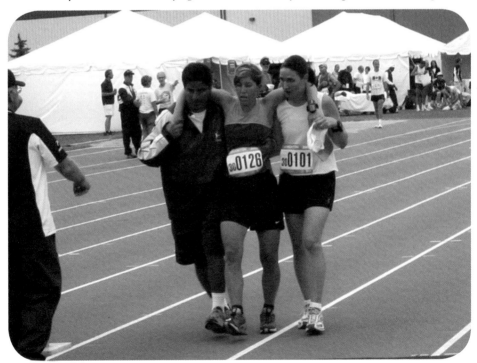

by the athlete. Swelling and tenderness may also affect the area. One of a physician's best methods in determining a stress fracture is if pain is felt when pressure is applied from above and below. X-rays of the injured site should be taken, though the fracture may not show up for the first 5 to 10 days after the injury. When stress fractures are ignored the results can be serious. Complete breaks in the bone, especially in the hip area, may necessitate surgery or prolonged disability.

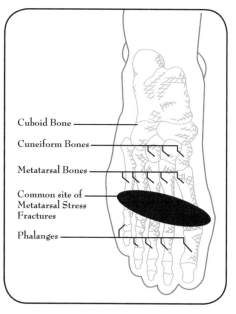

Cuboid Bone

Cuneiform Bones

Metatarsal Bones

Common site of Metatarsal Stress Fractures

Phalanges

Causes of Injury

- Switching to a harder running surface.
- Rapid increase of speed or distance.
- Returning to intense activity after a layoff.
- Inadequate rest and excessive stress.
- A change in footwear without proper adjustment period.
- Improper shoe selection to accommodate foot type.

Most athletes who incur stress fractures are in good physical condition and lack previous systemic ailments which may predispose them to the injury.

Short-term Treatment

- Discontinue the injurious activity immediately.
- Rest.
- Ice.
- Elevation.

If pain and swelling do not subside after a few days of self-prescribed care, and if athletic as well as normal activities become difficult, professional help should be sought.

Long-term Treatment

- Nonimpact aerobic activity, such as swimming, rowing, cross-country skiing, walking or bicycling, to maintain cardiovascular fitness.

- A cast may be used in tibial (lower leg) stress fractures. Metatarsal (foot) stress fractures may require casting for four to six weeks because these bones are more difficult to immobilize.
- A heel cup or special protective padding for heel fractures.
- Crutches to relieve the pressure and weight from the leg.
- Oral nonsteroidal anti-inflammatory medications to alleviate pain and swelling.

The return to athletic activity should be delayed for as long as possible—from four to eight weeks—depending on the location and severity of the injury. Though the pain may subside after the second week of treatment, returning to a normal exercise routine can delay healing and can cause permanent damage.

Shin Splints

Definition

The lower leg pain resulting from shin splints is caused by very small tears in the leg muscles at their point of attachment to the shin. There are two types:

Anterior shin splints occur in the front portion of the shin bone (tibia).

Posterior shin splints occur on the inside (medial) part of the leg along the tibia.

Anterior shin splints are due to muscle imbalances, insufficient shock absorption or toe running. Excessive pronation contributes to both anterior and posterior shin splints.

Symptoms

The pain may begin as a dull aching sensation after running. The aching may become more intense, even during walking, if ignored. Tender areas are often felt as one or more small bumps along either side of the shin bone.

Causes of Injury

- Tightness in the pos-terior muscles, which propel the body forward, places additional strain on the muscles in the front part of the lower leg, which work to lift the foot upward and also prepare the foot to strike the running surface.

- Hard surface running or worn or improper shoes increase the stress on the anterior leg muscles. Softer surfaces and shoe cushioning materials absorb more shock and less is transferred to the shins.
- The lower leg muscles suffer a tremendous amount of stress when a runner lands only on the balls of the feet (toe running), without the normal heel contact.
- The muscles of the foot and leg overwork in an attempt to stabilize the pronated foot and the repeated stress can cause the muscles to tear where they attach to the tibia.
- Rapid increase of speed or distance.

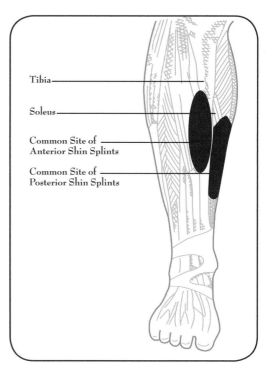

Tibia

Soleus

Common Site of Anterior Shin Splints

Common Site of Posterior Shin Splints

Short-term Treatment

- Aspirin or ibuprofen to reduce inflammation and relieve pain.
- Ice immediately after running, never before.
- Reduce distance and intensity for 7 to 10 days; never run through pain.
- Avoid hills and hard running surfaces.
- A varus wedge to support the inside of the foot and reduce the amount of pronation.
- Gentle stretching of the posterior leg and thigh muscles.

Self-enforced treatment of shin splints, as with most overuse injuries, is successful in most cases.

Long-term Treatment

Persistent problems may warrant a visit to a sports medicine specialist who may prescribe the following treatments:
- Strengthening and flexibility programs to correct muscle imbalance. These exercises should only be done in the absence of pain.
- Orthotic devices.
- Anti-inflammatory medications.

- Physical therapy involving ice, massage, ultrasound, electro-stimuli and heat to reduce inflammation and pain.

The best means of prevention of serious athletic injuries is to maintain good muscle strength and flexibility.

Runner's Knee

Definition

Chondromalacia patella, or "Runner's Knee," occurs when repeated stress on the knee causes inflammation and a gradual softening of the cartilage under the kneecap (patella). The inflammation of the cartilage prevents the kneecap from gliding smoothly over the end of the thigh bone (femur) therefore causing pain and swelling of the knee. The underside of the kneecap should be smooth and move within the femoral groove (a groove on the thigh bone). If the kneecap is pulled sideways, it becomes rough like sandpaper and the symptoms appear.

Symptoms

Runner's knee is typically associated with a pain that increases gradually over a period of time, often a year or longer, until it is severe enough that the athlete seeks medical attention. Symptoms usually occur beneath or on both sides of the kneecap. Pain may be intensified with activities such as a short run, squatting or jumping. Stiffness may occur simply from prolonged sitting or descending stairs.

Causes of Injury

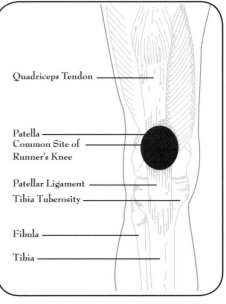

- Overpronation causes the lower leg to rotate inward because of the unstable pronated foot. The kneecap moves in an abnormal side-to-side motion instead of gliding within the normal track of the femoral groove on the thigh bone.
- Weak quadriceps may contribute to injury because the thigh muscles normally aid in proper tracking of the kneecap.
- Muscle imbalance.
- Direct or repeated trauma.

Quadriceps Tendon

Patella
Common Site of
Runner's Knee

Patellar Ligament
Tibia Tuberosity

Fibula

Tibia

- An untreated ligament injury.
- Some athletes may experience pain in one knee if they continually run along the same side of the road. The tilt in the road accentuates the pronation of the foot, thus resulting in the abnormal tracking of the knee.
- History of trauma.

Short-term Treatment

- Decrease activity and consider swimming. When recovering, avoid any exercise that puts weight on a bent knee.
- Rest if the knee is painful and swollen.
- Ice treatment for 15 minutes twice daily after activity to reduce pain and inflammation.
- Aspirin or ibuprofen. Or consult your physician about more sophisticated and effective anti-inflammatory medication.

Long-term Treatment

- Physiotherapy, including stretching and strengthening exercises for the quadriceps, hamstrings and calves.
- Orthotic devices to correct abnormal foot mechanics.
- Once the causes are determined and the appropriate steps have been taken to treat the condition, runner's knee should not keep the athlete from activity.

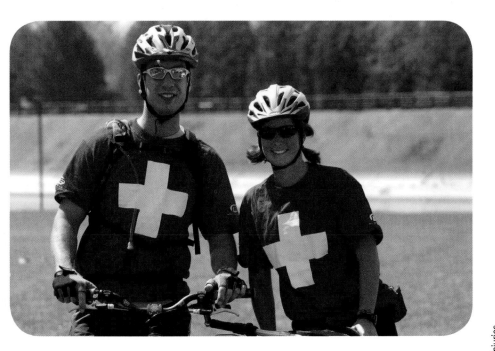

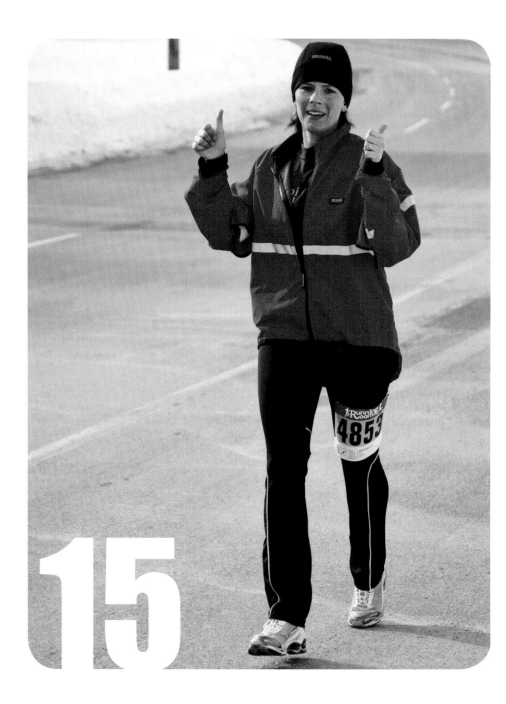

15

The popularity of the 5 K and 10 K road races over the years comes from the fact that it requires only a limited amount of training, which can fit into most busy schedules, and you recover quickly after the race. For most of us it is a fun event—you usually end up with a new T-shirt, great conversations with fellow runners, some food and a sense of accomplishment. The 5 K or 10 K race can be a simple benchmark to judge your current fitness, or it can be a real test of athletic and competitive abilities. The distance is short enough that most runners can enter the event with only simple modifications in their normal training.

You will find that running the occasional 5 K or 10 K will add some spark to your running. It can also serve as a motivational force to get you out the door on a regular basis.

For those days when you really do not feel like running, the thought of running with a buddy in a weekend race will keep you out on those training runs during the week. Most runners can comfortably run a 5 K or 10 K every couple of weeks. Combining races with an intelligent training program that is in line with your current fitness level allows you to improve your running times. Sometimes, staying a couple of footsteps in front of a training buddy can be the motivating force to push you that extra little bit. If a time goal is not high on your priorities, then running more comfortably and enjoying the race may be your goal. Keeping it fun and intelligent usually leads to satisfying results.

The training schedules on the following pages will help you prepare for a 5 K or 10 K race. Choose the schedule that best reflects your targeted finish time.

If you are running your very first 5 K or 10 K, finishing in a smiling upright position should be foremost in your mind—smiling, and upright makes for the best photos. For all runners, the best advice for the 5 K or 10 K is to keep it fun! The more relaxed and focused you are at the start of the race, the more likely you are to achieve your goal for the race.

Going into your first 5 K or 10 K, it is a great confidence builder if you have already run the distance. If you have not been able to achieve the distance in training, be sure to add in walking breaks of 1 minute for every 10 minutes of running if on the 10 K program and shorter run intervals for the 5 K program.

5 K Tune-up

The following schedules should include a run at least three times per week. All running should be done at a conversation pace, and all walking should be done briskly. Of course a proper warm-up and cooldown are required.

Your goal is to prepare yourself for a 5 K run that will be interspersed with some walking breaks.

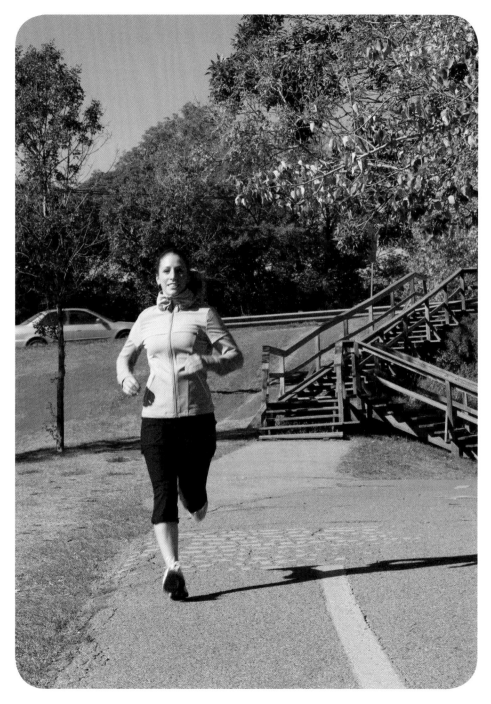

5 K Conditioning Program

Week	Sun	Mon	Tue	Wed	Thu	Fri	Sat	Total Time
1	0:25 mins	Off	Off	0:25 mins	Off	0:25 mins	Off	Walk/Run 1:15
	Workout: walk 1 min, run 5 min, x4 sets, plus walk 1 min = 25 mins							
2	0:25 mins	Off	Off	0:25 mins	Off	0:25 mins	Off	Walk/Run 1:15
	Workout: walk 1 min, run 7 min, x3 sets, plus walk 1 min = 25 mins							
3	0:23 mins	Off	Off	0:23 mins	Off	0:23 mins	Off	Walk/Run 1:09
	Workout: walk 1 min, run 10 min, x2 sets, plus walk 1 min = 23 mins							
4	0:23 mins	Off	Off	0:23 mins	Off	0:23 mins	Off	Walk/Run 1:09
	Workout: walk 1 min, run 10 min, x2 sets, plus walk 1 min = 23 mins							
5	0:26 mins	Off	Off	0:26 mins	Off	0:26 mins	Off	Walk/Run 1:18
	Workout: walk 1 min, run 10 min, x2 sets, walk 1 min, run 2 min, plus walk 1 min = 26 mins							
6	0:28 mins	Off	Off	0:28 mins	Off	0:28 mins	Off	Walk/Run 1:24
	Workout: walk 1 min, run 10 min, x2 sets, walk 1 min, run 4 min, plus walk 1 min = 28 mins							
7	0:29 mins	Off	Off	0:29 mins	Off	0:29 mins	Off	Walk/Run 1:27
	Workout: walk 1 min, run 10 min, x2 sets, walk 1 min, run 5 min, plus walk 1 min = 29 mins							
8	0:30 mins	Off	Off	0:30 mins	Off	0:30 mins	Off	Walk/Run 1:30
	Workout: walk 1 min, run 10 min, x2 sets, walk 1 min, run 6 min, plus walk 1 min = 30 mins							
9	0:32 mins	Off	Off	0:32 mins	Off	0:32 mins	Off	Walk/Run 1:36
	Workout: walk 1 min, run 10 min, x2 sets, walk 1 min, run 8 min, plus walk 1 min = 32 mins							
10	0:23 mins	Off	0:34 mins	0:34 mins	Off	0:34 mins	Off	Walk/Run 2:05
	Workout: walk 1 min, run 10 min, x2 sets, plus walk 1 min = 23 mins							
	Workout: walk 1 min, run 10 min, x3 sets, plus walk 1 min = 34 mins							
11	Race Day 5K Walk 1/Run 10							Walk/Run 0:30-0:40

Pace Schedule	Don't worry about pace or distance as the goal is to increase the interval of time running/walking. Week 1 will incorporate 1 min walk/5 min run. Week 2 will increase to 1 min walk/7 min run. All other weeks will progress to the formula of 1 min walk/10 min run.

15 · 5 Km & 10 Km Events

5 K Advanced Program

Week	Sun	Mon	Tue	Wed	Thu	Fri	Sat	Total Time
1	0:23 mins	Off	Off	0:23 mins	Off	0:23 mins	Off	Walk/Run 1:09

Workout: walk 1 min, run 10 min, x2 sets, plus walk 1 min = 23 mins

Week	Sun	Mon	Tue	Wed	Thu	Fri	Sat	Total Time
2	0:23 mins	Off	Off	0:23 mins	Off	0:23 mins	Off	Walk/Run 1:09

Workout: walk 1 min, run 10 min, x2 sets, plus walk 1 min = 23 mins

| 3 | 0:29 mins | Off | Off | 0:29 mins | Off | 0:29 mins | Off | Walk/Run 1:27 |

Workout: walk 1 min, run 10 min, x2 sets, walk 1 min, run 5 min, plus walk 1 min = 29 mins

| 4 | 0:36 mins | Off | Off | 0:36 mins | Off | 0:36 mins | Off | Walk/Run 1:48 |

Workout: walk 1 min, run 10 min, x3 sets, walk 1 min, run 1 min, plus walk 1 min = 36 mins

| 5 | 0:32 mins | Off | Off | 0:32 mins | Off | 0:32 mins | Off | Walk/Run 1:36 |

Workout: walk 1 min, run 10 min, x2 sets, walk 1 min, run 8 min, plus walk 1 min = 32 mins

| 6 | 0:34 mins | Off | 0:34 mins | 0:23 mins | Off | 0:34 mins | Off | Walk/Run 2:05 |

Workout: walk 1 min, run 10 min, x2 sets, plus walk 1 min = 23 mins
Workout: walk 1 min, run 10 min, x3 sets, plus walk 1 min = 34 mins

| 7 | 0:34 mins | Off | 0:34 mins | 0:23 mins | Off | 0:34 mins | Off | Walk/Run 2:05 |

Workout: walk 1 min, run 10 min, x3 sets, plus walk 1 min = 34 mins

| 8 | 0:34 mins | Off | 0:34 mins | 0:23 mins | Off | 0:34 mins | Off | Walk/Run 2:05 |

Workout: walk 1 min, run 10 min, x2 sets, plus walk 1 min = 23 mins
Workout: walk 1 min, run 10 min, x3 sets, plus walk 1 min = 34 mins

| 9 | 0:34 mins | Off | 0:34 mins | 0:29 mins | Off | 0:34 mins | Off | Walk/Run 2:11 |

Workout: walk 1 min, run 10 min, x3 sets, plus walk 1 min = 34 mins
Workout: walk 1 min, run 10 min, x2 sets, walk 1 min, run 5 min, plus walk 1 min = 29 mins

| 10 | 0:23 mins | Off | 0:34 mins | 0:26 mins | Off | 0:34 mins | 0:26 mins | Walk/Run 2:23 |

Workout: walk 1 min, run 10 min, x2 sets, plus walk 1 min = 23 mins
Workout: walk 1 min, run 10 min, x3 sets, plus walk 1 min = 34 mins
Workout: walk 1 min, run 10 min, x2 sets, walk 1 min, run 2 min, plus walk 1 min = 26 mins

| 11 | Race Day 5K Walk 1/Run 10 | | | | | | | Walk/Run 0:25-0:35 |

Pace Schedule Pace and distance are not a concern. This program goal is to increase the duration of running to walking and to slowly add in additional training days. All training uses the 1 min walk/10 min run principle.

10 K Tune-up

Many runners find that when the local 10 K race season arrives, they are left wondering how they can improve their race times when they just never seem to have time to go to the track for speed work. Here is a very simple workout that you can use once a week for eight weeks to sharpen your times for that 10 K season.

Odd Weeks

+ Warm up with 10 to 15 minutes of easy running.
+ Do some light strides to pick up the speed.
+ Run for four minutes at a pace that is slightly faster than your current 10 K race pace.
+ Recover with five minutes of easy running.
+ Start with four intervals: add one interval a week; hold at a maximum of eight intervals.

Even Weeks

+ Warm up with 10 to 15 minutes of easy running.
+ Do some light strides to pick up the speed.
+ Run for eight minutes at your current 5 K race pace.
+ Recover with five minutes of easy running.
+ Start with four intervals: add one interval a week; hold at a maximum of eight intervals.

If you have selected your parents well enough that you are able to run a 10 K in under 38 minutes (for which there is no schedule), follow the 80% rule: once you can run 80% of the race distance at your targeted race pace, you are ready to race the distance and achieve that target pace on race day. Start with once-a-week running sessions at race pace, progressively increasing the distance of these runs until you are running 80% of the race distance at your targeted race pace.

10 K Training Program Details

On the following pages you will find a variety of suggested training schedules. These schedules have been designed to help runners to complete the event and or to achieve specific time goals. The programs all follow the progressive structure as outlined in *Chapter 2, Building Your Program*. Long runs incorporate the 10/1 run/walk principle that has made the Running Room programs so successful. In addition you will see at the bottom of every training schedule a pace chart outlining the pace requirements for each run. Below you will find a description of the various types of workouts as reflected in the training schedules. You can refer to *Chapter 2, Building Your Program* for a more details description of *'Training Methods'*. In addition *Chapter 9, Types of Training* provides a nice review of the various workout requirements of a successful running program.

10 K Training Program Workouts

Workouts Long Slow Distance (LSD–Run/Walk)

Long Slow Distance runs are the cornerstone of any distance training program. Take a full minute to walk for every 10 minutes of running. These runs are meant to be done much slower than race pace (60– 70% of maximum heart rate), so don't be overly concerned with your pace. These runs work to increase the capillary network in your body and raise your anaerobic threshold. They also mentally prepare you for long races.

A note on LSD Pace

The pace for the long run on the chart includes the walk time. This program provides an upper end (slow) and bottom end (fast) pace to use as a guideline. The upper end pace is preferable because it will keep you injury free. Running at the bottom end pace is a common mistake made by many runners. They try to run at the maximum pace, which is an open invitation to injury. I know of very few runners who have been injured from running too slowly, but loads of runners who incurred injuries by running too fast. In the early stages of the program it is very easy to run the long runs too fast, but like the marathon or half marathon the long runs require discipline and patience. Practice your sense of pace by slowing the long runs down. You will recover faster and remain injury free.

Steady Run

The steady run is a run below targeted race pace (70% maximum heart rate). Run at comfortable speed; if in doubt, go slowly. The run is broken down into components of running and walking. We encourage you to use the run/walk approach. Walk breaks are a great way to keep you consistent in your training.

Hills

Distance for the day is calculated as the approximate distance covered up and down the hill. Now, you will no doubt have to run to the hill and back from the hill unless of course you drive to the hill. You will need to add your total warm-up and warm-down distance to the totals noted on the training schedule. I recommend a distance of 3 km both ways to ensure adequate warm-up and recovery because hills put a lot of stress on the body. Hills are run at tempo pace (80%

maximum heart rate) and must include a heart rate recovery to 120 bpm at the bottom of each hill repeat.

VO2 Max

VO2 max is the volume of oxygen your body can obtain while training at your maximum hear rate. High VO2 levels indicate high fitness levels, allowing these fit athletes to train more intensely than beginners. Interval training of tempo, fartlek and speed sessions improves the efficiency of your body to transfer oxygen-rich blood to your working muscles.

Tempo

Before starting tempo runs, include several weeks of hill running to improve your strength, form and confidence. For the tempo runs, run at 80% of your maximum heart rate for 60–80% of your planned race distance to improve your coordination and leg turnover rate. Include a warm-up and cooldown of about three to five minutes. These runs simulate race conditions and the effort required on race day.

Fartlek (Speed Play)

Fartlek runs are spontaneous runs over varying distances and intensity. Run the short bursts at 70–80% of your maximum heart rate, if you are wearing a monitor. From a perceived effort, conversation is possible but you notice increased breathing, heart rate and perspiration. Between these short bursts of hard effort, but no longer than three minutes, add in recovery periods of easy running to bring your heart rate down to 120 beats per minute. Speed play fires up your performance with a burst of speed. The added recovery/rest interval keeps the session attainable and fun.

Speed

Going back to our training analogy of "Building the House," speed training is nailing down the roof and one of the last things we do. You must have a sufficient base training and strength training period before tackling speed. Speed is simply fast runs over short distances, e.g., 5 x 400 m., usually with a relatively long period of recovery to allow the unpleasant side effects of the anaerobic activity to diminish. In our training programs we factor in a 3 km warm-up and 3 km warm-down into the total distance to run. I have seen many runners come up injured when attempting speed work and inevitably as a result of running too fast. In the training programs I have purposefully lowered the pace of your speed works (95% maximum heart rate) as opposed to a much higher rate (110%

maximum heart rate), which is commonly used but results in many injuries. In these programs we use speed to fine tune not to damage, and it has proven very successful in all our programs.

Walk Adjusted Race Pace

How do we arrive at a "Walk Adjusted" race pace? When you are walking, you are moving slower than your "average run pace." When you are running, you are moving faster than your "average walk pace." The walk adjusted race pace factors in the variation in walking and running speed. The challenge is knowing the average speed of your walking pace. We have devised a formula to calculate moderate walk pace, which allows us to determine the exact splits including running and walking pace. The effect of this calculation is that the "Walk Adjusted" run pace is faster per kilometer than the average race pace. However when calculated with your walk pace you will end up with your target race pace. You can go on-line at runningroom.com and print out your "Walk Adjusted" pace bands for race day.

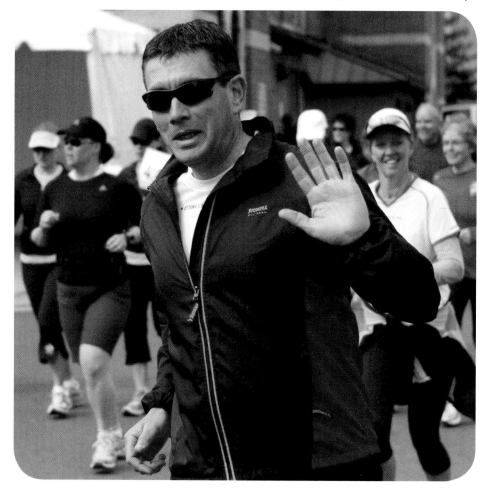

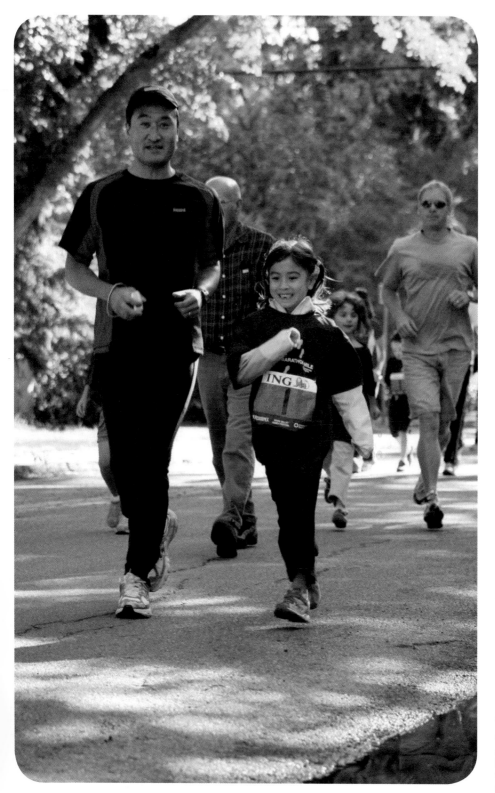

10 K Gradual Build
(Recorded in Kilometers)

Week	Sun	Mon	Tue	Wed	Thu	Fri	Sat	Total
1	Off	Off	3 Run/Walk	4 Run/Walk	Off	3 Run/Walk	Off	Run/Walk 10
2	5 LSD Run/Walk	Off	3 Run/Walk	4 Run/Walk	Off	3 Run/Walk	Off	Run/Walk 15
3	6 LSD Run/Walk	Off	4 Run/Walk	4 Run/Walk	Off	4 Run/Walk	Off	Run/Walk 18
4	7 LSD Run/Walk	Off	4 Run/Walk	4 Run/Walk	Off	4 Run/Walk	Off	Run/Walk 19
5	8 LSD Run/Walk	Off	3 Run/Walk	3 Hills (400 m hills) 2.5 km	Off	4 Run/Walk	Off	Run/Walk 17.5
6	8 LSD Run/Walk	Off	3 Run/Walk	4 Hills (400 m hills) 3 km	Off	4 Run/Walk	Off	Run/Walk 18
7	8 LSD Run/Walk	Off	3 Run/Walk	5 Hills (400 m hills) 4 km	Off	5 Run/Walk	Off	Run/Walk 20
8	9 LSD Run/Walk	Off	3 Run/Walk	6 Hills (400 m hills) 5 km	Off	5 Run/Walk	Off	Run/Walk 22
9	10 LSD Run/Walk	Off	4 Run/Walk	5 Run/Walk	Off	4 Run/Walk	Off	Run/Walk 23
10	6 LSD Run/Walk	Off	3 Run/Walk	5 Run/Walk	Off	3 Run/Walk	Off	Run/Walk 17
11	10 km Race							Run/Walk 10
Pace Schedule	Don't worry about pace here. The goal is simply to build your training base.							
	Run/Walk Interval = 10 min Running/1 min Walking							

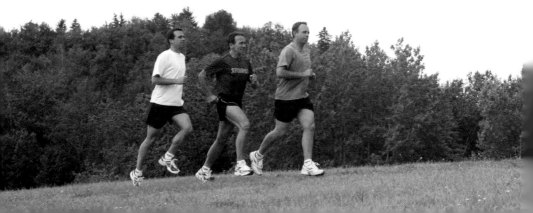

10 K To Complete
(Recorded in Kilometers)

Week	Sun	Mon	Tue	Wed	Thu	Fri	Sat	Total
1	Off	Off	6 Steady Run	Off	5 Steady Run	Off	3 Steady Run	Run/Walk 14
2	6 LSD Run/Walk	Off	6 Steady Run	Off	6 Steady Run	Off	3 Steady Run	Run/Walk 21
3	6 LSD Run/Walk	Off	6 Steady Run	Off	6 Steady Run	Off	3 Steady Run	Run/Walk 21
4	8 LSD Run/Walk	Off	6 Steady Run	3 Steady Run	6 Steady Run	Off	3 Steady Run	Run/Walk 26
5	8 LSD Run/Walk	Off	6 Steady Run	3 Hills (400 m hills) 2.5 km	6 Steady Run	5 Steady Run	Off	Run/Walk 27.5
6	10 LSD Run/Walk	Off	6 Steady Run	4 Hills (400 m hills) 3 km	5 Steady Run	6 Steady Run	Off	Run/Walk 30
7	10 LSD Run/Walk	Off	8 Steady Run	5 Hills (400 m hills) 4 km	5 Steady Run	Off	6 Steady Run	Run/Walk 33
8	11 LSD Run/Walk	Off	6 Steady Run	6 Hills (400 m hills) 5 km	8 Steady Run	5 Steady Run	Off	Run/Walk 35
9	11 LSD Run/Walk	Off	8 Steady Run	8 Tempo	5 Steady Run	Off	6 Steady Run	Run/Walk 38
10	13 LSD Run/Walk	Off	8 Steady Run	5 Tempo	Off	3 Race Pace	Off	Run/Walk 29
11	10 Km Race							Run/Walk 10
Pace Schedule	Pacing is not used here. The goal is to "complete," so adapting to the increased distance is the focus.							
	Run/Walk Interval and Steady Runs = 10 min Running/1 min Walking							

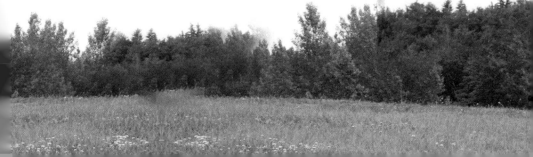

Week	Sun	Mon	Tue	Wed	Thu	Fri	Sat	Total
1	Off	Off	6 Steady Run	4 Hills 3 km	6 Steady Run	5 Steady Run	Off	20
2	6 LSD Run/Walk	Off	6 Steady Run	5 Hills 4 km	6 Steady Run	5 Steady Run	Off	27
3	10 LSD Run/Walk	Off	6 Steady Run	6 Hills 5 km	6 Steady Run	6 Steady Run	Off	33
4	10 LSD Run/Walk	Off	6 Steady Run	7 Hills 5.5 km	6 Steady Run	6 Steady Run	Off	33.5
5	13 LSD Run/Walk	Off	8 Steady Run	8 Hills 6 km	8 Steady Run	8 Steady Run	Off	43
6	16 LSD Run/Walk	Off	8 Steady Run	9 Hills 7 km	8 Steady Run	8 Steady Run	Off	47
7	13 LSD Run/Walk	Off	8 Steady Run	10 Hills 8 km	6 Steady Run	6 Steady Run	Off	41
8	16 LSD Run/Walk	Off	8 Steady Run	Speed 4 X 400 m 8 km	8 Steady Run	8 Steady Run	Off	48
9	16 LSD Run/Walk	Off	8 Steady Run	Speed 5 X 400 m 8 km	8 Steady Run	8 Steady Run	Off	48
10	13 LSD Run/Walk	Off	8 Steady Run	Speed 6 X 400 m 8.5 km	8 Steady Run	8 Steady Run	Off	45.5
11	16 LSD Run/Walk	Off	8 Steady Run	Speed 7 X 400 m 9 km	13 Steady Run	8 Steady Run	Off	54
12	16 LSD Run/Walk	Off	6 Race Pace	6 Race Pace	3 Steady Run	Off	3 Steady Run	34
13	10 Km Race							10

Pace Schedule	Long Run (LSD)	Steady Run	Tempo/ Hill (400 m)	Speed	Race	Walk Adjusted Race Pace
To Complete 0:55	6:40–7:30	6:40	6:00	5:15	5:30	5:14

Run/Walk Interval and Steady Runs = 10 min Running/1 min Walking

10 K To Complete in 50 Minutes
(Recorded in Kilometers)

Week	Sun	Mon	Tue	Wed	Thu	Fri	Sat	Total
1	Off	Off	6 Steady Run	4 Hills 3 km	6 Steady Run	5 Tempo	Off	20
2	6 LSD Run/Walk	Off	6 Steady Run	5 Hills 4 km	6 Steady Run	5 Tempo	Off	27
3	10 LSD Run/Walk	Off	6 Steady Run	6 Hills 5 km	6 Steady Run	6 Tempo	Off	33
4	10 LSD Run/Walk	Off	6 Steady Run	7 Hills 5.5 km	6 Steady Run	6 Tempo	Off	33.5
5	13 LSD Run/Walk	Off	8 Steady Run	8 Hills 6 km	8 Steady Run	8 Tempo	Off	43
6	16 LSD Run/Walk	Off	8 Steady Run	9 Hills 7 km	8 Steady Run	8 Tempo	Off	47
7	13 LSD Run/Walk	Off	8 Steady Run	10 Hills 7 km	6 Steady Run	6 Tempo	Off	40
8	16 LSD Run/Walk	Off	8 Steady Run	Speed 4 X 400 m 8 km	8 Steady Run	8 Tempo	Off	48
9	16 LSD Run/Walk	Off	8 Steady Run	Speed 5 X 400 m 8 km	8 Steady Run	8 Tempo	Off	48
10	13 LSD Run/Walk	Off	8 Steady Run	Speed 6 X 400 m 8.5 km	8 Steady Run	8 Tempo	Off	45.5
11	16 LSD Run/Walk	Off	8 Steady Run	Speed 7 X 400 m 9 km	13 Steady Run	8 Tempo	Off	54
12	16 Run/Walk	Off	6 RacePace	6 Race Pace	3 Steady run	Off	3 Steady run	34
13	10 Km Race							10

Pace Schedule	Long Run (LSD)	Steady Run	Tempo/ Hill (400 m)	Speed	Race	Walk Adjusted Race Pace
To Complete 0:50	6:07–6:53	6:07	5:30	4:47	5:00	4:46

Run/Walk Interval and Steady Runs = 10 min Running/1 min Walking

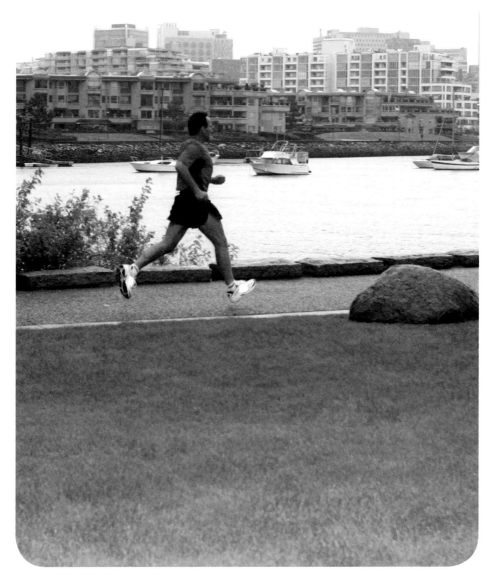

10 K To Complete in 48 Minutes
(Recorded in Kilometers)

Week	Sun	Mon	Tue	Wed	Thu	Fri	Sat	Total
1	Off	Off	6 Steady Run	4 Hills 3 km	6 Steady Run	5 Tempo	5 Steady Run	25
2	6 LSD Run/Walk	Off	6 Steady Run	5 Hills 4 km	6 Steady Run	5 Tempo	5 Steady Run	32
3	10 LSD Run/Walk	Off	6 Steady Run	6 Hills 5 km	6 Steady Run	6 Tempo	5 Steady Run	38
4	10 LSD Run/Walk	Off	6 Steady Run	7 Hills 5.5 km	6 Steady Run	6 Tempo	5 Steady Run	38.5
5	13 LSD Run/Walk	Off	8 Steady Run	8 Hills 6 km	8 Steady Run	8 Tempo	Off	43
6	16 LSD Run/Walk	Off	8 Steady Run	9 Hills 7 km	8 Steady Run	8 Tempo	5 Steady Run	52
7	13 LSD Run/Walk	Off	6 Steady Run	10 Hills 8 km	8 Steady Run	6 Tempo	Off	41
8	16 LSD Run/Walk	Off	8 Steady Run	Speed 4 X 400 m 8 km	8 Steady Run	8 Tempo	5 Steady Run	53
9	19 LSD Run/Walk	Off	8 Steady Run	Speed 5 X 400 m 8 km	8 Steady Run	8 Tempo	5 Steady Run	56
10	22 LSD Run/Walk	Off	8 Steady Run	Speed 6 X 400 m 8.5 km	8 Steady Run	8 Tempo	5 Steady Run	59.5
11	26 LSD Run/Walk	Off	8 Steady Run	Speed 7 X 400 m 9 km	8 Steady Run	8 Tempo	6 Steady Run	65
12	13 LSD Run/Walk	Off	6 Race Pace	6 Race Pace	3 Steady Run	Off	3 Steady Run	31
13	10 Km Race							10

Pace Schedule	Long Run (LSD)	Steady Run	Tempo/ Hill (400 m)	Speed	Race	Walk Adjusted Race Pace
To Complete 0:48	5:53–6:38	5:53	5:18	4:37	4:48	4:34

Run/Walk Interval and Steady Runs = 10 min Running/1 min Walking

15 5 Km & 10 Km Events

10 K To Complete in 44 Minutes
(Recorded in Kilometers)

Week	Sun	Mon	Tue	Wed	Thu	Fri	Sat	Total
1	Off	Off	6 Steady Run	4 Hills 3 km	5 Steady Run	6 Tempo	5 Steady Run	25
2	10 LSD Run/Walk	Off	6 Steady Run	5 Hills 4 km	5 Steady Run	6 Tempo	5 Steady Run	36
3	10 LSD Run/Walk	Off	6 Steady Run	6 Hills 5 km	6 Steady Run	5 Tempo	6 Steady Run	38
4	13 LSD Run/Walk	Off	6 Steady Run	7 Hills 5.5 km	5 Steady Run	6 Tempo	6 Steady Run	41.5
5	16 LSD Run/Walk	Off	8 Steady Run	8 Hills 6 km	8 Steady Run	8 Tempo	Off	46
6	16 LSD Run/Walk	Off	8 Steady Run	9 Hills 7 km	8 Steady Run	8 Tempo	5 Steady Run	52
7	19 LSD Run/Walk	Off	8 Steady Run	10 Hills 8 km	6 Steady Run	6 Tempo	Off	47
8	16 LSD Run/Walk	Off	8 Steady Run	Speed 4 x 400 m 8 km	8 Steady Run	8 Tempo	5 Steady Run	53
9	19 LSD Run/Walk	Off	8 Steady Run	Speed 5 x 400 m 8 km	8 Steady Run	8 Tempo	5 Steady Run	56
10	22 LSD Run/Walk	Off	8 Steady Run	Speed 6 x 400 m 8.5 km	6 Steady Run	8 Tempo	5 Steady Run	57.5
11	26 LSD Run/Walk	Off	8 Steady Run	Speed 7 x 400 m 9 km	8 Steady Run	8 Tempo	6 Steady Run	65
12	13 LSD Run/Walk	Off	6 Steady Run	6 Race Pace	3 Steady Run	Off	3 Steady Run	31
13	10 Km Race							10

Pace Schedule	Long Run (LSD)	Steady Run	Tempo/ Hill (400 m)	Speed	Race	Walk Adjusted Race Pace
To Complete 0:44	5:26–6:08	5:26	4:53	4:15	4:24	4:09

Run/Walk Interval and Steady Runs = 10 min Running/1 min Walking

10 K To Complete in 40 Minutes

(Recorded in Kilometers)

Week	Sun	Mon	Tue	Wed	Thu	Fri	Sat	Total
1	Off	Off	6 Steady Run	5 Hills 4 km	8 Steady Run	8 Tempo	8 Steady Run	34
2	10 LSD Run/Walk	Off	6 Steady Run	6 Hills 5 km	8 Steady Run	8 Tempo	8 Steady Run	45
3	13 LSD Run/Walk	Off	6 Steady Run	7 Hills 5.5 km	13 Steady Run	13 Tempo	6 Steady Run	56.5
4	16 LSD Run/Walk	Off	6 Steady Run	8 Hills 6 km	8 Steady Run	8 Tempo	8 Steady Run	52
5	19 LSD Run/Walk	Off	8 Steady Run	9 Hills 7 km	13 Steady Run	13 Tempo	8 Steady Run	68
6	22 LSD Run/Walk	Off	10 Steady Run	10 Hills 8 km	16 Steady Run	13 Tempo	8 Steady Run	77
7	26 LSD Run/Walk	Off	8 Steady Run	Speed 4 X 400 m 8 km	16 Steady Run	13 Tempo	8 Steady Run	79
8	19 LSD Run/Walk	Off	8 Steady Run	Speed 5 X 400 m 8 km	16 Steady Run	13 Tempo	8 Steady Run	72
9	26 LSD Run/Walk	Off	8 Steady Run	Speed 6 X 400 m 8.5 km	16 Steady Run	10 Tempo	Off	68.5
10	26 LSD Run/Walk	Off	8 Steady Run	Speed 7 X 400 m 9 km	16 Steady Run	8 Tempo	8 Steady Run	75
11	26 LSD Run/Walk	Off	8 Steady Run	Speed 8 X 400 m 9 km	8 Steady Run	8 Tempo	Off	59
12	16 LSD Run/Walk	Off	6 Race Pace	6 Race Pace	6 Steady Run	Off	3 Steady Run	37
13	10 Km Race							10

Pace Schedule	Long Run (LSD)	Steady Run	Tempo/ Hill (400 m)	Speed	Race	Walk Adjusted Race Pace
To Complete 0:40	4:58–5:37	4:58	4:27	3:53	4:00	3:48

Run/Walk Interval and Steady Runs = 10 min Running/1 min Walking

10 K To Complete in 38 Minutes
(Recorded in Kilometers)

Week	Sun	Mon	Tue	Wed	Thu	Fri	Sat	Total
1	Off	Off	6 Steady Run	5 Hills 4 km	8 Steady Run	8 Tempo	8 Steady Run	34
2	10 LSD Run/Walk	Off	6 Steady Run	6 Hills 5 km	8 Steady Run	8 Tempo	8 Steady Run	45
3	13 LSD Run/Walk	Off	6 Steady Run	7 Hills 5.5 km	13 Steady Run	13 Tempo	6 Steady Run	56.5
4	16 LSD Run/Walk	Off	6 Steady Run	8 Hills 6 km	13 Steady Run	13 Tempo	8 Steady Run	62
5	19 LSD Run/Walk	Off	8 Steady Run	9 Hills 7 km	13 Steady Run	13 Tempo	8 Steady Run	68
6	22 LSD Run/Walk	Off	10 Steady Run	10 Hills 8 km	16 Steady Run	16 Tempo	6 Steady Run	78
7	24 LSD Run/Walk	Off	10 Steady Run	Speed 4 x 400 m 8 km	16 Steady Run	16 Tempo	8 Steady Run	82
8	19 LSD Run/Walk	Off	10 Steady Run	Speed 5 x 400 m 8 km	16 Steady Run	16 Tempo	8 Steady Run	77
9	29 LSD Run/Walk	Off	13 Steady Run	Speed 6 x 400 m 8.5 km	13 Steady Run	16 Tempo	8 Steady Run	87.5
10	29 LSD Run/Walk	Off	13 Steady Run	Speed 7 x 400 m 9 km	13 Run/Walk	16 Tempo	8 Steady Run	88
11	29 LSD Run/Walk	Off	8 Steady Run	Speed 8 x 400 m 9 km	13 Steady Run	13 Tempo	Off	72
12	16 LSD Run/Walk	Off	6 Race Pace	6 Race Pace	6 Steady Run	Off	3 Steady Run	37
13	10 Km Race							10

Pace Schedule	Long Run (LSD)	Steady Run	Tempo/ Hill (400 m)	Speed	Race	Walk Adjusted Race Pace
To Complete 0:38	4:44–5:21	4:44	4:15	3:42	3:48	3:36

Run/Walk Interval and Steady Runs = 10 min Running/1 min Walking

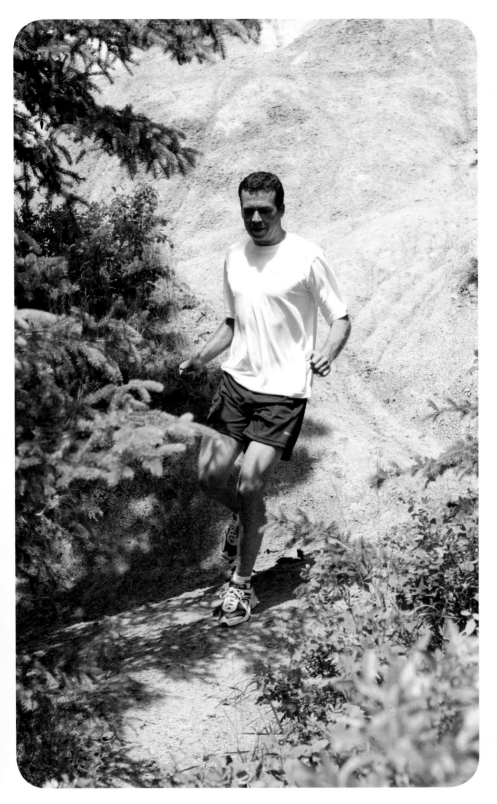

10 K Gradual Build
(Recorded in Miles)

Week	Sun	Mon	Tue	Wed	Thu	Fri	Sat	Total
1	Off	Off	2 Run/Walk	2.5 Run/Walk	Off	2 Run/Walk	Off	Run/Walk 6.5
2	3 LSD Run/Walk	Off	2 Run/Walk	2.5 Run/Walk	Off	2 Run/Walk	Off	Run/Walk 9.5
3	4 LSD Run/Walk	Off	2.5 Run/Walk	2.5 Run/Walk	Off	2.5 Run/Walk	Off	Run/Walk 11.5
4	4.5 LSD Run/Walk	Off	2.5 Run/Walk	2.5 Run/Walk	Off	2.5 Run/Walk	Off	Run/Walk 12
5	5 LSD Run/Walk	Off	2 Run/Walk	3 Hills (400 m hills) 1.5 mi	Off	2.5 Run/Walk	Off	Run/Walk 11
6	3.5 LSD Run/Walk	Off	2 Run/Walk	4 Hills (400 m hills) 2 mi	Off	2.5 Run/Walk	Off	Run/Walk 10
7	5 LSD Run/Walk	Off	2 Run/Walk	5 Hills (400 m hills) 2.5 mi	Off	3 Run/Walk	Off	Run/Walk 12.5
8	5.5 LSD Run/Walk	Off	2 Run/Walk	6 Hills (400 m hills) 3 mi	Off	3 Run/Walk	Off	Run/Walk 13.5
9	6 LSD Run/Walk	Off	2.5 Run/Walk	3 Run/Walk	Off	2.5 Run/Walk	Off	Run/Walk 14
10	4 LSD Run/Walk	Off	2 Run/Walk	3 Run/Walk	Off	2 Run/Walk	Off	Run/Walk 11
11	10 K Race							Run/Walk 6

Pace Schedule	Don't worry about pace here. The goal is simply to build your training base.

Run/Walk Interval = 10 min Running/1 min Walking

10 K To Complete
(Recorded in Miles)

Week	Sun	Mon	Tue	Wed	Thu	Fri	Sat	Total
1	Off	Off	4 Steady Run	Off	3 Steady Run	Off	2 Steady Run	Run/Walk 9
2	4 LSD Run/Walk	Off	4 Steady Run	Off	4 Steady Run	Off	2 Steady Run	Run/Walk 14
3	4 LSD Run/Walk	Off	4 Steady Run	Off	4 Steady Run	Off	2 Steady Run	Run/Walk 14
4	5 LSD Run/Walk	Off	4 Steady Run	2 Steady Run	4 Steady Run	Off	2 Steady Run	Run/Walk 17
5	5 LSD Run/Walk	Off	4 Steady Run	3 Hills (400 m hills) 1.5 mi	4 Steady Run	3 Steady Run	Off	Run/Walk 17.5
6	6 LSD Run/Walk	Off	4 Steady Run	4 Hills (400 m hills) 2 mi	3 Steady Run	4 Steady Run	Off	Run/Walk 19
7	6 LSD Run/Walk	Off	5 Steady Run	5 Hills (400 m hills) 2.5 mi	3 Steady Run	Off	4 Steady Run	Run/Walk 20.5
8	7 LSD Run/Walk	Off	4 Steady Run	6 Hills (400 m hills) 3 mi	5 Steady Run	3 Steady Run	Off	Run/Walk 22
9	7 LSD Run/Walk	Off	5 Steady Run	5 Tempo	3 Steady Run	Off	4 Steady Run	Run/Walk 24
10	8 LSD Run/Walk	Off	5 Steady Run	3 Tempo	Off	2 Race Pace	Off	Run/Walk 18
11	10 K Race							Run/Walk 6
Pace Schedule	Pacing is not used here. The goal is to "complete" so adapting to the increased distance is the focus.							
	Run/Walk Interval and Steady Run = 10 min Running/1 min Walking							

10 K To Complete in 55 Minutes
(Recorded in Miles)

Week	Sun	Mon	Tue	Wed	Thu	Fri	Sat	Total
1	Off	Off	4 Steady Run	4 Hills 2 mi	4 Steady Run	3 Steady Run	Off	13
2	4 Steady Run	Off	4 Steady Run	5 Hills 2.5 mi	4 Steady Run	3 Steady Run	Off	17.5
3	6 Steady Run	Off	4 Steady Run	6 Hills 3 mi	4 Steady Run	4 Steady Run	Off	21
4	6 LSD Run/Walk	Off	4 Steady Run	7 Hills 3.5 mi	4 Steady Run	4 Steady Run	Off	21.5
5	8 LSD Run/Walk	Off	5 Steady Run	8 Hills 4 mi	5 Steady Run	5 Steady Run	Off	27
6	10 LSD Run/Walk	Off	5 Steady Run	9 Hills 4.5 mi	5 Steady Run	5 Steady Run	Off	29.5
7	8 LSD Run/Walk	Off	5 Steady Run	10 Hills 5 mi	4 Steady Run	4 Steady Run	Off	26
8	10 LSD Run/Walk	Off	5 Steady Run	Speed 4 x 400 m 5 mi	5 Steady Run	5 Steady Run	Off	30
9	10 LSD Run/Walk	Off	5 Steady Run	Speed 5 x 400 m 5 mi	5 Steady Run	5 Steady Run	Off	30
10	8 LSD Run/Walk	Off	5 Steady Run	Speed 6 x 400 m 5 mi	8 Steady Run	5 Steady Run	Off	31
11	10 LSD Run/Walk	Off	5 Steady Run	Speed 7 x 400 m 5.5 mi	5 Steady Run	5 Steady Run	Off	30.5
12	10 LSD Run/Walk	Off	4 Race Pace	4 Race Pace	2 Steady Run	Off	2 Steady Run	22
13	10 K Race							6

Pace Schedule	Long Run (LSD)	Steady Run	Tempo/ Hill (400 m)	Speed	Race	Walk Adjusted Race Pace
To Complete 0:55	10:44–12:04	10:44	9:40	8:26	8:51	8:26
	Run/Walk Interval and Steady Run = 10 min Running/1 min Walking					

10 K To Complete in 50 Minutes
(Recorded in Miles)

Week	Sun	Mon	Tue	Wed	Thu	Fri	Sat	Total
1	Off	Off	4 Steady Run	4 Hills 2 mi	4 Steady Run	3 Tempo	Off	13
2	4 LSD Run/Walk	Off	4 Steady Run	5 Hills 2.5 mi	4 Steady Run	3 Tempo	Off	17.5
3	6 LSD Run/Walk	Off	4 Steady Run	6 Hills 3 mi	4 Steady Run	4 Tempo	Off	21
4	6 LSD Run/Walk	Off	4 Steady Run	7 Hills 3.5 mi	4 Steady Run	4 Tempo	Off	21.5
5	8 LSD Run/Walk	Off	5 Steady Run	8 Hills 4 mi	5 Steady Run	5 Tempo	Off	27
6	10 LSD Run/Walk	Off	5 Steady Run	9 Hills 4.5 mi	5 Steady Run	5 Tempo	Off	29.5
7	8 LSD Run/Walk	Off	5 Steady Run	10 Hills 4.5 mi	4 Steady Run	4 Tempo	Off	25.5
8	10 LSD Run/Walk	Off	5 Steady Run	Speed 4 X 400 m 5 mi	5 Steady Run	5 Tempo	Off	30
9	10 LSD Run/Walk	Off	5 Steady Run	Speed 5 X 400 m 5 mi	5 Steady Run	5 Tempo	Off	30
10	8 LSD Run/Walk	Off	5 Steady Run	Speed 6 X 400 m 5 mi	8 Steady Run	5 Tempo	Off	31
11	10 LSD Run/Walk	Off	5 Steady Run	Speed 7 X 400 m 5.5 mi	5 Steady Run	5 Tempo	Off	30.5
12	10 Run/Walk	Off	4 RacePace	4 RacePace	2 Steady Run	Off	2 Steady run	22
13	10 K Race							6

Pace Schedule	Long Run (LSD)	Steady Run	Tempo/ Hill (400 m)	Speed	Race	Walk Adjusted Race Pace
To Complete 0:50	9:50–11:05	9:50	8:51	7:43	8:03	7:41

Run/Walk Interval and Steady Run = 10 min Running/1 min Walking

10 K To Complete in 48 Minutes
(Recorded in Miles)

Week	Sun	Mon	Tue	Wed	Thu	Fri	Sat	Total
1	Off	Off	4 Steady Run	4 Hills 2 mi	4 Steady Run	3 Tempo	3 Steady Run	16
2	4 LSD Run/Walk	Off	4 Steady Run	5 Hills 2.5 mi	4 Steady Run	3 Tempo	3 Steady Run	20.5
3	6 LSD Run/Walk	Off	4 Steady Run	6 Hills 3 mi	4 Steady Run	4 Tempo	3 Steady Run	24
4	6 LSD Run/Walk	Off	4 Steady Run	7 Hills 3.5 mi	4 Steady Run	4 Tempo	3 Steady Run	24.5
5	8 LSD Run/Walk	Off	5 Steady Run	8 Hills 4 mi	5 Steady Run	5 Tempo	Off	27
6	10 LSD Run/Walk	Off	5 Steady Run	9 Hills 4.5 mi	5 Steady Run	5 Tempo	3 Steady Run	32.5
7	8 LSD Run/Walk	Off	4 Steady Run	10 Hills 5 mi	5 Steady Run	4 Tempo	Off	26
8	10 LSD Run/Walk	Off	5 Steady Run	Speed 4 X 400 m 5 mi	5 Steady Run	5 Tempo	3 Steady Run	33
9	12 LSD Run/Walk	Off	5 Steady Run	Speed 5 X 400 m 5 mi	5 Steady Run	5 Tempo	3 Steady Run	35
10	14 LSD Run/Walk	Off	5 Steady Run	Speed 6 X 400 m 5 mi	5 Steady Run	5 Tempo	3 Steady Run	37
11	16 LSD Run/Walk	Off	5 Steady Run	Speed 7 X 400 m 5.5 mi	5 Steady Run	5 Tempo	4 Steady Run	40.5
12	8 LSD Run/Walk	Off	4 Race Pace	4 Race Pace	2 Steady Run	Off	2 Steady Run	20
13	10 K Race							6

Pace Schedule	Long Run (LSD)	Steady Run	Tempo/ Hill (400 m)	Speed	Race	Walk Adjusted Race Pace
To Complete 0:48	9:28–10:41	9:28	8:31	7:25	7:43	7:21
	Run/Walk Interval and Steady Run = 10 min Running/1 min Walking					

10 K To Complete in 44 Minutes
(Recorded in Miles)

Week	Sun	Mon	Tue	Wed	Thu	Fri	Sat	Total
1	Off	Off	4 Steady Run	4 Hills 2 mi	3 Steady Run	4 Tempo	3 Steady Run	16
2	6 LSD Run/Walk	Off	4 Steady Run	5 Hills 2.5 mi	3 Steady Run	4 Tempo	3 Steady Run	22.5
3	6 LSD Run/Walk	Off	4 Steady Run	6 Hills 3 mi	4 Steady Run	3 Tempo	4 Steady Run	24
4	8 LSD Run/Walk	Off	4 Steady Run	7 Hills 3.5 mi	3 Steady Run	4 Tempo	4 Steady Run	26.5
5	10 LSD Run/Walk	Off	5 Steady Run	8 Hills 4 mi	5 Steady Run	5 Tempo	Off	29
6	10 LSD Run/Walk	Off	5 Steady Run	9 Hills 4.5 mi	5 Steady Run	5 Tempo	3 Steady Run	32.5
7	12 LSD Run/Walk	Off	5 Steady Run	10 Hills 5 mi	4 Steady Run	4 Tempo	Off	30
8	10 LSD Run/Walk	Off	5 Steady Run	Speed 4 x 400 m 5 mi	5 Steady Run	5 Tempo	3 Steady Run	33
9	12 LSD Run/Walk	Off	5 Steady Run	Speed 5 x 400 m 5 mi	5 Steady Run	5 Tempo	3 Steady Run	35
10	14 LSD Run/Walk	Off	5 Steady Run	Speed 6 x 400 m 5 mi	4 Steady Run	5 Tempo	3 Steady Run	36
11	16 LSD Run/Walk	Off	5 Steady Run	Speed 7 x 400 m 5.5 mi	5 Steady Run	5 Tempo	4 Steady Run	40.5
12	8 LSD Run/Walk	Off	4 Race Pace	4 Race Pace	2 Steady Run	Off	2 Steady Run	20
13	10 K Race							6

Pace Schedule	Long Run (LSD)	Steady Run	Tempo/ Hill (400 m)	Speed	Race	Walk Adjusted Race Pace
To Complete 0:44	8:44–9:52	8:44	7:51	6:50	7:05	6:41

Run/Walk Interval and Steady Run = 10 min Running/1 min Walking

10 K To Complete in 40 Minutes
(Recorded in Miles)

Week	Sun	Mon	Tue	Wed	Thu	Fri	Sat	Total
1	Off	Off	4 Steady Run	5 Hills 2.5 mi	5 Steady Run	5 Tempo	5 Steady Run	21.5
2	6 LSD Run/Walk	Off	4 Steady Run	6 Hills 3 mi	5 Steady Run	5 Tempo	5 Steady Run	28
3	8 LSD Run/Walk	Off	4 Steady Run	7 Hills 3.5 mi	8 Steady Run	8 Tempo	4 Steady Run	35.5
4	10 LSD Run/Walk	Off	4 Steady Run	8 Hills 4 mi	5 Steady Run	5 Tempo	5 Steady Run	33
5	12 LSD Run/Walk	Off	5 Steady Run	9 Hills 4.5 mi	8 Steady Run	8 Tempo	5 Steady Run	42.5
6	14 LSD Run/Walk	Off	6 Steady Run	10 Hills 5 mi	10 Steady Run	8 Tempo	5 Steady Run	48
7	16 LSD Run/Walk	Off	5 Steady Run	Speed 4 x 400 m 5 mi	10 Steady Run	8 Tempo	5 Steady Run	49
8	12 LSD Run/Walk	Off	5 Steady Run	Speed 5 x 400 m 4.5 mi	10 Steady Run	8 Tempo	5 Steady Run	45
9	16 LSD Run/Walk	Off	5 Steady Run	Speed 6 x 400 m 5 mi	10 Steady Run	6 Tempo	Off	42
10	16 LSD Run/Walk	Off	5 Steady Run	Speed 7 x 400 m 5.5 mi	10 Steady Run	5 Tempo	5 Steady Run	46.5
11	16 LSD Run/Walk	Off	5 Steady Run	Speed 8 x 400 m 6 mi	5 Steady Run	5 Tempo	Off	37
12	10 LSD Run/Walk	Off	4 Race Pace	4 Race Pace	4 Steady Run	Off	2 Steady Run	24
13	10 K Race							6

Pace Schedule	Long Run (LSD)	Steady Run	Tempo/ Hill (400 m)	Speed	Race	Walk Adjusted Race Pace
To Complete 0:40	7:59–9:02	7:59	7:10	6:14	6:26	6:07

Run/Walk Interval and Steady Run = 10 min Running/1 min Walking

10 K To Complete in 38 Minutes
(Recorded in Miles)

Week	Sun	Mon	Tue	Wed	Thu	Fri	Sat	Total
1	Off	Off	4 Steady Run	5 Hills 2.5 mi	5 Steady Run	5 Tempo	5 Steady Run	21.5
2	6 LSD Run/Walk	Off	4 Steady Run	6 Hills 3 mi	5 Steady Run	5 Tempo	5 Steady Run	28
3	8 LSD Run/Walk	Off	4 Steady Run	7 Hills 3.5 mi	8 Steady Run	8 Tempo	4 Steady Run	35.5
4	10 LSD Run/Walk	Off	4 Steady Run	8 Hills 4 mi	8 Steady Run	8 Tempo	5 Steady Run	39
5	12 LSD Run/Walk	Off	5 Steady Run	9 Hills 4.5 mi	8 Steady Run	8 Tempo	5 Steady Run	42.5
6	14 LSD Run/Walk	Off	6 Steady Run	10 Hills 5 mi	10 Steady Run	10 Tempo	4 Steady Run	49
7	15 LSD Run/Walk	Off	6 Steady Run	Speed 4 x 400 m 5 mi	10 Steady Run	10 Tempo	5 Steady Run	51
8	12 LSD Run/Walk	Off	6 Steady Run	Speed 5 x 400 m 5 mi	10 Steady Run	10 Tempo	5 Steady Run	48
9	18 LSD Run/Walk	Off	8 Steady Run	Speed 6 x 400 m 5 mi	8 Steady Run	10 Tempo	5 Steady Run	54
10	18 LSD Run/Walk	Off	8 Steady Run	Speed 7 x 400 m 5.5 mi	8 Run/Walk	10 Tempo	5 Steady Run	54.5
11	18 LSD Run/Walk	Off	5 Steady Run	Speed 8 x 400 m 6 mi	8 Steady Run	8 Tempo	Off	45
12	10 LSD Run/Walk	Off	4 Race Pace	4 Race Pace	4 Race Pace	Off	2 Steady Run	24
13	10 K Race							6

Pace Schedule	Long Run (LSD)	Steady Run	Tempo/ Hill (400 m)	Speed	Race	Walk Adjusted Race Pace
To Complete 0:38	7:37–8:37	7:37	6:50	5:57	6:07	5:48

Run/Walk Interval and Steady Run = 10 min Running/1 min Walking

5 Km & 10 Km Events

15

"The Full" Half Marathon

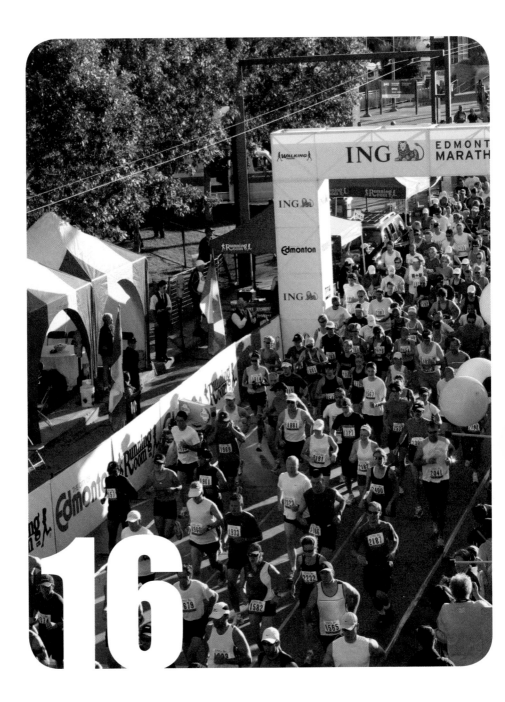

16

"I'm only running the half marathon," is a familiar quote I hear the day before many marathons across the country. Let's set the record straight: the half marathon is not half a race, and it is not called "only the half-marathon"; it is a challenging distance that gives most folks an equal sense of accomplishment as the full marathon. I like to call this event the full half marathon.

Occasionally, I would like to tell runners not to run half marathons that are attached to full marathons for the very reason that the runners often think they have only run half a race. There are, however, many positive reasons to run them: in most cases, the half marathon and the marathon start and finish at the same spot, and for running half the distance you get the same goodies at the finish, the same cheering finish-line crowd, the same T-shirt and the same good company to share your celebration.

Some folks really enjoy the half marathon distance, it challenges them but requires far less training and recovery than the marathon. Training for a half marathon requires going beyond normal fitness running—it requires some additional time and commitment—but the celebration of the finish line is well worth the effort. The introduction into longer runs gets us back to the basics of long slow runs and the delights that come from doing them. We discover that running can be social, is great for burning fat and awakens us both mentally and physically.

Half Marathon Training Program Details

The training schedules on the following pages will help you prepare for a half marathon. Choose the schedule that best reflects your targeted finish time. There are two schedules for each time goal: the first one presents the training distances in kilometers; the second in miles. The half marathon is a serious distance, you must take your training seriously—so stick to the program. More is not necessarily better.

These schedules have been designed to help runners to complete the event and or to achieve specific time goals. The programs all follow the progressive structure as outlined in Chapter 2, Building Your Program. Long runs incorporate the 10/1 run/walk principle that has made the Running Room programs so successful. In addition you will see at the bottom of every training schedule a pace chart outlining the pace requirements for each run. Below you will find a description of the various types of workouts as reflected in the training schedules. You can refer to *Chapter 2, Building Your Program* for a more detailed description of "*Training Methods.*" In addition *Chapter 9, Types of Training* provides a nice review of the various workout requirements of a successful running program.

Workouts Long Slow Distance (LSD—Run/Walk)

Long Slow Distance runs are the cornerstone of any distance training program. Take a full minute to walk for every 10 minutes of running. These runs are meant to be done much slower than race pace (60– 70% of maximum heart rate), so don't be overly concerned with your pace. These runs work to increase the capillary network in your body and raise your anaerobic threshold. They also mentally prepare you for long races.

A note on LSD Pace

The pace for the long run on the chart includes the walk time. This program provides an upper end (slow) and bottom end (fast) pace to use as a guideline. The upper end pace is preferable because it will keep you injury free. Running at the bottom end pace is a common mistake made by many runners. They try to run at the maximum pace, which is an open invitation to injury. I know of very few runners who have been injured from running too slowly, but loads of runners who incurred injuries by running too fast. In the early stages of the program it is very easy to run the long runs too fast, but like the marathon or half marathon the long runs require discipline and patience. Practice your sense of pace by slowing the long runs down. You will recover faster and remain injury free.

Steady Run

The steady run is a run below targeted race pace (70% maximum heart rate). Run at comfortable speed; if in doubt, go slowly. The run is broken down into components of running and walking. We encourage you to use the run/walk approach. Walk breaks are a great way to keep you consistent in your training.

Hills

Distance for the day is calculated as the approximate distance covered up and down the hill. Now, you will no doubt have to run to the hill and back from the hill unless of course you drive to the hill. You will need to add your total warm-up and warm-down distance to the totals noted on the training schedule. I recommend a distance of 3 km both ways to ensure adequate warm-up and recovery because hills put a lot of stress on the body. Hills are run at tempo pace (80% maximum heart rate) and must include a heart rate recovery to 120 bpm at the bottom of each hill repeat.

VO2 Max

VO2 max is the volume of oxygen your body can obtain while training at your maximum hear rate. High VO2 levels indicate high fitness levels, allowing these fit athletes to train more intensely than beginners. Interval training of tempo, fartlek and speed sessions improves the efficiency of your body to transfer oxygen-rich blood to your working muscles.

Tempo

Before starting tempo runs, include several weeks of hill running to improve your strength, form and confidence. For the tempo runs, run at 80% of your maximum heart rate for 60–80% of your planned race distance to improve your coordination and leg turnover rate. Include a warm-up and cooldown of about three to five minutes. These runs simulate race conditions and the effort required on race day.

Fartlek (Speed Play)

Fartlek runs are spontaneous runs over varying distances and intensity. Run the short bursts at 70–80% of your maximum heart rate, if you are wearing a monitor. From a perceived effort, conversation is possible but you notice increased breathing, heart rate and perspiration. Between these short bursts of hard effort, but no longer than three minutes, add in recovery periods of easy running to bring your heart rate down to 120 beats per minute. Speed play fires up your performance with a burst of speed. The added recovery/rest interval keeps the session attainable and fun.

Speed

Going back to our training analogy of "Building the House," speed training is nailing down the roof and one of the last things we do. You must have a sufficient base training and strength training period before tackling speed. Speed is simply fast runs over short distances, e.g., 5 x 400 m, usually with a relatively long period of recovery to allow the unpleasant side effects of the anaerobic activity to diminish. In our training programs we factor in a 3 km warm-up and 3 km warm-down into the total distance to run. I have seen many runners come up injured when attempting speed work and inevitably as a result of running too fast. In the training programs I have purposefully lowered the pace of your speed works (95% maximum heart rate) as opposed to a much higher rate (110% maximum heart rate), which is commonly used but results in many injuries. In these programs we use speed to fine tune not to damage, and it has proven very successful in all our programs.

Walk Adjusted Race Pace

How do we arrive at a "Walk Adjusted" race pace? When you are walking, you are moving slower than your "average run pace." When you are running, you are moving faster than your "average walk pace." The walk adjusted race pace factors in the variation in walking and running speed. The challenge is knowing the average speed of your walking pace. We have devised a formula to calculate moderate walk pace, which allows us to determine the exact splits including running and walking pace. The effect of this calculation is that the "Walk Adjusted" run pace is faster per kilometer than the average race pace. However when calculated with your walk pace you will end up with your target race pace. You can go on-line at Runningroom.com and print out your "Walk Adjusted" pace bands for race day!

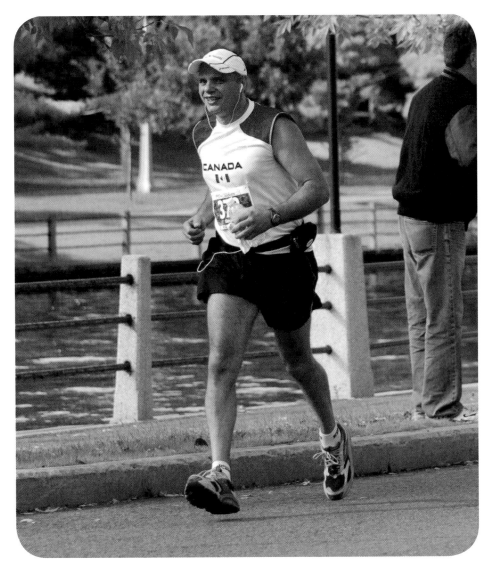

Half Marathon To Complete
(Recorded in Kilometers)

Week	Sun	Mon	Tue	Wed	Thu	Fri	Sat	Total
1	Off	Off	Off	3 Steady Run	3 Steady Run	Off	3 Steady Run	9
2	7 LSD Run/Walk	Off	4 Steady Run	3 Steady Run	3 Steady Run	Off	3 Steady Run	20
3	7 LSD Run/Walk	Off	4 Steady Run	3 Steady Run	4 Steady Run	Off	3 Steady Run	21
4	7 LSD Run/Walk	Off	3 Steady Run	4 Steady Run	3 Steady Run	Off	4 Steady Run	21
5	9 LSD Run/Walk	Off	4 Steady Run	3 Steady Run	3 Steady Run	Off	3 Steady Run	22
6	9 LSD Run/Walk	Off	5 Steady Run	3 Steady Run	4 Steady Run	Off	3 Steady Run	24
7	10 LSD Run/Walk	Off	4 Steady Run	3 Hills 2.5 km	5 Steady Run	Off	3 Steady Run	24.5
8	10 LSD Run/Walk	Off	4 Steady Run	4 Hills 3 km	5 Steady Run	Off	4 Steady Run	26
9	12 LSD Run/Walk	Off	4 Steady Run	5 Hills 4 km	6 Steady Run	Off	4 Steady Run	30
10	14 LSD Run/Walk	Off	4 Steady Run	6 Hills 5 km	6 Steady Run	Off	5 Steady Run	34
11	16 LSD Run/Walk	Off	5 Steady Run	7 Hills 5.5 km	7 Steady Run	Off	5 Steady Run	38.5
12	16 LSD Run/Walk	Off	5 Steady Run	8 Hills 6 km	7 Steady Run	Off	6 Steady Run	40
13	12 LSD Run/Walk	Off	5 Steady Run	9 Hills 7 km	8 Steady Run	Off	6 Steady Run	38
14	18 LSD Run/Walk	Off	6 Steady Run	6 Fartlek	8 Steady Run	Off	6 Steady Run	44
15	18 LSD Run/Walk	Off	6 Steady Run	4 Fartlek	8 Steady Run	Off	6 Steady Run	42
16	20 LSD Run/Walk	Off	6 Steady Run	4 Fartlek	8 Steady Run	Off	6 Steady Run	44
17	6 LSD Run/Wak	Off	10 Steady Run	6 Steady Run	Off	Off	3 Steady Run	25
18	Race - Half Marathon							21.1

Pace Schedule	Long Run (LSD)	Steady Run	Tempo/Fartlek/Hills	Speed	Race	Walk Adjusted Race Pace
To Complete	9:29–10:33	9:29	8:37	7:36	8:32	8:21

Run/Walk Interval = 10 min Running/1 min Walking
Hills are a distance of 400 m

16 Half Marathon

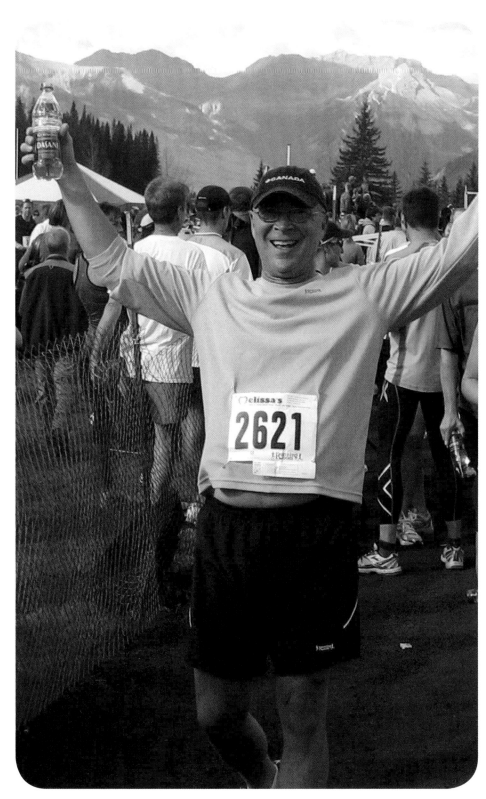

Half Marathon To Complete in 2:30
(Recorded in Kilometers)

Week	Sun	Mon	Tue	Wed	Thu	Fri	Sat	Total
1	Off	Off	Off	3 Tempo	3 Steady Run	Off	3 Steady Run	9
2	7 LSD Run/Walk	Off	4 Tempo	3 Tempo	3 Steady Run	Off	3 Steady Run	20
3	7 LSD Run/Walk	Off	4 Tempo	3 Tempo	4 Steady Run	Off	3 Steady Run	21
4	7 LSD Run/Walk	Off	3 Tempo	4 Tempo	3 Steady Run	Off	4 Steady Run	21
5	9 LSD Run/Walk	Off	4 Tempo	4 Tempo	3 Steady Run	Off	3 Steady Run	23
6	9 LSD Run/Walk	Off	5 Tempo	3 Tempo	4 Steady Run	Off	3 Steady Run	24
7	10 LSD Run/Walk	Off	4 Tempo	3 Hills 2.5 km	5 Steady Run	Off	3 Steady Run	24.5
8	10 LSD Run/Walk	Off	4 Tempo	4 Hills 3 km	5 Steady Run	Off	4 Steady Run	26
9	12 LSD Run/Walk	Off	4 Tempo	5 Hills 4 km	6 Steady Run	Off	4 Steady Run	30
10	14 LSD Run/Walk	Off	4 Tempo	6 Hills 5 km	6 Steady Run	Off	5 Steady Run	34
11	16 LSD Run/Walk	Off	5 Tempo	7 Hills 5.5 km	7 Steady Run	Off	5 Steady Run	38.5
12	16 LSD Run/Walk	Off	5 Tempo	8 Hills 6 km	7 Steady Run	Off	6 Steady Run	40
13	12 LSD Run/Walk	Off	5 Tempo	9 Hills 7 km	8 Steady Run	Off	6 Steady Run	38
14	18 LSD Run/Walk	Off	6 Tempo	6 Fartlek	8 Steady Run	Off	6 Steady Run	44
15	18 LSD Run/Walk	Off	6 Tempo	4 Fartlek	8 Steady Run	Off	6 Steady Run	42
16	20 LSD Run/Walk	Off	6 Tempo	6 Fartlek	8 Steady Run	Off	6 Race Pace	46
17	6 LSD Run/Walk	Off	10 Race Pace	6 Race Pace	Off	Off	3 Steady Run	25
18	Race - Half Marathon							21.1

Pace Schedule	Long Run (LSD)	Steady Run	Tempo/Fartlek/Hills	Speed	Race	Walk Adjusted Race Pace
To Complete 2:30	8:03–9:00	8:03	7:17	6:23	7:07	6:53

Run/Walk Interval = 10 min Running/1 min Walking
Hills are a distance of 400 m

Half Marathon To Complete in 2:15
(Recorded in Kilometers)

Week	Sun	Mon	Tue	Wed	Thu	Fri	Sat	Total
1	Off	Off	Off	3 Tempo	3 Steady Run	Off	3 Steady Run	9
2	7 LSD Run/Walk	Off	4 Tempo	3 Tempo	3 Steady Run	Off	3 Steady Run	20
3	7 LSD Run/Walk	Off	4 Tempo	3 Tempo	4 Steady Run	Off	3 Steady Run	21
4	7 LSD Run/Walk	Off	3 Tempo	4 Tempo	3 Steady Run	Off	4 Steady Run	21
5	9 LSD Run/Walk	Off	4 Tempo	4 Tempo	3 Steady Run	Off	3 Steady Run	23
6	9 LSD Run/Walk	Off	5 Tempo	3 Tempo	4 Steady Run	Off	3 Steady Run	24
7	10 LSD Run/Walk	Off	4 Tempo	3 Hills 2.5 km	5 Steady Run	Off	3 Steady Run	24.5
8	10 LSD Run/Walk	Off	4 Tempo	4 Hills 3 km	5 Steady Run	Off	4 Steady Run	26
9	12 LSD Run/Walk	Off	4 Tempo	5 Hills 4 km	6 Steady Run	Off	4 Steady Run	30
10	14 LSD Run/Walk	Off	4 Tempo	6 Hills 5 km	6 Steady Run	Off	5 Steady Run	34
11	16 LSD Run/Walk	Off	5 Tempo	7 Hills 5.5 km	7 Steady Run	Off	5 Steady Run	38.5
12	16 LSD Run/Walk	Off	5 Tempo	8 Hills 6 km	7 Steady Run	Off	6 Steady Run	40
13	12 LSD Run/Walk	Off	5 Tempo	9 Hills 7 km	8 Steady Run	Off	6 Steady Run	38
14	18 LSD Run/Walk	Off	6 Tempo	Speed 2 x 1.6 km 9 km	8 Steady Run	Off	6 Steady Run	47
15	18 LSD Run/Walk	Off	6 Tempo	Speed 3 x 1.6 km 11 km	8 Steady Run	Off	6 Steady Run	49
16	20 LSD Run/Walk	Off	6 Tempo	Speed 4 x 1.6 km 12 km	8 Steady Run	Off	6 Race Pace	52
17	6 LSD Run/Walk	Off	10 Race Pace	6 Race Pace	Off	Off	3 Steady Run	25
18	Race - Half Marathon							21.1

Pace Schedule	Long Run (LSD)	Steady Run	Tempo/Far-tlek/Hills	Speed	Race	Walk Adjusted Race Pace
To Complete 2:15	7:19–8:12	7:19	6:36	5:46	6:24	6:09

Run/Walk Interval = 10 min Running/1 min Walking
Hills are a distance of 400 m

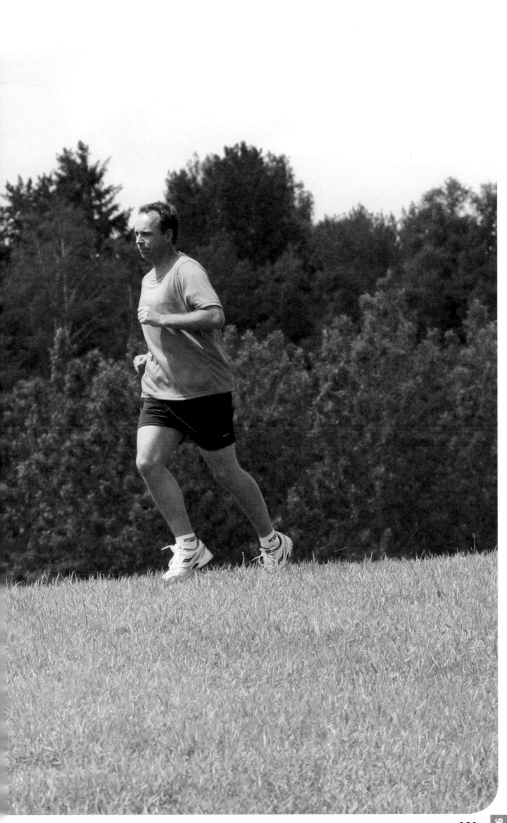

Half Marathon To Complete in 2:00
(Recorded in Kilometers)

Week	Sun	Mon	Tue	Wed	Thu	Fri	Sat	Total
1	Off	Off	Off	3 Tempo	3 Steady Run	Off	3 Steady Run	9
2	7 LSD Run/Walk	Off	4 Tempo	3 Tempo	3 Steady Run	Off	3 Steady Run	20
3	7 LSD Run/Walk	Off	4 Tempo	3 Tempo	4 Steady Run	Off	3 Steady Run	21
4	7 LSD Run/Walk	Off	3 Tempo	4 Tempo	3 Steady Run	Off	4 Steady Run	21
5	9 LSD Run/Walk	Off	4 Tempo	4 Tempo	3 Steady Run	Off	3 Steady Run	23
6	9 LSD Run/Walk	Off	5 Tempo	3 Tempo	4 Steady Run	Off	3 Steady Run	24
7	10 LSD Run/Walk	Off	4 Tempo	3 Hills 2.5 km	5 Steady Run	Off	3 Steady Run	24.5
8	10 LSD Run/Walk	Off	4 Tempo	4 Hills 3 km	5 Steady Run	Off	4 Steady Run	26
9	12 LSD Run/Walk	Off	4 Tempo	5 Hills 4 km	6 Steady Run	Off	4 Steady Run	30
10	14 LSD Run/Walk	Off	4 Tempo	6 Hills 5 km	6 Steady Run	Off	5 Steady Run	34
11	16 LSD Run/Walk	Off	5 Tempo	7 Hills 5.5 km	7 Steady Run	Off	5 Steady Run	38.5
12	16 LSD Run/Walk	Off	5 Tempo	8 Hills 6 km	7 Steady Run	Off	6 Steady Run	40
13	12 LSD Run/Walk	Off	5 Tempo	9 Hills 7 km	8 Steady Run	Off	6 Steady Run	38
14	18 LSD Run/Walk	Off	6 Tempo	Speed 2 X 1.6 km 9 km	8 Steady Run	Off	6 Steady Run	47
15	18 LSD Run/Walk	Off	6 Tempo	Speed 3 X 1.6 km 11 km	8 Steady Run	Off	6 Steady Run	49
16	20 LSD Run/Walk	Off	6 Tempo	Speed 4 X 1.6 km 12 km	8 Steady Run	Off	6 Race Pace	52
17	6 LSD Run/Walk	Off	10 Race Pace	6 Race Pace	Off	Off	3 Steady Run	25
18	Race - Half Marathon							21.1

Pace Schedule	Long Run (LSD)	Steady Run	Tempo/Fartlek/Hills	Speed	Race	Walk Adjusted Race Pace
To Complete 2:00	6:34–7:23	6:34	5:55	5:10	5:41	5:27

Run/Walk Interval = 10 min Running/1 min Walking
Hills are a distance of 400 m

Week	Sun	Mon	Tue	Wed	Thu	Fri	Sat	Total
1	Off	Off	Off	3 Tempo	3 Steady Run	Off	3 Steady Run	9
2	7 LSD Run/Walk	Off	4 Tempo	3 Tempo	3 Steady Run	Off	3 Steady Run	20
3	7 LSD Run/Walk	Off	4 Tempo	3 Tempo	4 Steady Run	Off	3 Steady Run	21
4	7 LSD Run/Walk	Off	3 Tempo	4 Tempo	3 Steady Run	Off	4 Steady Run	21
5	9 LSD Run/Walk	Off	4 Tempo	4 Tempo	3 Steady Run	Off	3 Steady Run	23
6	9 LSD Run/Walk	Off	5 Tempo	3 Tempo	4 Steady Run	Off	3 Steady Run	24
7	10 LSD Run/Walk	Off	4 Tempo	3 Hills 2.5 km	5 Steady Run	Off	3 Steady Run	24.5
8	10 LSD Run/Walk	Off	4 Tempo	4 Hills 3 km	5 Steady Run	Off	4 Steady Run	26
9	12 LSD Run/Walk	Off	4 Tempo	5 Hills 4 km	6 Steady Run	Off	4 Steady Run	30
10	14 LSD Run/Walk	Off	4 Tempo	6 Hills 5 km	6 Steady Run	Off	5 Steady Run	34
11	16 LSD Run/Walk	Off	5 Tempo	7 Hills 5.5 km	7 Steady Run	Off	5 Steady Run	38.5
12	16 LSD Run/Walk	Off	5 Tempo	8 Hills 6 km	7 Steady Run	Off	6 Steady Run	40
13	12 LSD Run/Walk	Off	5 Tempo	9 Hills 7 km	8 Steady Run	Off	6 Steady Run	38
14	18 LSD Run/Walk	Off	6 Tempo	Speed 2 X 1.6 km 9 km	8 Steady Run	Off	6 Steady Run	47
15	18 LSD Run/Walk	Off	6 Tempo	Speed 3 X 1.6 km 11 km	8 Steady Run	Off	6 Steady Run	49
16	20 LSD Run/Walk	Off	6 Tempo	Speed 4 X 1.6 km 12 km	8 Steady Run	Off	6 Race Pace	52
17	6 LSD Run/Walk	Off	10 Race Pace	6 Race Pace	Off	Off	3 Steady Run	25
18	Race - Half Marathon							21.1

Pace Schedule	Long Run (LSD)	Steady Run	Tempo/Far- tlek/Hills	Speed	Race	Walk Adjusted Race Pace
To Complete 1:50	6:04–6:50	6:04	5:27	4:45	5:13	4:57

Run/Walk Interval = 10 min Running/1 min Walking
Hills are a distance of 400 m

Half Marathon To Complete in 1:45
(Recorded in Kilometers)

week	Sun	Mon	Tue	Wed	Thu	Fri	Sat	Total
1	Off	Off	Off	3 Tempo	3 Steady Run	Off	3 Steady Run	9
2	7 LSD Run/Walk	Off	4 Tempo	3 Tempo	3 Steady Run	Off	3 Steady Run	20
3	7 LSD Run/Walk	Off	4 Tempo	3 Tempo	4 Steady Run	Off	3 Steady Run	21
4	7 LSD Run/Walk	Off	3 Tempo	4 Tempo	3 Steady Run	Off	4 Steady Run	21
5	9 LSD Run/Walk	Off	4 Tempo	4 Tempo	3 Steady Run	Off	3 Steady Run	23
6	9 LSD Run/Walk	Off	5 Tempo	3 Tempo	4 Steady Run	Off	3 Steady Run	24
7	10 LSD Run/Walk	Off	4 Tempo	3 Hills 2.5 km	5 Steady Run	Off	3 Steady Run	24.5
8	10 LSD Run/Walk	Off	4 Tempo	4 Hills 3 km	5 Steady Run	Off	4 Steady Run	26
9	12 LSD Run/Walk	Off	4 Tempo	5 Hills 4 km	6 Steady Run	Off	4 Steady Run	30
10	14 LSD Run/Walk	Off	4 Fartlek	6 Hills 5 km	6 Steady Run	Off	5 Steady Run	34
11	16 LSD Run/Walk	Off	5 Fartlek	7 Hills 5.5 km	7 Steady Run	Off	5 Steady Run	38.5
12	16 LSD Run/Walk	Off	5 Fartlek	8 Hills 6 km	7 Steady Run	Off	6 Steady Run	40
13	12 LSD Run/Walk	Off	5 Fartlek	9 Hills 7 km	8 Steady Run	Off	6 Steady Run	38
14	18 LSD Run/Walk	Off	6 Fartlek	Speed 2 X 1.6 km 9 km	8 Steady Run	Off	6 Steady Run	47
15	18 LSD Run/Walk	Off	6 Fartlek	Speed 3 X 1.6 km 11 km	8 Steady Run	Off	6 Steady Run	49
16	20 LSD Run/Walk	Off	6 Fartlek	Speed 4 X 1.6 km 12 km	8 Steady Run	Off	6 Race Pace	52
17	6 LSD Run/Walk	Off	10 Race Pace	6 Race Pace	Off	Off	3 Steady Run	25
18	Race - Half Marathon							21.1

Pace Schedule	Long Run (LSD)	Steady Run	Tempo/Far-tlek/Hills	Speed	Race	Walk Adjusted Race Pace
To Complete 1:45	5:49–6:33	5:49	5:14	4:33	4:59	4:44

Run/Walk Interval = 10 min Running/1 min Walking
Hills are a distance of 400 m

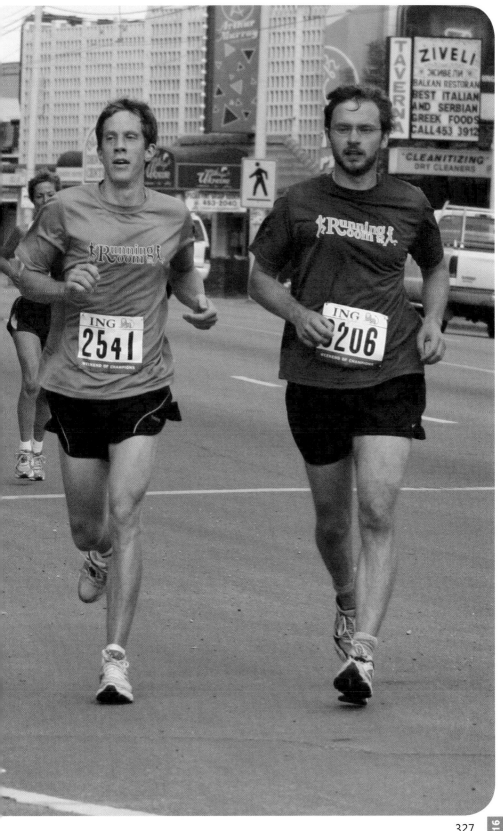

Half Marathon To Complete in 1:40
(Recorded in Kilometers)

Week	Sun	Mon	Tue	Wed	Thu	Fri	Sat	Total
1	Off	Off	Off	3 Tempo	3 Steady Run	Off	3 Steady Run	9
2	7 LSD Run/Walk	Off	4 Tempo	3 Tempo	3 Steady Run	Off	3 Steady Run	20
3	7 LSD Run/Walk	Off	4 Tempo	3 Tempo	4 Steady Run	Off	3 Steady Run	21
4	7 LSD Run/Walk	Off	3 Tempo	4 Tempo	3 Steady Run	Off	4 Steady Run	21
5	9 LSD Run/Walk	Off	4 Tempo	4 Tempo	3 Steady Run	Off	3 Steady Run	23
6	9 LSD Run/Walk	Off	5 Tempo	3 Tempo	4 Steady Run	Off	3 Steady Run	24
7	10 LSD Run/Walk	Off	4 Tempo	3 Hills 2.5 km	5 Steady Run	Off	3 Steady Run	24.5
8	10 LSD Run/Walk	Off	4 Tempo	4 Hills 3 km	5 Steady Run	Off	4 Steady Run	26
9	12 LSD Run/Walk	Off	4 Tempo	5 Hills 4 km	6 Steady Run	Off	4 Steady Run	30
10	14 LSD Run/Walk	Off	4 Fartlek	6 Hills 5 km	6 Steady Run	Off	5 Steady Run	34
11	16 LSD Run/Walk	Off	5 Fartlek	7 Hills 5.5 km	7 Steady Run	Off	5 Steady Run	38.5
12	16 LSD Run/Walk	Off	5 Fartlek	8 Hills 6 km	7 Steady Run	Off	6 Steady Run	40
13	12 LSD Run/Walk	Off	5 Fartlek	9 Hills 7 km	8 Steady Run	Off	6 Steady Run	38
14	18 LSD Run/Walk	Off	6 Fartlek	Speed 2 X 1.6 km 9 km	8 Steady Run	Off	6 Steady Run	47
15	18 LSD Run/Walk	Off	6 Fartlek	Speed 3 X 1.6 km 11 km	8 Steady Run	Off	6 Steady Run	49
16	20 LSD Run/Walk	Off	6 Fartlek	Speed 4 X 1.6 km 12 km	8 Steady Run	Off	6 Race Pace	52
17	6 LSD Run/Walk	Off	10 Race Pace	6 Race Pace	Off	Off	3 Steady Run	25
18	Race - Half Marathon							21.1

Pace Schedule	Long Run (LSD)	Steady Run	Tempo/Far-tlek/Hills	Speed	Race	Walk Adjusted Race Pace
To Complete 1:40	5:33–6:16	5:33	5:00	4:21	4:44	4:29

Run/Walk Interval = 10 min Running/1 min Walking
Hills are a distance of 400 m

Half Marathon To Complete in 1:30

(Recorded in Kilometers)

Week	Sun	Mon	Tue	Wed	Thu	Fri	Sat	Total
1	Off	Off	Off	Off	Off	10 Steady Run	6 Steady Run	16
2	11 LSD Run/Walk	Off	8 Tempo	10 Tempo	12 Steady Run	13 Steady Run	6 Steady Run	60
3	13 LSD Run/Walk	Off	8 Tempo	10 Tempo	12 Steady Run	13 Steady Run	6 Steady Run	62
4	13 LSD Run/Walk	Off	8 Tempo	10 Tempo	12 Steady Run	13 Steady Run	6 Steady Run	62
5	16 LSD Run/Walk	Off	8 Tempo	10 Tempo	12 Steady Run	13 Steady Run	6 Steady Run	65
6	16 LSD Run/Walk	Off	8 Tempo	3 Hills 2.5 km	8 Steady Run	13 Steady Run	6 Steady Run	53.5
7	13 LSD Run/Walk	Off	8 Tempo	4 Hills 3 km	8 Steady Run	13 Steady Run	6 Steady Run	51
8	16 LSD Run/Walk	Off	8 Tempo	5 Hills 4 km	8 Steady Run	13 Steady Run	6 Steady Run	55
9	19 LSD Run/Walk	Off	8 Tempo	6 Hills 5 km	8 Steady Run	13 Steady Run	6 Steady Run	59
10	19 LSD Run/Walk	Off	8 Fartlek	7 Hills 5.5 km	8 Steady Run	13 Steady Run	6 Steady Run	59.5
11	21 LSD Run/Walk	Off	8 Fartlek	8 Hills 6 km	8 Steady Run	13 Steady Run	6 Steady Run	62
12	16 LSD Run/Walk	Off	8 Fartlek	9 Hills 7 km	8 Steady Run	13 Steady Run	6 Steady Run	58
13	22 LSD Run/Walk	Off	8 Fartlek	Speed 2 X 1.6 km 9 km	8 Steady Run	13 Steady Run	6 Steady Run	66
14	26 LSD Run/Walk	Off	8 Fartlek	Speed 3 X 1.6 km 11 km	8 Steady Run	13 Steady Run	6 Steady Run	72
15	16 LSD Run/Walk	Off	8 Fartlek	Speed 4 X 1.6 km 12 km	8 Steady Run	13 Steady Run	6 Race Pace	63
16	6 LSD Run/Walk	Off	10 Race Pace	6 Race Pace	Off	Off	3 Steady Run	25
17	Race - Half Marathon							21.1

Pace Schedule	Long Run (LSD)	Steady Run	Tempo/Far-tlek/Hills	Speed	Race	Walk Adjusted Race Pace
To Complete 1:30	5:02–5:42	5:02	4:32	3:56	4:16	4:02

Run/Walk Interval = 10 min Running/1 min Walking
Hills are a distance of 400 m

Half Marathon To Complete
(Recorded in Miles)

Week	Sun	Mon	Tue	Wed	Thu	Fri	Sat	Total
1	Off	Off	Off	2 Steady Run	2 Steady Run	Off	2 Steady Run	6
2	4.5 LSD Run/Walk	Off	2.5 Steady Run	2 Steady Run	2 Steady Run	Off	2 Steady Run	13
3	4.5 LSD Run/Walk	Off	2.5 Steady Run	2 Steady Run	2.5 Steady Run	Off	2 Steady Run	13.5
4	4.5 LSD Run/Walk	Off	2 Steady Run	2.5 Steady Run	2 Steady Run	Off	2.5 Steady Run	13.5
5	5.5 LSD Run/Walk	Off	2.5 Steady Run	2 Steady Run	2 Steady Run	Off	2 Steady Run	14
6	5.5 LSD Run/Walk	Off	3 Steady Run	2 Steady Run	2.5 Steady Run	Off	2 Steady Run	15
7	6 LSD Run/Walk	Off	2.5 Steady Run	3 Hills 1.5 mi	3 Steady Run	Off	2 Steady Run	15
8	6 LSD Run/Walk	Off	2.5 Steady Run	4 Hills 2 mi	3 Steady Run	Off	2.5 Steady Run	16
9	7.5 LSD Run/Walk	Off	2.5 Steady Run	5 Hills 2.5 mi	4 Steady Run	Off	2.5 Steady Run	19
10	8.5 LSD Run/Walk	Off	2.5 Steady Run	6 Hills 3 mi	4 Steady Run	Off	3 Steady Run	21
11	10 LSD Run/Walk	Off	3 Steady Run	7 Hills 3.5 mi	4.5 Steady Run	Off	3 Steady Run	24.5
12	10 LSD Run/Walk	Off	3 Steady Run	8 Hills 4 mi	4.5 Steady Run	Off	4 Steady Run	25.5
13	7.5 LSD Run/Walk	Off	3 Steady Run	9 Hills 4.5 mi	5 Steady Run	Off	4 Steady Run	24
14	11 LSD Run/Walk	Off	4 Steady Run	2.5 Fartlek	5 Steady Run	Off	4 Steady Run	26.5
15	11 LSD Run/Walk	Off	4 Steady Run	2.5 Fartlek	5 Steady Run	Off	4 Steady Run	26.5
16	12.5 LSD Run/Walk	Off	4 Steady Run	2.5 Fartlek	5 Steady Run	Off	4 Steady Run	28
17	4 Steady Run	Off	6 Steady Run	4 Steady Run	Off	Off	2 Steady Run	16
18	Race - Half Marathon							13

Pace Schedule	Long Run (LSD)	Steady Run	Tempo/Far-tlek/Hills	Speed	Race	Walk Adjusted Race Pace
To Complete	15:16–16:58	15:16	13:52	12:13	13:44	13:19

Run/Walk Interval = 10 min Running/1 min Walking
Hills are a distance of 400 m

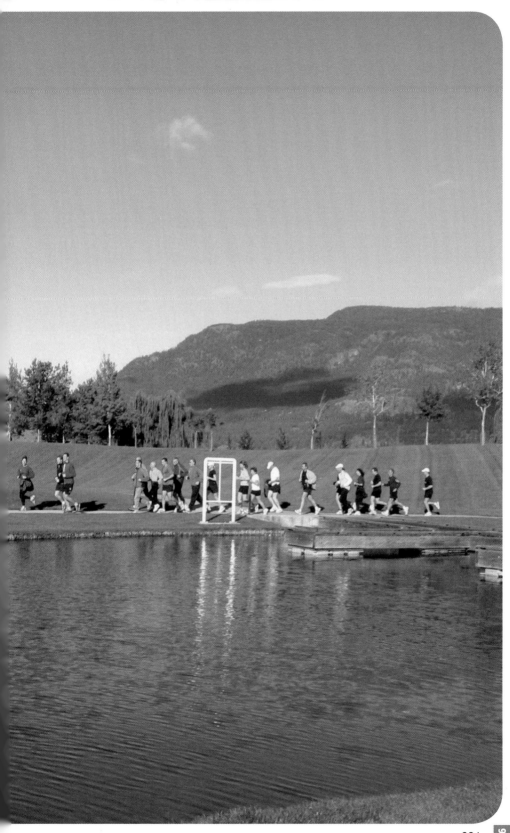

Half Marathon To Complete in 2:30
(Recorded in Miles)

Week	Sun	Mon	Tue	Wed	Thu	Fri	Sat	Total
1	Off	Off	Off	2 Tempo	2 Steady Run	Off	2 Steady Run	6
2	4.5 LSD Run/Walk	Off	2.5 Tempo	2 Tempo	2 Steady Run	Off	2 Steady Run	13
3	4.5 LSD Run/Walk	Off	2.5 Tempo	2 Tempo	2.5 Steady Run	Off	2 Steady Run	13.5
4	4.5 LSD Run/Walk	Off	2 Tempo	2.5 Tempo	2 Steady Run	Off	2.5 Steady Run	13.5
5	5.5 LSD Run/Walk	Off	2.5 Tempo	2.5 Tempo	2 Steady Run	Off	2 Steady Run	14.5
6	5.5 LSD Run/Walk	Off	3 Tempo	2 Tempo	2.5 Steady Run	Off	2 Steady Run	15
7	6 LSD Run/Walk	Off	2.5 Tempo	3 Hills 1.5 mi	3 Steady Run	Off	2 Steady Run	15
8	6 LSD Run/Walk	Off	2.5 Tempo	4 Hills 2 mi	3 Steady Run	Off	2.5 Steady Run	16
9	7.5 LSD Run/Walk	Off	2.5 Tempo	5 Hills 2.5 mi	4 Steady Run	Off	2.5 Steady Run	19
10	8.5 LSD Run/Walk	Off	2.5 Tempo	6 Hills 3 mi	4 Steady Run	Off	3 Steady Run	21
11	10 LSD Run/Walk	Off	3 Tempo	7 Hills 3.5 mi	4.5 Steady Run	Off	3 Steady Run	24
12	10 LSD Run/Walk	Off	3 Tempo	8 Hills 4 mi	4.5 Steady Run	Off	4 Steady Run	25.5
13	7.5 LSD Run/Walk	Off	3 Tempo	9 Hills 4.5 mi	5 Steady Run	Off	4 Steady Run	24
14	11 LSD Run/Walk	Off	4 Tempo	4 Fartlek	5 Steady Run	Off	4 Steady Run	28
15	11 LSD Run/Walk	Off	4 Tempo	4 Fartlek	5 Steady Run	Off	4 Steady Run	28
16	12.5 LSD Run/Walk	Off	4 Tempo	4 Fartlek	5 Steady Run	Off	4 Race Pace	29.5
17	4 LSD Steady Run	Off	6 Race Pace	4 Race Pace	Off	Off	2 Steady Run	16
18	Race - Half Marathon							13

Pace Schedule	Long Run (LSD)	Steady Run	Tempo/Far-tlek/Hills	Speed	Race	Walk Adjusted Race Pace
To Complete 2:30	12:57–14:29	12:57	11:43	10:16	11:27	11:02

Run/Walk Interval = 10 min Running/1 min Walking
Hills are a distance of 400 m

Half Marathon To Complete in 2:15
(Recorded in Miles)

Week	Sun	Mon	Tue	Wed	Thu	Fri	Sat	Total
1	Off	Off	Off	2 Tempo	2 Steady Run	Off	2 Steady Run	6
2	4.5 LSD Run/Walk	Off	2.5 Tempo	2 Tempo	2 Steady Run	Off	2 Steady Run	13
3	4.5 LSD Run/Walk	Off	2.5 Tempo	2 Tempo	2.5 Steady Run	Off	2 Steady Run	13.5
4	4.5 LSD Run/Walk	Off	2 Tempo	2.5 Tempo	2 Steady Run	Off	2.5 Steady Run	13.5
5	5.5 LSD Run/Walk	Off	2.5 Tempo	2.5 Tempo	2 Steady Run	Off	2 Steady Run	14.5
6	5.5 LSD Run/Walk	Off	3 Tempo	2 Tempo	2.5 Steady Run	Off	2 Steady Run	15
7	6 LSD Run/Walk	Off	2.5 Tempo	3 Hills 1.5 mi	3 Steady Run	Off	2 Steady Run	15
8	6 LSD Run/Walk	Off	2.5 Tempo	4 Hills 2 mi	3 Steady Run	Off	2.5 Steady Run	16
9	7.5 LSD Run/Walk	Off	2.5 Tempo	5 Hills 2.5 mi	4 Steady Run	Off	2.5 Steady Run	19
10	8.5 LSD Run/Walk	Off	2.5 Tempo	6 Hills 3 mi	4 Steady Run	Off	3 Steady Run	21
11	10 LSD Run/Walk	Off	3 Tempo	7 Hills 3.5 mi	4.5 Steady Run	Off	3 Steady Run	24
12	10 LSD Run/Walk	Off	3 Tempo	8 Hills 4 mi	4.5 Steady Run	Off	4 Steady Run	25.5
13	7.5 LSD Run/Walk	Off	3 Tempo	9 Hills 4.5 mi	5 Steady Run	Off	4 Steady Run	24
14	11 LSD Run/Walk	Off	4 Tempo	Speed 2 X 1 mi 6 mi	5 Steady Run	Off	4 Steady Run	30
15	11 LSD Run/Walk	Off	4 Tempo	Speed 3 X 1 mi 7 mi	5 Steady Run	Off	4 Steady Run	31
16	12.5 LSD Run/Walk	Off	4 Tempo	Speed 4 X 1 mi 8 mi	5 Steady Run	Off	4 Race Pace	33.5
17	4 Steady Run	Off	6 Race Pace	4 Race Pace	Off	Off	2 Steady Run	16
18	Race - Half Marathon							13

Pace Schedule	Long Run (LSD)	Steady Run	Tempo/Far-tlek/Hills	Speed	Race	Walk Adjusted Race Pace
To Complete 2:15	11:46–13:12	11:46	10:37	9:17	10:18	9:54

Run/Walk Interval = 10 min Running/1 min Walking
Hills are a distance of 400 m

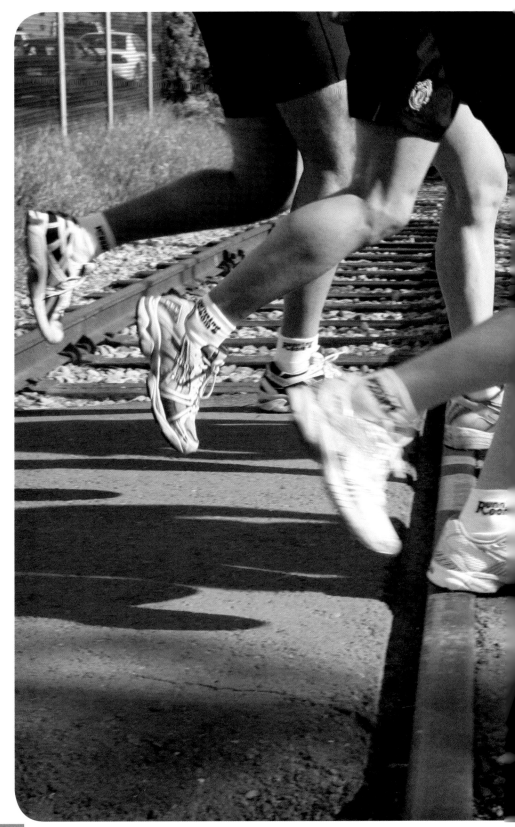

Half Marathon To Complete in 2:00
(Recorded in Miles)

Week	Sun	Mon	Tue	Wed	Thu	Fri	Sat	Total
1	Off	Off	Off	2 Tempo	2 Steady Run	Off	2 Steady Run	6
2	4.5 LSD Run/Walk	Off	2.5 Tempo	2 Tempo	2 Steady Run	Off	2 Steady Run	13
3	4.5 LSD Run/Walk	Off	2.5 Tempo	2 Tempo	2.5 Steady Run	Off	2 Steady Run	13.5
4	4.5LSD Run/Walk	Off	2 Tempo	2.5 Tempo	2 Steady Run	Off	2.5 Steady Run	13.5
5	5.5 LSD Run/Walk	Off	2.5 Tempo	2.5 Tempo	2 Steady Run	Off	2 Steady Run	14.5
6	5.5 LSD Run/Walk	Off	3 Tempo	2 Tempo	2.5 Steady Run	Off	2 Steady Run	15
7	6 LSD Run/Walk	Off	2.5 Tempo	3 Hills 1.5 mi	3 Steady Run	Off	2 Steady Run	15
8	6 LSD Run/Walk	Off	2.5 Tempo	4 Hills 2 mi	3 Steady Run	Off	2.5 Steady Run	16
9	7.5 LSD Run/Walk	Off	2.5 Tempo	5 Hills 2.5 mi	4 Steady Run	Off	2.5 Steady Run	19
10	8.5 LSD Run/Walk	Off	2.5 Tempo	6 Hills 3 mi	4 Steady Run	Off	3 Steady Run	21
11	10 LSD Run/Walk	Off	3 Tempo	7 Hills 3.5 mi	4.5 Steady Run	Off	3 Steady Run	24
12	10 LSD Run/Walk	Off	3 Tempo	8 Hills 4 mi	4.5 Steady Run	Off	4 Steady Run	25.5
13	7.5. LSD Run/Walk	Off	3 Tempo	9 Hills 4.5 mi	5 Steady Run	Off	4 Steady Run	24
14	11 LSD Run/Walk	Off	4 Tempo	Speed 2 X 1 mi 6 mi	5 Steady Run	Off	4 Steady Run	30
15	11 LSD Run/Walk	Off	4 Tempo	Speed 3 X 1 mi 7 mi	5 Steady Run	Off	4 Steady Run	31
16	12.5 LSD Run/Walk	Off	4 Tempo	Speed 4 X 1 mi 8 mi	5 Steady Run	Off	4 Race Pace	33.5
17	4 Steady Run	Off	6 Race Pace	4 Race Pace	Off	Off	2 Steady Run	16
18	Race - Half Marathon							13

Pace Schedule	Long Run (LSD)	Steady Run	Tempo/Far-tlek/Hills	Speed	Race	Walk Adjusted Race Pace
To Complete 2:00	10:35–11:54	10:35	9:31	8:19	9:09	8:46

Run/Walk Interval = 10 min Running/1 min Walking
Hills are a distance of 400 m

Half Marathon To Complete in 1:50
(Recorded in Miles)

Week	Sun	Mon	Tue	Wed	Thu	Fri	Sat	Total
1	Off	Off	Off	2 Tempo	2 Steady Run	Off	2 Steady Run	6
2	4.5 LSD Run/Walk	Off	2.5 Tempo	2 Tempo	2 Steady Run	Off	2 Steady Run	13
3	4.5 LSD Run/Walk	Off	2.5 Tempo	2 Tempo	2.5 Steady Run	Off	2 Steady Run	13.5
4	4.5 LSD Run/Walk	Off	2 Tempo	2.5 Tempo	2 Steady Run	Off	2.5 Steady Run	13.5
5	5.5 LSD Run/Walk	Off	2.5 Tempo	2.5 Tempo	2 Steady Run	Off	2 Steady Run	14.5
6	5.5 LSD Run/Walk	Off	3 Tempo	2 Tempo	2.5 Steady Run	Off	2 Steady Run	15
7	6 LSD Run/Walk	Off	2.5 Tempo	3 Hills 1.5 mi	3 Steady Run	Off	2 Steady Run	15
8	6 LSD Run/Walk	Off	2.5 Tempo	4 Hills 2 mi	3 Steady Run	Off	2.5 Steady Run	16
9	7.5 LSD Run/Walk	Off	2.5 Tempo	5 Hills 2.5 mi	4 Steady Run	Off	2.5 Steady Run	19
10	8.5 LSD Run/Walk	Off	2.5 Tempo	6 Hills 3 mi	4 Steady Run	Off	3 Steady Run	21
11	10 LSD Run/Walk	Off	3 Tempo	7 Hills 3.5 mi	4.5 Steady Run	Off	3 Steady Run	24
12	10 LSD Run/Walk	Off	3 Tempo	8 Hills 4 mi	4.5 Steady Run	Off	4 Steady Run	25.5
13	7.5 LSD Run/Walk	Off	3 Tempo	9 Hills 4.5 mi	5 Steady Run	Off	4 Steady Run	24
14	11 LSD Run/Walk	Off	4 Tempo	Speed 2 X 1 mi 6 mi	5 Steady Run	Off	4 Steady Run	30
15	11 LSD Run/Walk	Off	4 Tempo	Speed 3 X 1 mi 7 mi	5 Steady Run	Off	4 Steady Run	31
16	12.5 LSD Run/Walk	Off	4 Tempo	Speed 4 X 1 mi 8 mi	5 Steady Run	Off	4 Race Pace	33.5
17	4 LSD Run/Walk	Off	6 Race Pace	4 Race Pace	Off	Off	2 Steady Run	16
18	Race - Half Marathon							13

Pace Schedule	Long Run (LSD)	Steady Run	Tempo/Far-tlek/Hills	Speed	Race	Walk Adjusted Race Pace
To Complete 1:50	9:46–11:00	9:46	8:47	7:39	8:23	7:58

Run/Walk Interval = 10 min Running/1 min Walking
Hills are a distance of 400 m

Half Marathon To Complete in 1:45
(Recorded in Miles)

Week	Sun	Mon	Tue	Wed	Thu	Fri	Sat	Total
1	Off	Off	Off	2 Tempo	2 Steady Run	Off	2 Steady Run	6
2	4.5 LSD Run/Walk	Off	2.5 Tempo	2 Tempo	2 Steady Run	Off	2 Steady Run	13
3	4.5 LSD Run/Walk	Off	2.5 Tempo	2 Tempo	2.5 Steady Run	Off	2 Steady Run	13.5
4	4.5 LSD Run/Walk	Off	2 Tempo	2.5 Tempo	2 Steady Run	Off	2.5 Steady Run	13.5
5	5.5 LSD Run/Walk	Off	2.5 Tempo	2.5 Tempo	2 Steady Run	Off	2 Steady Run	14.5
6	5.5 LSD Run/Walk	Off	3 Tempo	2 Tempo	2.5 Steady Run	Off	2 Steady Run	15
7	6 LSD Run/Walk	Off	2.5 Tempo	3 Hills 1.5 mi	3 Steady Run	Off	2 Steady Run	15
8	6 LSD Run/Walk	Off	2.5 Tempo	4 Hills 2 mi	3 Steady Run	Off	2.5 Steady Run	16
9	7.5 LSD Run/Walk	Off	2.5 Tempo	5 Hills 2.5 mi	4 Steady Run	Off	2.5 Steady Run	19
10	8.5 LSD Run/Walk	Off	2.5 Fartlek	6 Hills 3 mi	4 Steady Run	Off	3 Steady Run	21
11	10 LSD Run/Walk	Off	3 Fartlek	7 Hills 3.5 mi	4.5 Steady Run	Off	3 Steady Run	24
12	10 LSD Run/Walk	Off	3 Fartlek	8 Hills 4 mi	4.5 Steady Run	Off	4 Steady Run	25.5
13	7.5 LSD Run/Walk	Off	3 Fartlek	9 Hills 4.5 mi	5 Steady Run	Off	4 Steady Run	24
14	11 LSD Run/Walk	Off	4 Fartlek	Speed 2 X 1 mi 6 mi	5 Steady Run	Off	4 Steady Run	30
15	11 LSD Run/Walk	Off	4 Fartlek	Speed 3 X 1 mi 7 mi	5 Steady Run	Off	4 Steady Run	31
16	12.5 LSD Run/Walk	Off	4 Fartlek	Speed 4 X 1 mi 8 mi	5 Steady Run	Off	4 Race Pace	33.5
17	4 LSD Run/Walk	Off	6 Race Pace	4 Race Pace	Off	Off	2 Steady Run	16
18	Race - Half Marathon							13

Pace Schedule	Long Run (LSD)	Steady Run	Tempo/Far-tlek/Hills	Speed	Race	Walk Adjusted Race Pace
To Complete 1:45	9:21–10:33	9:21	8:25	7:20	8:01	7:37

Run/Walk Interval = 10 min Running/1 min Walking
Hills are a distance of 400 m

16 Half Marathon

Week	Sun	Mon	Tue	Wed	Thu	Fri	Sat	Total
1	Off	Off	Off	2 Tempo	2 Steady Run	Off	2 Steady Run	6
2	4.5 LSD Run/Walk	Off	2.5 Tempo	2 Tempo	2 Steady Run	Off	2 Steady Run	13
3	4.5 LSD Run/Walk	Off	2.5 Tempo	2 Tempo	2.5 Steady Run	Off	2 Steady Run	13.5
4	4.5 LSD Run/Walk	Off	2 Tempo	2.5 Tempo	2 Steady Run	Off	2.5 Steady Run	13.5
5	5.5 LSD Run/Walk	Off	2.5 Tempo	2.5 Tempo	2 Steady Run	Off	2 Steady Run	14.5
6	5.5 LSD Run/Walk	Off	3 Tempo	2 Tempo	2.5 Steady Run	Off	2 Steady Run	15
7	6 LSD Run/Walk	Off	2.5 Tempo	3 Hills 1.5 mi	3 Steady Run	Off	2 Steady Run	15
8	6 LSD Run/Walk	Off	2.5 Tempo	4 Hills 2 mi	3 Steady Run	Off	2.5 Steady Run	16
9	7.5 LSD Run/Walk	Off	2.5 Tempo	5 Hills 2.5 mi	4 Steady Run	Off	2.5 Steady Run	19
10	8.5 LSD Run/Walk	Off	2.5 Fartlek	6 Hills 3 mi	4 Steady Run	Off	3 Steady Run	21
11	10 LSD Run/Walk	Off	3 Fartlek	7 Hills 3.5 mi	4.5 Steady Run	Off	3 Steady Run	24
12	10 LSD Run/Walk	Off	3 Fartlek	8 Hills 4 mi	4.5 Steady Run	Off	4 Steady Run	25.5
13	7.5 LSD Run/Walk	Off	3 Fartlek	9 Hills 4.5 mi	5 Steady Run	Off	4 Steady Run	24
14	11 LSD Run/Walk	Off	4 Fartlek	Speed 2 X 1 mi 6 mi	5 Steady Run	Off	4 Steady Run	30
15	11 LSD Run/Walk	Off	4 Fartlek	Speed 3 X 1 mi 7 mi	5 Steady Run	Off	4 Steady Run	31
16	12.5 LSD Run/Walk	Off	4 Fartlek	Speed 4 X 1 mi 8 mi	5 Steady Run	Off	4 Race Pace	33.5
17	4 LSD Run/Walk	Off	6 Race Pace	4 Race Pace	Off	Off	2 Steady Run	16
18	Race - Half Marathon							13

Pace Schedule	Long Run (LSD)	Steady Run	Tempo/Far-tlek/Hills	Speed	Race	Walk Adjusted Race Pace
To Complete 1:40	8:57–10:06	8:57	8:02	7:00	7:38	7:13

Run/Walk Interval = 10 min Running/1 min Walking
Hills are a distance of 400 m

Half Marathon To Complete in 1:30
(Recorded in Miles)

Week	Sun	Mon	Tue	Wed	Thu	Fri	Sat	Total
1	Off	Off	Off	Off	Off	6 Steady Run	4 Steady Run	10
2	7 LSD Run/Walk	Off	5 Tempo	6 Tempo	7.5 Steady Run	8 Steady Run	4 Steady Run	37.5
3	8 LSD Run/Walk	Off	5 Tempo	6 Tempo	7.5 Steady Run	8 Steady Run	4 Steady Run	38.5
4	8 LSD Run/Walk	Off	5 Tempo	6 Tempo	7.5 Steady Run	8 Steady Run	4 Steady Run	38.5
5	10 LSD Run/Walk	Off	5 Tempo	6 Tempo	7.5 Steady Run	8 Steady Run	4 Steady Run	40.5
6	10 LSD Run/Walk	Off	5 Tempo	3 Hills 1.5 mi	5 Steady Run	8 Steady Run	4 Steady Run	33.5
7	8 LSD Run/Walk	Off	5 Tempo	4 Hills 2 mi	5 Steady Run	8 Steady Run	4 Steady Run	32
8	10 LSD Run/Walk	Off	5 Tempo	5 Hills 2.5 mi	5 Steady Run	8 Steady Run	4 Steady Run	34.5
9	12 LSD Run/Walk	Off	5 Tempo	6 Hills 3 mi	5 Steady Run	8 Steady Run	4 Steady Run	37
10	12 LSD Run/Walk	Off	5 Fartlek	7 Hills 3.5 mi	5 Steady Run	8 Steady Run	4 Steady Run	37.5
11	13 LSD Run/Walk	Off	5 Fartlek	8 Hills 4 mi	5 Steady Run	8 Steady Run	4 Steady Run	39
12	10 LSD Run/Walk	Off	5 Fartlek	9 Hills 4.5 mi	5 Steady Run	8 Steady Run	4 Steady Run	36.5
13	13.5 LSD Run/Walk	Off	5 Fartlek	Speed 2 X 1 mi 6 mi	5 Steady Run	8 Steady Run	4 Steady Run	41.5
14	16 LSD Run/Walk	Off	5 Fartlek	Speed 3 X 1 mi 7 mi	5 Steady Run	8 Steady Run	4 Steady Run	45
15	10 LSD Run/Walk	Off	5 Fartlek	Speed 4 X 1 mi 8 mi	5 Steady Run	8 Steady Run	4 Race Pace	40
16	4 LSD Run/Walk	Off	6 Race Pace	4 Race Pace	Off	Off	2 Steady Run	16
17	Race - Half Marathon							13

Pace Schedule	Long Run (LSD)	Steady Run	Tempo/Far-tlek/Hills	Speed	Race	Walk Adjusted Race Pace
To Complete 1:30	8:07–9:10	8:07	7:17	6:20	6:52	6:29

Run/Walk Interval = 10 min Running/1 min Walking
Hills are a distance of 400 m

The Marathon

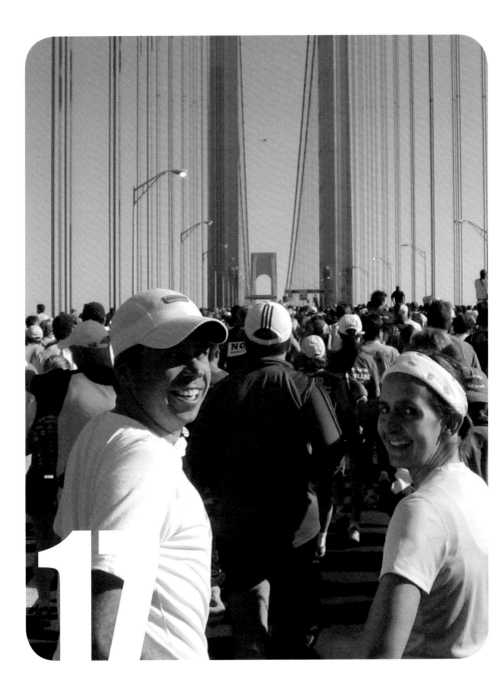

17

Are you ready for the ultimate running challenge? You'll find it in the marathon.

Training for the marathon can positively change the way you look at the rest of your life, you will experience a dramatic change in your physical and mental outlook on life and you will gain the self-confidence to achieve both your athletic and personal goals. By training to run a marathon, you'll find personal resources you didn't know were there.

The largest-growing group in the modern marathon is composed of people who just want to complete the 42.2-km (26.2-mi) course. Over the years it has become obvious that not all of us can be competitive marathoners. Just as our fingerprints are unique to each of us, so are our other attributes, such as body type, resting heart rate, maximum heart rate and requirements put on us by family, work, friends and commitments to the community.

If you decide the marathon is your event, don't plan on doing more than two in a year. This gives you lots of time to rest, recover and start training for the next race.

Hitting the Wall

The biggest problem runners usually have to contend with during the marathon is "hitting the wall," a catchy phrase for depleting the glycogen stores in their muscles. Much of your success in the marathon will depend on energy conservation and efficient fuel utilization. If your glycogen runs out, the race is over, whether you have reached the finish line or not. Long slow training runs teach your body how to use its fuel more efficiently, and they promote the utilization of fat (you probably have enough to run dozens of marathons), which conserves glycogen. With proper long training runs, the "wall" will move farther and farther away, until finally it does not appear at all during the marathon. People often ask why it is necessary to do the weekly long runs at such an agonizingly slow pace. Quite simply, you are running them for endurance, not speed, and if you train too fast, you will not only be too tired to benefit from your other runs that week, you will also greatly increase your risk of injury.

First-time marathoners should take a walking break of 1 minute for every 10 minutes of running on their long runs (and during the race itself). These walking breaks will only slow you down by about 15 seconds a kilometer (25 seconds a mile), which is less than 7 minutes for the entire marathon. By not taking these short breaks, especially at the beginning, you may end up going slower rather than faster because of the accumulate fatigue.

Experienced marathoners should be running their long runs at 1 to 1½ minutes a mile (½ to 1 minute a kilometer) slower than their planned race pace. Everyone should be able to pass the talk test, which means you should be able to carry on a conversation without gasping for breath. If you can't talk, you are running to fast.

Where is the Wall?

+ It starts at the length of your longest continuous run in the last two to three weeks.
+ You can bring it closer by running too fast.
+ You can move it farther away it by running slower or inserting 1-minute walking breaks every 10 minutes.

Tapering for a Marathon

Many experienced marathoners will tell you that you'll only perform as well as you've tapered. Many people forget that training is hard work and you can't just jump into an event and perform well without proper planning. Everyone's performance can benefit from a good taper, which is a carefully planned period of reduced training. This gradual easing up allows your body to disperse the residual fatigue products that have been carried from one workout to another. The extra recovery and regeneration that can occur during a taper result in what is called peaking. Come race day, your legs will have that extra snap to ensure your best performance.

The biggest complaint I get about tapering is that people often feel extremely restless during this period—they feel like they should be doing more. Don't. The beginning of the taper period signifies the end of training—and the beginning of competition preparation—and any hard training done during this period will do more to hurt your performance than help it because you won't recover fast enough. A good taper will make you feel like a horse in the gate at the start of the race for the few days before your event. It is the feeling of peak fitness; use it to your advantage.

A taper for a marathon should generally take up the last two to three weeks before the event—your last long run should take place no later than two weeks before the event. During the taper period, you should run only 30–50% of your regular weekly distance. The best tapers have runners maintaining their training intensity while gradually reducing their training distance to practically zero a few days before the event. Focus on keeping the intensity up on your continuous runs and reducing their length significantly. Forget speed training if you have any planned.

Your last quality workout should be on the second Saturday before the race. Run 16 km (10 mi) at your target pace for the marathon. This run is a high-quality workout that requires your discipline, so it is best to run it alone and concentrate on your form and setting your targeted pace. Do not race or get in a race with one of your training partners. Work at your race pace, include your 10:1's.

Starting on Monday, you will begin to cut back your distance in the tapering phase of the program. Some people feel very heavy and their disposition suffers during the tapering phase. Concentrate on the joy of less distance and the fact that you have all this extra time to relax and enjoy the tapering phase.

The most important day is two days prior to the race. Take the day off, go to bed early and enjoy as much sleep as possible. Stay in bed, read and relax. Even if you can't sleep, stay lying down—it's the best way to get you ready for race day. Remember, nothing you do in the final week will help you, but everything you do can hinder your performance. Quality training takes at least two weeks to improve your performance, but overtraining can affect your performance the next day.

Visualization is a key part of the week as you relax and think about your training and the goals you have set for the marathon. Read or listen to some of your favorite music to motivate yourself.

Marathon Training Questions

How can I race 42 km (26 mi.) when my long run is only 32 km (20 mi.)?

Over the years, there have been a variety of training programs that overextend the long run beyond the marathon distance. My experience is that the frequency of injury increases as we extend the long run beyond the 32-km. (20-mi) distance. I have seen too many folks run a great long run of 40–45 km. (25–28 mi) and then on marathon day come up with a disappointing time. The reason is that they did not give themselves enough time to recover from the long extended run.

Your training program is made up of base training, strength training and speed training. You train specifically in each phase; then on race day you put It all together and run the marathon. Your distances should be looked at over a four-week period, not on one individual day. The taper phase of your training allows you to rest and recover from training and to perform to a higher standard on race day.

Another key ingredient on race day is your adrenaline level, which, together with the group support and the crowd, will carry you the extra distance.

How can I run my targeted pace in the marathon when I have run my long training runs slower?

Slowing the long runs down helps you recover faster and gives you the desired endurance training effect while dramatically lowering your injury risk. You have plenty of hills, intervals and fartlek sessions to run at race pace or faster to give you the speed. If you ran your long runs at nearly race pace, you would need one day per mile to recover. It would take you 20 days to recover from a 32-km (20 mi.) training run. By slowing your pace by 15–20%, you will find that within a day or two you are ready to train hard, allowing you to do quality strength or speed work. This approach is called specified training.

How can I prevent injury and be sure I take it to the start line?

Many talented runners who approach their training in an overzealous manner end up sidelined by injury. Keep your training fun, keep it specific, keep it to the program and do not add to the program. Your training program is planned so that you will continually improve and get stronger. More is not necessarily better, fatigue will rob you of energy, both mentally and physically. Remember, running is playtime; don't make it feel like work!

How much of my total weekly distance should be speed?

Speed work should account for no more than 10–15% of your total weekly distance. Stick to the program and don't add any speed to your endurance training sessions. Training faster too often won't give your body enough time to recover between sessions.

For the long slow runs, is the recommended pace only for the running portion or does it include the walk break?

The pace includes the walk time. For example: The race pace time of 5:00 includes the total run time plus walk break. If your projected finish time is 5 hours, your race pace is 7:07 min/km. To achieve this overall pace while adding in walks requires that you run at a pace of 6.52 min/km. Running at this pace added to your walking pace will equal 7:07 min/km.

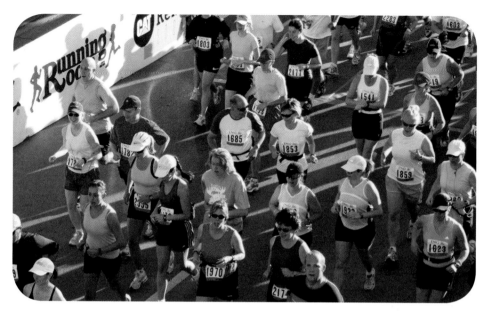

Marathon Training Program Details

On the following pages you will find a variety of suggested training schedules. These schedules have been designed to help runners to complete the event and to achieve specific time goals. The programs all follow the progressive structure as outlined in Chapter 2, Building Your Program. Long runs incorporate the 10/1 run/walk principle that has made the Running Room programs so successful. In addition you will see at the bottom of every training schedule a pace chart outlining the pace requirements for each run. Below you will find a description of the various types of workouts as reflected in the training schedules. You can refer to Chapter 2, Building Your Program for a more details description of 'Training Methods'. In addition Chapter 9, Types of Training provides a nice review of the various workout requirements of a successful running program.

Marathon Training Program Workouts

Workouts Long Slow Distance (LSD–Run/Walk)

Long Slow Distance runs are the cornerstone of any distance training program. Take a full minute to walk for every 10 minutes of running. These runs are meant to be done much slower than race pace (60– 70% of maximum heart rate), so don't be overly concerned with your pace. These runs work to increase the capillary network in your body and raise your anaerobic threshold. They also mentally prepare you for long races.

A note on LSD Pace

The pace for the long run on the chart includes the walk time. This program provides an upper end (slow) and bottom end (fast) pace to use as a guideline. The upper end pace is preferable because it will keep you injury free. Running at the bottom end pace is a common mistake made by many runners. They try to run at the maximum pace, which is an open invitation to injury. I know of very few runners who have been injured from running too slowly, but loads of runners who incurred injuries by running too fast. In the early stages of the program it is very easy to run the long runs too fast, but like the marathon or half marathon the long runs require discipline and patience. Practice your sense of pace by slowing the long runs down. You will recover faster and remain injury free.

Steady Run

The steady run is a run below targeted race pace (70% maximum heart rate). Run at comfortable speed; if in doubt, go slowly. The run is broken down into components of running and walking. We encourage you to use the run/walk approach. Walk breaks are a great way to keep you consistent in your training.

Hills

Distance for the day is calculated as the approximate distance covered up and down the hill. Now, you will no doubt have to run to the hill and back from the hill unless of course you drive to the hill. You will need to add your total warm-up and warm-down distance to the totals noted on the training schedule. I recommend a distance of 3 km both ways to ensure adequate warm-up and recovery because hills put a lot of stress on the body. Hills are run at tempo pace (80% maximum heart rate) and must include a heart rate recovery to 120 bpm at the bottom of each hill repeat.

VO2 Max

VO2 max is the volume of oxygen your body can obtain while training at your maximum hear rate. High VO2 levels indicate high fitness levels, allowing these fit athletes to train more intensely than beginners. Interval training of tempo, fartlek and speed sessions improves the efficiency of your body to transfer oxygen-rich blood to your working muscles.

Tempo

Before starting tempo runs, include several weeks of hill running to improve your strength, form and confidence. For the tempo runs, run at 80% of your maximum heart rate for 60–80% of your planned race distance to improve your coordination and leg turnover rate. Include a warm-up and cooldown of about three to five minutes. These runs simulate race conditions and the effort required on race day.

Fartlek (Speed Play)

Fartlek runs are spontaneous runs over varying distances and intensity. Run the short bursts at 70–80% of your maximum heart rate, if you are wearing a monitor. From a perceived effort, conversation is possible but you notice increased breathing, heart rate and perspiration. Between these short bursts of hard effort, but no longer than three minutes, add in recovery periods of easy running to bring your heart rate down to 120 beats per minute. Speed play fires up your performance with a burst of speed. The added recovery/rest interval keeps the session attainable and fun.

Speed

Going back to our training analogy of "Building the House," speed training is nailing down the roof and one of the last things we do. You must have a sufficient base training and strength training period before tackling speed. Speed is simply fast runs over short distances, e.g., 5 x 400 m, usually with a relatively long period of recovery to allow the unpleasant side effects of the anaerobic activity to diminish. In our training programs we factor in a 3 km warm-up and 3 km warm-down into the total distance to run. I have seen many runners come up injured when attempting speed work and inevitably as a result of running too fast. In the training programs I have purposefully lowered the pace of your speed works (95% maximum heart rate) as opposed to a much higher rate (110% maximum heart rate), which is commonly used but results in many injuries. In these programs we use speed to fine tune not to damage, and it has proven very successful in all our programs.

Walk Adjusted Race Pace

How do we arrive at a "Walk Adjusted" race pace? When you are walking, you are moving slower than your "average run pace." When you are running, you are moving faster than your "average walk pace." The walk adjusted race pace factors in the variation in walking and running speed. The challenge is knowing the average speed of your walking pace. We have devised a formula to calculate moderate walk pace, which allows us to determine the exact splits including running and walking pace. The effect of this calculation is that the "Walk Adjusted" run pace is faster per kilometer than the average race pace. However when calculated with your walk pace you will end up with your target race pace. You can go on-line at Runningroom.com and print out your "Walk Adjusted" pace bands for race day!

Choosing Your Marathon Training Program

Before you start training for a marathon, you should have a reasonable, intelligent goal for the race. Take a look at the following summaries and choose the level that best suits your needs and abilities. Take all the elements into consideration: your 1.6 km (1 mi.) pace, the weekly training distance required, the training pace for the long run and the race pace for the marathon.

Target Requirements to Complete the Marathon
Race pace: 7.49 min./km (12.36 min./mi.)
Walk adjusted race pace: 7.36 min./km (12.10 min/mi.)
Long run pace: 8.37–9.37 min./km (13.52–15.28 min./mi.)
1 km time trial: 6.25, 1 mi.: 10.20
10 K time trial: 1:11.45
Base training: 24–32 km (15–20 mi.)

Target Requirements for a 5-hour Marathon
Race pace: 7.07 min./km (11.27 min./mi.)
Walk adjusted race pace: 6.52 min./km (11.02 min/mi.)
Long run pace: 7.52–8.49 min./km (12.40–14.11 min./mi.)
1 km time trial: 5.50, 1 mi.: 9.24
10 K time trial: 1:05.12
Base training: 24–32 km (15–20 mi.)

Target Requirements for a 4-hour-45-minute Marathon
Race pace: 6.45 min./km (10.52 min./mi.)
Walk adjusted race pace: 6.31 min./km (10.29 min/mi.)
Long run pace: 7.30–8.25 min./km (12.04–13.32 min./mi.)
1 km time trial: 5.33, 1 mi.: 8.56
10 K time trial: 1:01.57
Base training: 32–40 km (20–25 mi.)

Target Requirements for a 4-hour-30-minute Marathon
Race pace: 6.24 min./km (10.18 min./mi.)
Walk adjusted race pace: 6.09 min./km (9.54 min/mi.)
Long run pace: 7.08–8.00 min./km (11.28–12.53 min./mi.)
1 km time trial: 5.15, 1 mi.: 8.27
10 K time trial: 58.41
Base training: 35–48 km (22–30 mi.)

Target Requirements for a 4-hour-15-minute Marathon
Race pace: 6.03 min./km (9.44 min./mi.)
Walk adjusted race pace: 5.47 min./km (9.19 min/mi.)
Long run pace: 6.45–7.35 min./km (10.52–12.13 min./mi.)
1 km time trial: 4.58, 1 mi.: 7.59
10 K time trial: 55.25
Base training: 40–48 km (25–30 mi.)

Target Requirements for a 4-hour Marathon
Race pace: 5.41 min./km (9.09 min./mi.)
Walk adjusted race pace: 5.26 min./km (8.45 min/mi.)
Long run pace: 6.22–7.11 min./km (10.15–11.33 min./mi.)
1 km time trial: 4.40, 1 mi.: 7.31
10 K time trial: 52.10
Base training: 48–56 km (30–35 mi.)

Target Requirements for a 3-hour-45-minute Marathon
Race pace: 5.20 min./km (8.35 min./mi.)
Walk adjusted race pace: 5.05 min./km (8.10 min/mi.)
Long run pace: 5.59–6.45 min./km (9.39–10.52 min./mi.)
1 km time trial: 4.23, 1 mi.: 7.03
10 K time trial: 48.54
Base training: 56–64 km (35–40 mi.)

Target Requirements for a 3-hour-30-minute Marathon
Race pace: 4.59 min./km (8.01 min./mi.)
Walk adjusted race pace: 4.43 min./km (7.36 min/mi.)
Long run pace: 5.37–6.20 min./km (9.02–10.12 min./mi.)
1 km time trial: 4.05, 1 mi.: 6.34
10 K time trial: 45.39
Base training: 64–72 km (40–45 mi.)

Target Requirements for a 3-hour-10-minute Marathon
Race pace: 4.30 min./km (7.15 min./mi.)
Walk adjusted race pace: 4.15 min./km (6.51 min/mi.)
Long run pace: 5.06–5.46 min./km (8.13–9.17 min./mi.)
1 km time trial: 3.42, 1 mi.: 5.57
10 K time trial: 41.18
Base training: 64–72 km (40–45 mi.)

Week	Sun	Mon	Tue	Wed	Thu	Fri	Sat	Total
1	10 LSD Run/Walk	Off	6 Tempo	10 Tempo	6 Steady Run	Off	6 Steady Run	38
2	10 LSD Run/Walk	Off	6 Tempo	10 Tempo	6 Steady Run	Off	6 Steady Run	38
3	13 LSD Run/Walk	Off	6 Tempo	10 Tempo	8 Steady Run	Off	6 Steady Run	43
4	13 LSD Run/Walk	Off	6 Tempo	10 Tempo	8 Steady Run	Off	6 Steady Run	43
5	16 LSD Run/Walk	Off	6 Tempo	10 Tempo	8 Steady Run	Off	6 Steady Run	46
6	16 LSD Run/Walk	Off	6 Tempo	10 Tempo	8 Steady Run	Off	6 Steady Run	46
7	19 LSD Run/Walk	Off	6 Tempo	4 Hills 5 km	8 Steady Run	Off	6 Steady Run	44
8	23 LSD Run/Walk	Off	6 Tempo	5 Hills 6 km	8 Steady Run	Off	6 Steady Run	49
9	26 LSD Run/Walk	Off	6 Tempo	6 Hills 7 km	8 Steady Run	Off	6 Steady Run	53
10	19 LSD Run/Walk	Off	6 Tempo	7 Hills 8.5 km	8 Steady Run	Off	6 Steady Run	47.5
11	29 LSD Run/Walk	Off	6 Tempo	8 Hills 9.5 km	8 Steady Run	Off	6 Steady Run	58.5
12	29 LSD Run/Walk	Off	6 Tempo	9 Hills 11 km	8 Steady Run	Off	6 Steady Run	60
13	32 LSD Run/Walk	Off	6 Tempo	10 Hills 12 km	8 Steady Run	Off	6 Steady Run	64
14	23 LSD Run/Walk	Off	6 Tempo	10 Fartlek	8 Steady Run	Off	6 Steady Run	53
15	29 LSD Run/Walk	Off	6 Tempo	10 Fartlek	10 Steady Run	Off	6 Steady Run	61
16	32 LSD Run/Walk	Off	6 Tempo	10 Fartlek	10 Steady Run	Off	6 Steady Run	64
17	23 LSD Run/Walk	Off	6 Tempo	10 Fartlek	10 Steady Run	Off	16 Race Pace	65
18	6 Run/Walk	Off	6 Tempo	10 Steady Run	Off	Off	3 Steady Run	25
19	Race - Marathon							42.2

Pace Schedule	Long Run (LSD)	Steady Run	Tempo/ Hills/Fartlek	Speed	Race	Walk Adjusted Race Pace
To Complete	8:37–9:37	8:37	7:48	6:51	7:49	7:36

Run/Walk Interval = 10 min Running/1 min Walking
Hills are a distance of 600 m

Marathon To Complete in 5:00
(Recorded in Kilometers)

Week	Sun	Mon	Tue	Wed	Thu	Fri	Sat	Total
1	10 LSD Run/Walk	Off	6 Tempo	10 Tempo	6 Steady Run	Off	6 Steady Run	38
2	10 LSD Run/Walk	Off	6 Tempo	10 Tempo	6 Steady Run	Off	6 Steady Run	38
3	13 LSD Run/Walk	Off	6 Tempo	10 Tempo	8 Steady Run	Off	6 Steady	43
4	13 LSD Run/Walk	Off	6 Tempo	10 Tempo	8 Steady Run	Off	6 Steady	43
5	16 LSD Run/Walk	Off	6 Tempo	10 Tempo	8 Steady Run	Off	6 Steady	46
6	16 LSD Run/Walk	Off	6 Tempo	10 Tempo	8 Steady Run	Off	6 Steady Run	46
7	19 LSD Run/Walk	Off	6 Tempo	4 Hills 5 km	8 Steady Run	Off	6 Steady Run	44
8	23 LSD Run/Walk	Off	6 Tempo	5 Hills 6 km	8 Steady Run	Off	6 Steady Run	49
9	26 LSD Run/Walk	Off	6 Tempo	6 Hills 7 km	8 Steady Run	Off	6 Steady Run	53
10	19 LSD Run/Walk	Off	6 Tempo	7 Hills 8.5 km	8 Steady Run	Off	6 Steady Run	47.5
11	29 LSD Run/Walk	Off	6 Tempo	8 Hills 9.5 km	8 Steady Run	Off	6 Steady Run	58.5
12	29 LSD Run/Walk	Off	6 Tempo	9 Hills 11 km	8 Steady Run	Off	6 Steady Run	60
13	32 LSD Run/Walk	Off	6 Tempo	10 Hills 12 km	8 Steady Run	Off	6 Steady Run	64
14	23 LSD Run/Walk	Off	6 Tempo	10 Fartlek	8 Steady Run	Off	6 Steady Run	53
15	29 LSD Run/Walk	Off	6 Tempo	10 Fartlek	10 Steady Run	Off	6 Steady Run	61
16	32 LSD Run/Walk	Off	6 Tempo	10 Fartlek	10 Steady Run	Off	6 Steady Run	64
17	23 LSD Run/Walk	Off	6 Tempo	10 Fartlek	10 Steady Run	Off	16 Race Pace	65
18	6 Steady Run	Off	6 Race Pace	10 Race Pace	Off	Off	3 Steady Run	25
19	Race - Marathon							42.2

Pace Schedule	Long Run (LSD)	Steady Run	Tempo/ Hills/Fartlek	Speed	Race	Walk Adjusted Race Pace
To Complete 5:00	7:52–8:49	7:52	7:07	6:14	7:07	6:52

Run/Walk Interval = 10 min Running/1 min Walking
Hills are a distance of 600 m

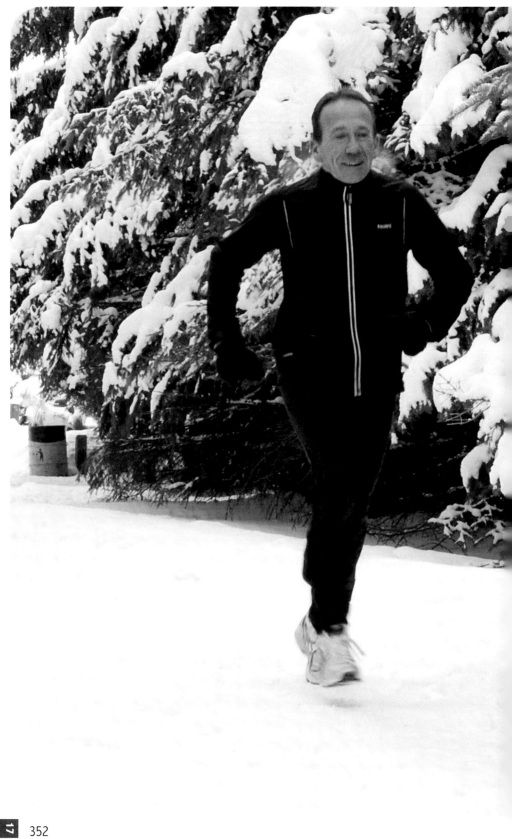

Marathon To Complete in 4:45
(Recorded in Kilometers)

Week	Sun	Mon	Tue	Wed	Thu	Fri	Sat	Total
1	10 LSD Run/Walk	Off	6 Tempo	10 Tempo	6 Steady Run	Off	6 Steady Run	38
2	10 LSD Run/Walk	Off	6 Tempo	10 Tempo	6 Steady Run	Off	6 Steady Run	38
3	13 LSD Run/Walk	Off	6 Tempo	10 Tempo	8 Steady Run	Off	6 Steady Run	43
4	13 LSD Run/Walk	Off	6 Tempo	10 Tempo	8 Steady Run	Off	6 Steady Run	43
5	16 LSD Run/Walk	Off	6 Tempo	10 Tempo	8 Steady Run	Off	6 Steady Run	46
6	16 LSD Run/Walk	Off	6 Tempo	10 Tempo	8 Steady Run	Off	6 Steady Run	46
7	19 LSD Run/Walk	Off	6 Tempo	4 Hills 5 km	8 Steady Run	Off	6 Steady Run	44
8	23 LSD Run/Walk	Off	6 Tempo	5 Hills 6 km	8 Steady Run	Off	6 Steady Run	49
9	26 LSD Run/Walk	Off	6 Tempo	6 Hills 7 km	8 Steady Run	Off	6 Steady Run	53
10	19 LSD Run/Walk	Off	6 Tempo	7 Hills 8.5 km	8 Steady Run	Off	6 Steady Run	47.5
11	29 LSD Run/Walk	Off	6 Tempo	8 Hills 9.5 km	8 Steady Run	Off	6 Steady Run	58.5
12	29 LSD Run/Walk	Off	6 Tempo	9 Hills 11 km	8 Steady Run	Off	6 Steady Run	60
13	32 LSD Run/Walk	Off	6 Tempo	10 Hills 12 km	8 Steady Run	Off	6 Steady Run	64
14	23 LSD Run/Walk	Off	6 Tempo	10 Fartlek	8 Steady Run	Off	6 Steady Run	53
15	29 LSD Run/Walk	Off	6 Tempo	10 Fartlek	10 Steady Run	Off	6 Steady Run	61
16	32 LSD Run/Walk	Off	6 Tempo	10 Fartlek	10 Steady Run	Off	6 Steady Run	64
17	23 LSD Run/Walk	Off	6 Tempo	10 Fartlek	10 Steady Run	Off	16 Race Pace	65
18	6 Steady Run	Off	6 Race Pace	10 Race Pace	Off	Off	3 Steady Run	25
19	Race - Marathon							42.2

Pace Schedule	Long Run (LSD)	Steady Run	Tempo/ Hills/Fartlek	Speed	Race	Walk Adjusted Race Pace
To Complete 4:45	7:30–8:25	7:30	6:47	5:56	6:45	6:31

Run/Walk Interval = 10 min Running/1 min Walking
Hills are a distance of 600 m

Week	Sun	Mon	Tue	Wed	Thu	Fri	Sat	Total
1	10 LSD Run/Walk	Off	6 Tempo	10 Tempo	6 Steady Run	Off	6 Steady Run	38
2	10 LSD Run/Walk	Off	6 Tempo	10 Tempo	6 Steady Run	Off	6 Steady Run	38
3	13 LSD Run/Walk	Off	6 Tempo	10 Tempo	8 Steady Run	Off	6 Steady Run	43
4	13 LSD Run/Walk	Off	6 Tempo	10 Tempo	8 Steady Run	Off	6 Steady Run	43
5	16 LSD Run/Walk	Off	6 Tempo	10 Tempo	8 Steady Run	Off	6 Steady Run	46
6	16 LSD Run/Walk	Off	6 Tempo	10 Tempo	8 Steady Run	Off	6 Steady Run	46
7	19 LSD Run/Walk	Off	6 Tempo	4 Hills 5 km	8 Steady Run	Off	6 Steady Run	44
8	23 LSD Run/Walk	Off	6 Tempo	5 Hills 6 km	8 Steady Run	Off	6 Steady Run	49
9	26 LSD Run/Walk	Off	6 Tempo	6 Hills 7 km	8 Steady Run	Off	6 Steady Run	53
10	19 LSD Run/Walk	Off	6 Tempo	7 Hills 8.5 km	8 Steady Run	Off	6 Steady Run	47.5
11	29 LSD Run/Walk	Off	6 Tempo	8 Hills 9.5 km	8 Steady Run	Off	6 Steady Run	58.5
12	29 LSD Run/Walk	Off	6 Tempo	9 Hills 11 km	8 Steady Run	Off	6 Steady Run	60
13	32 LSD Run/Walk	Off	6 Tempo	10 Hills 12 km	8 Steady Run	Off	6 Steady Run	64
14	23 LSD Run/Walk	Off	6 Tempo	10 Fartlek	8 Steady Run	Off	6 Steady Run	53
15	29 LSD Run/Walk	Off	6 Tempo	10 Fartlek	10 Steady Run	Off	6 Steady Run	61
16	32 LSD Run/Walk	Off	6 Tempo	10 Fartlek	10 Steady Run	Off	6 Steady Run	64
17	23 LSD Run/Walk	Off	6 Tempo	10 Fartlek	10 Steady Run	Off	16 Race Pace	65
18	6 LSD Run/Walk	Off	6 Race Pace	10 Race Pace	Off	Off	3 Steady Run	25
19	Race - Marathon							42.2

Pace Schedule	Long Run (LSD)	Steady Run	Tempo/ Hills/Fartlek	Speed	Race	Walk Adjusted Race Pace
To Complete 4:30	7:08–8:00	7:08	6:26	5:37	6:24	6:09

Run/Walk Interval = 10 min Running/1 min Walking
Hills are a distance of 600 m

Marathon To Complete in 4:15
(Recorded in Kilometers)

Week	Sun	Mon	Tue	Wed	Thu	Fri	Sat	Total
1	10 LSD Run/Walk	Off	6 Tempo	10 Tempo	6 Steady Run	Off	6 Steady Run	38
2	10 LSD Run/Walk	Off	6 Tempo	10 Tempo	6 Steady Run	Off	6 Steady Run	38
3	13 LSD Run/Walk	Off	6 Tempo	10 Tempo	8 Steady Run	Off	6 Steady Run	43
4	13 LSD Run/Walk	Off	6 Tempo	10 Tempo	8 Steady Run	Off	6 Steady Run	43
5	16 LSD Run/Walk	Off	6 Tempo	10 Tempo	8 Steady Run	Off	6 Steady Run	46
6	16 LSD Run/Walk	Off	6 Tempo	10 Tempo	8 Steady Run	Off	6 Steady Run	46
7	19 LSD Run/Walk	Off	6 Tempo	4 Hills 5 km	8 Steady Run	Off	6 Steady Run	44
8	23 LSD Run/Walk	Off	6 Tempo	5 Hills 6 km	8 Steady Run	Off	6 Steady Run	49
9	26 LSD Run/Walk	Off	6 Tempo	6 Hills 7 km	10 Steady Run	Off	6 Steady Run	55
10	19 LSD Run/Walk	Off	6 Tempo	7 Hills 8.5 km	10 Steady Run	Off	6 Steady Run	49.5
11	29 LSD Run/Walk	Off	6 Tempo	8 Hills 9.5 km	10 Steady Run	Off	6 Steady Run	60.5
12	29 LSD Run/Walk	Off	6 Tempo	9 Hills 11 km	10 Steady Run	Off	6 Steady Run	62
13	32 LSD Run/Walk	Off	6 Tempo	10 Hills 12 km	10 Steady Run	Off	6 Steady Run	66
14	23 LSD Run/Walk	Off	6 Tempo	10 Fartlek	10 Steady Run	Off	6 Steady Run	55
15	29 LSD Run/Walk	Off	6 Tempo	10 Fartlek	10 Steady Run	Off	6 Steady Run	61
16	32 LSD Run/Walk	Off	6 Tempo	10 Fartlek	10 Steady Run	Off	6 Steady Run	64
17	23 LSD Run/Walk	Off	6 Tempo	10 Fartlek	10 Steady Run	Off	16 Race Pace	65
18	6 LSD Run/Walk	Off	6 Race Pace	10 Race Pace	Off	Off	3 Steady Run	25
19	Race - Marathon							42.2

Pace Schedule	Long Run (LSD)	Steady Run	Tempo/ Hills/Fartlek	Speed	Race	Walk Adjusted Race Pace
To Complete 4:15	6:45–7:35	6:45	6:05	5:19	6:03	5:47

Run/Walk Interval = 10 min Running/1 min Walking
Hills are a distance of 600 m

Marathon To Complete in 4:00
(Recorded in Kilometers)

Week	Sun	Mon	Tue	Wed	Thu	Fri	Sat	Total
1	10 LSD Run/Walk	Off	6 Tempo	10 Tempo	6 Steady Run	Off	6 Steady Run	38
2	10 LSD Run/Walk	Off	6 Tempo	10 Tempo	6 Steady Run	Off	6 Steady Run	38
3	13 LSD Run/Walk	Off	6 Tempo	10 Tempo	8 Steady Run	Off	6 Steady Run	43
4	13 LSD Run/Walk	Off	6 Tempo	10 Tempo	8 Steady Run	Off	6 Steady Run	43
5	16 LSD Run/Walk	Off	6 Tempo	10 Tempo	8 Steady Run	Off	6 Steady Run	46
6	16 LSD Run/Walk	Off	6 Tempo	10 Tempo	8 Steady Run	Off	6 Stead Run	46
7	19 LSD Run/Walk	Off	6 Tempo	4 Hills 5 km	8 Steady Run	Off	6 Steady Run	44
8	23 LSD Run/Walk	Off	6 Tempo	5 Hills 6 km	8 Steady Run	Off	6 Steady Run	49
9	26 LSD Run/Walk	Off	6 Tempo	6 Hills 7 km	10 Steady Run	Off	6 Steady Run	55
10	19 LSD Run/Walk	Off	6 Tempo	7 Hills 8.5 km	10 Steady Run	Off	6 Steady Run	49.5
11	29 LSD Run/Walk	Off	6 Tempo	8 Hills 9.5 km	10 Steady Run	Off	6 Steady Run	60.5
12	29 LSD Run/Walk	Off	6 Tempo	9 Hills 11 km	10 Steady Run	Off	6 Steady Run	62
13	32 LSD Run/Walk	Off	6 Tempo	10 Hills 12 km	10 Steady Run	Off	6 Steady Run	66
14	23 LSD Run/Walk	Off	6 Tempo	10 Fartlek	10 Steady Run	Off	6 Steady Run	55
15	29 LSD Run/Walk	Off	6 Tempo	10 Fartlek	10 Steady Run	Off	6 Steady Run	61
16	32 LSD Run/Walk	Off	6 Tempo	10 Fartlek	10 Steady Run	Off	6 Steady Run	64
17	23 LSD Run/Walk	Off	6 Tempo	10 Fartlek	10 Steady Run	Off	16 Race Pace	65
18	6 Steady Run	Off	6 Race Pace	10 Race Pace	Off	Off	3 Steady Run	25
19	Race - Marathon							42.2

Pace Schedule	Long Run (LSD)	Steady Run	Tempo/ Hills/Fartlek	Speed	Race	Walk Adjusted Race Pace
To Complete 4:00	6:22–7:11	6:22	5:44	5:00	5:41	5:26

Run/Walk Interval = 10 min Running/1 min Walking
Hills are a distance of 600 m

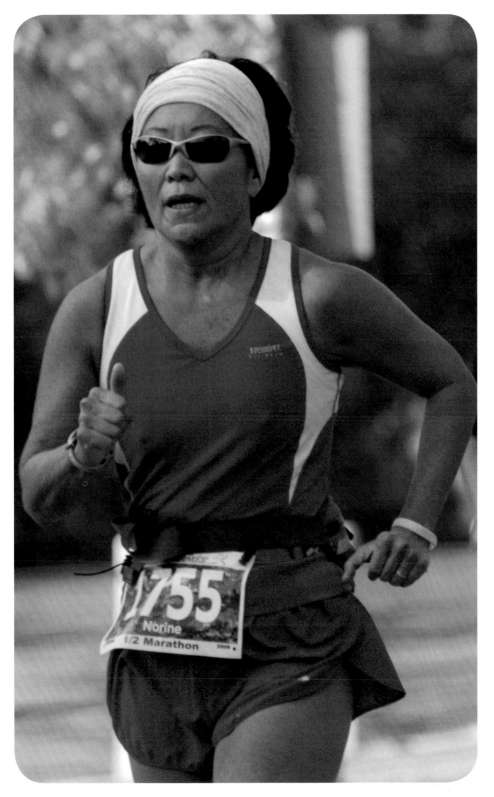

(Recorded in Kilometers)

Week	Sun	Mon	Tue	Wed	Thu	Fri	Sat	Total
1	10 LSD Run/Walk	Off	6 Tempo	10 Tempo	8 Steady Run	10 Steady Run	6 Steady Run	50
2	13 LSD Run/Walk	Off	6 Tempo	10 Tempo	8 Steady Run	10 Steady Run	6 Steady Run	53
3	13 LSD Run/Walk	Off	6 Tempo	10 Tempo	8 Steady Run	10 Steady Run	6 Steady Run	53
4	13 LSD Run/Walk	Off	6 Tempo	10 Tempo	8 Steady Run	10 Steady Run	6 Steady Run	53
5	16 LSD Run/Walk	Off	6 Tempo	10 Tempo	8 Steady Run	10 Steady Run	6 Steady Run	56
6	16 LSD Run/Walk	Off	6 Tempo	10 Tempo	8 Steady Run	10 Steady Run	6 Steady Run	56
7	19 LSD Run/Walk	Off	6 Tempo	4 Hills 5 km	8 Steady Run	10 Steady Run	6 Steady Run	54
8	23 LSD Run/Walk	Off	10 Tempo	5 Hills 6 km	6 Steady Run	10 Steady Run	6 Steady Run	61
9	26 LSD Run/Walk	Off	10 Tempo	6 Hills 7 km	6 Steady Run	10 Steady Run	6 Steady Run	65
10	19 LSD Run/Walk	Off	10 Tempo	7 Hills 8.5 km	6 Steady Run	10 Steady Run	6 Steady Run	59.5
11	29 LSD Run/Walk	Off	6 Tempo	8 Hills 9.5 km	8 Steady Run	10 Steady Run	6 Steady Run	68.5
12	29 LSD Run/Walk	Off	6 Tempo	9 Hills 11 km	6 Steady Run	10 Steady Run	6 Steady Run	68
13	32 LSD Run/Walk	Off	6 Tempo	10 Hills 12 km	6 Steady Run	10 Steady Run	6 Steady Run	72
14	23 LSD Run/Walk	Off	6 Tempo	Speed 2 X 1.6 km 9 km	8 Steady Run	10 Steady Run	6 Steady Run	62
15	29 LSD Run/Walk	Off	6 Tempo	Speed 3 X 1.6 km 11 km	6 Steady Run	10 Steady Run	6 Steady Run	68
16	32 LSD Run/Walk	Off	6 Tempo	Speed 4 X 1.6 km 12 km	6 Steady Run	10 Steady Run	6 Steady Run	72
17	23 LSD Run/Walk	Off	6 Tempo	Speed 5 X 1.6 km 14 km	6 Steady Run	10 Steady Run	16 Race Pace	75
18	6 LSD Run/Walk	Off	6 Race Pace	10 Race Pace	Off	Off	3 Steady Run	25
19	Race - Marathon							42.2

Pace Schedule	Long Run (LSD)	Steady Run	Tempo/ Hills/Fartlek	Speed	Race	Walk Adjusted Race Pace
To Complete 3:45	6:00–6:45	6:00	5:24	4:42	5:20	5:05

Run/Walk Interval = 10 min Running/1 min Walking
Hills are a distance of 600 m

Marathon To Complete in 3:30
(Recorded in Kilometers)

Week	Sun	Mon	Tue	Wed	Thu	Fri	Sat	Total
1	10 LSD Run/Walk	Off	8 Tempo	10 Steady Run	10 Fartlek	8 Steady Run	8 Steady Run	54
2	13 LSD Run/Walk	Off	8 Tempo	10 Steady Run	10 Fartlek	8 Steady Run	8 Steady Run	57
3	13 LSD Run/Walk	Off	8 Tempo	10 Steady Run	10 Fartlek	8 Steady Run	8 Steady Run	57
4	13 LSD Run/Walk	Off	8 Tempo	10 Steady Run	10 Fartlek	8 Steady Run	8 Steady Run	57
5	16 LSD Run/Walk	Off	8 Tempo	10 Steady Run	10 Fartlek	8 Steady Run	8 Steady Run	60
6	16 LSD Run/Walk	Off	8 Tempo	10 Steady Run	10 Fartlek	8 Steady Run	8 Steady Run	60
7	19 LSD Run/Walk	Off	8 Tempo	4 Hills 5 km	8 Steady Run	10 Fartlek	8 Steady Run	58
8	23 LSD Run/Walk	Off	8 Tempo	5 Hills 6 km	8 Steady Run	10 Fartlek	8 Steady Run	63
9	26 LSD Run/Walk	Off	8 Tempo	6 Hills 7 km	8 Steady Run	10 Fartlek	8 Steady Run	67
10	19 LSD Run/Walk	Off	8 Tempo	7 Hills 8.5 km	8 Steady Run	10 Fartlek	8 Steady Run	61.5
11	29 LSD Run/Walk	Off	8 Tempo	8 Hills 9.5 km	8 Steady Run	10 Fartlek	8 Steady Run	72.5
12	29 LSD Run/Walk	Off	8 Tempo	9 Hills 11 km	8 Steady Run	10 Fartlek	8 Steady Run	74
13	32 LSD Run/Walk	Off	8 Tempo	10 Hills 12 km	8 Steady Run	10 Fartlek	8 Steady Run	78
14	23 LSD Run/Walk	Off	8 Tempo	Speed 2 X 1.6 km 9 km	8 Steady Run	10 Fartlek	8 Steady Run	66
15	29 LSD Run/Walk	Off	8 Tempo	Speed 3 X 1.6 km 11 km	8 Steady Run	10 Fartlek	8 Steady Run	74
16	32 LSD Run/Walk	Off	8 Tempo	Speed 4 X 1.6 km 12 km	8 Steady Run	10 Fartlek	8 Steady Run	78
17	23 LSD Run/Walk	Off	8 Tempo	Speed 5 X 1.6 km 14 km	8 Steady Run	10 Fartlek	16 Race Pace	79
18	6 Steady Run	Off	8 Race Pace	10 Race Pace	Off	Off	3 Steady Run	27
19	Race - Marathon							42.2

Pace Schedule	Long Run (LSD)	Steady Run	Tempo/ Hills/Fartlek	Speed	Race	Walk Adjusted Race Pace
To Complete 3:30	5:37–6:20	5:37	5:03	4:24	4:59	4:43

Run/Walk Interval = 10 min Running/1 min Walking
Hills are a distance of 600 m

Marathon To Complete in 3:10
(Recorded in Kilometers)

Week	Sun	Mon	Tue	Wed	Thu	Fri	Sat	Total
1	10 LSD Steady	Off	8 Tempo	10 Steady Run	13 Fartlek	13 Steady Run	8 Steady Run	62
2	13 LSD Steady	Off	8 Tempo	10 Steady Run	13 Fartlek	13 Steady Run	8 Steady Run	65
3	16 LSD Steady	Off	8 Tempo	10 Steady Run	13 Fartlek	13 Steady Run	8 Steady Run	68
4	16 LSD Steady	Off	8 Tempo	10 Steady Run	13 Fartlek	13 Steady Run	8 Steady Run	68
5	19 LSD Steady	Off	8 Tempo	10 Steady Run	13 Fartlek	13 Steady Run	8 Steady Run	71
6	23 LSD Steady	Off	8 Tempo	10 Steady Run	13 Fartlek	13 Steady Run	8 Steady Run	75
7	26 LSD Steady	Off	8 Tempo	4 Hills 5 km	8 Steady Run	13 Fartlek	8 Steady Run	68
8	26 LSD Steady	Off	11 Tempo	5 Hills 6 km	8 Steady Run	13 Fartlek	8 Steady Run	72
9	29 LSD Steady	Off	11 Tempo	6 Hills 7 km	8 Steady Run	13 Fartlek	8 Steady Run	76
10	23 LSD Steady	Off	11 Tempo	7 Hills 8.5 km	8 Steady Run	13 Fartlek	8 Steady Run	71.5
11	29 LSD Steady	Off	8 Tempo	8 Hills 9.5 km	8 Steady Run	13 Fartlek	8 Steady Run	75.5
12	32 LSD Steady	Off	8 Tempo	9 Hills 11 km	8 Steady Run	13 Fartlek	8 Steady Run	80
13	32 LSD Steady	Off	8 Tempo	10 Hills 12 km	8 Steady Run	13 Fartlek	8 Steady Run	81
14	22 LSD Steady	Off	8 Tempo	Speed 2 x 1.6 km 9 km	8 Steady Run	13 Fartlek	8 Steady Run	68
15	32 LSD Steady	Off	8 Tempo	Speed 3 x 1.6 km 11 km	8 Steady Run	13 Fartlek	8 Steady Run	80
16	32 LSD Steady	Off	8 Tempo	Speed 4 x 1.6 km 12 km	8 Steady Run	13 Fartlek	8 Steady Run	81
17	23 LSD Steady	Off	8 Tempo	Speed 5 x 1.6 km 14 km	8 Steady Run	13 Fartlek	16 Race Pace	82
18	6 LSD Steady	Off	8 Race Pace	10 Race Pace	Off	Off	3 Steady Run	27
19	Race - Marathon							42.2

Pace Schedule	Long Run (LSD)	Steady Run	Tempo/ Hills/Fartlek	Speed	Race	Walk Adjusted Race Pace
To Complete 3:10	5:06–5:46	5:06	4:35	3:59	4:30	4:15

Run/Walk Interval = 10 min Running/1 min Walking
Hills are a distance of 600 m

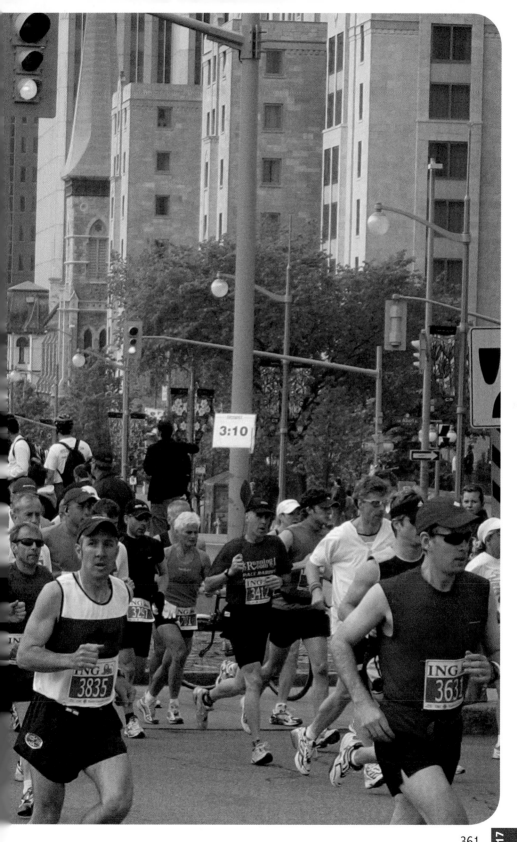

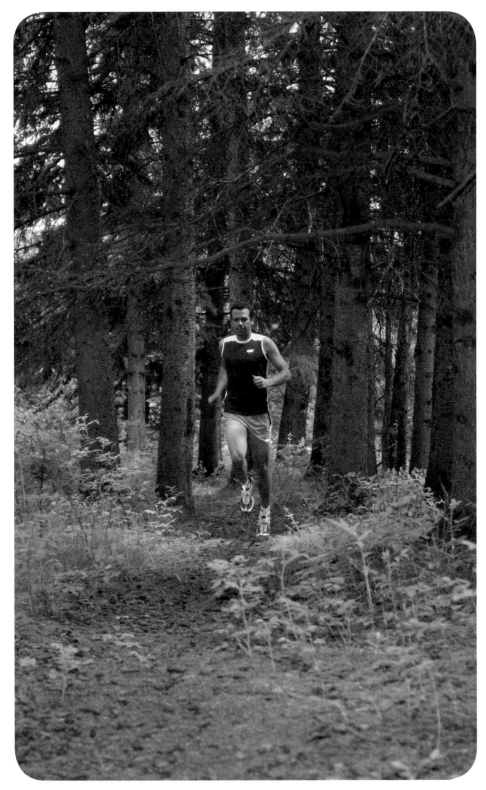

Marathon To Complete in 3:00
(Recorded in Kilometers)

Week	Sun	Mon	Tue	Wed	Thu	Fri	Sat	Total
1	16 LSD Steady	Off	13 Tempo	10 Steady Run	13 Fartlek	13 Steady Run	8 Steady Run	73
2	16 LSD Steady	8 Steady Run	13 Tempo	10 Steady Run	13 Fartlek	13 Steady Run	8 Steady Run	81
3	19 LSD Steady	8 Steady Run	13 Tempo	10 Steady Run	13 Fartlek	13 Steady Run	8 Steady Run	84
4	19 LSD Steady	Off	13 Tempo	4 Hills 5 km	8 Steady Run	13 Fartlek	8 Steady Run	66
5	23 LSD Steady	8 Steady Run	13 Tempo	5 Hills 6 km	8 Steady Run	13 Fartlek	8 Steady Run	79
6	23 LSD Steady	8 Steady Run	13 Tempo	5 Hills 6 km	8 Steady Run	13 Fartlek	8 Steady Run	79
7	26 LSD Steady	Off	13 Tempo	6 Hills 7 km	8 Steady Run	13 Fartlek	8 Steady Run	75
8	29 LSD Steady	8 Steady Run	13 Tempo	6 Hills 7 km	8 Steady Run	13 Fartlek	8 Steady Run	86
9	23 LSD Steady	8 Steady Run	13 Tempo	7 Hills 8.5 km	8 Steady Run	13 Fartlek	8 Steady Run	81.5
10	29 LSD Steady	8 Steady Run	13 Tempo	7 Hills 8.5 km	8 Steady Run	13 Fartlek	8 Steady Run	87.5
11	32 LSD Steady	Off	13 Tempo	8 Hills 9.5 km	8 Steady Run	13 Fartlek	8 Steady Run	83.5
12	32 LSD Steady	8 Steady Run	13 Tempo	9 Hills 11 km	8 Steady Run	13 Fartlek	8 Steady Run	93
13	32 LSD Steady	8 Steady Run	13 Tempo	10 Hills 12 km	8 Steady Run	13 Fartlek	8 Steady Run	94
14	22 LSD Steady	8 Steady Run	13 Tempo	Speed 2 X 1.6 km 9 km	8 Steady Run	13 Fartlek	8 Steady Run	81
15	32 LSD Steady	8 Steady Run	13 Tempo	Speed 3 X 1.6 km 11 km	8 Steady Run	13 Fartlek	8 Steady Run	93
16	32 LSD Steady	8 Steady Run	13 Tempo	Speed 4 X 1.6 km 12 km	8 Steady Run	13 Fartlek	8 Steady Run	94
17	23 LSD Steady	8 Steady Run	13 Tempo	Speed 5 X 1.6 km 14 km	8 Steady Run	13 Fartlek	16 Race Pace	95
18	6 Steady Run	Off	13 Race Pace	10 Race Pace	Off	Off	3 Steady Run	32
19	Race - Marathon							42.2

Pace Schedule	Long Run (LSD)	Steady Run	Tempo/ Hills/Fartlek	Speed	Race	Walk Adjusted Race Pace
To Complete 3:00	4:51–5:29	4:51	4:21	3:47	4:16	4:02

Run/Walk Interval = 10 min Running/1 min Walking
Hills are a distance of 600 m

Week	Sun	Mon	Tue	Wed	Thu	Fri	Sat	Total
1	6 LSD Run/Walk	Off	4 Tempo	6 Tempo	4 Steady Run	Off	4 Steady Run	24
2	6 LSD Run/Walk	Off	4 Tempo	6 Tempo	4 Steady Run	Off	4 Steady Run	24
3	8 LSD Run/Walk	Off	4 Tempo	6 Tempo	5 Steady Run	Off	4 Steady Run	27
4	8 LSD Run/Walk	Off	4 Tempo	6 Tempo	5 Steady Run	Off	4 Steady Run	27
5	10 LSD Run/Walk	Off	4 Tempo	6 Tempo	5 Steady Run	Off	4 Steady Run	29
6	10 LSD Run/Walk	Off	4 Tempo	6 Tempo	5 Steady Run	Off	4 Steady Run	29
7	12 LSD Run/Walk	Off	4 Tempo	4 Hills 3 mi	5 Steady Run	Off	4 Steady Run	28
8	14 LSD Run/Walk	Off	4 Tempo	5 Hills 4 mi	5 Steady Run	Off	4 Steady Run	31
9	16 LSD Run/Walk	Off	4 Tempo	6 Hills 4.5 mi	5 Steady Run	Off	4 Steady Run	33.5
10	12 LSD Run/Walk	Off	4 Tempo	7 Hills 5 mi	5 Steady Run	Off	4 Steady Run	30
11	18 LSD Run/Walk	Off	4 Tempo	8 Hills 6 mi	5 Steady Run	Off	4 Steady Run	37
12	18 LSD Run/Walk	Off	4 Tempo	9 Hills 7 mi	5 Steady Run	Off	4 Steady Run	38
13	20 LSD Run/Walk	Off	4 Tempo	10 Hills 7.5 mi	5 Steady Run	Off	4 Steady Run	40.5
14	14 LSD Run/Walk	Off	4 Tempo	6 Fartlek	5 Steady Runl	Off	4 Steady Run	33
15	18 LSD Run/Walk	Off	4 Tempo	6 Fartlek	6 Steady Run	Off	4 Steady Run	38
16	20 LSD Run/Walk	Off	4 Tempo	6 Fartlek	6 Steady Run	Off	4 Steady Run	40
17	14 LSD Run/Walk	Off	4 Tempo	6 Fartlek	6 Steady Run	Off	10 Race Pace	40
18	4 LSD Run/Walk	Off	4 Tempo	6 Steady Run	Off	Off	2 Steady Run	16
19	Race - Marathon							26.2

Pace Schedule	Long Run (LSD)	Steady Run	Tempo/ Hills/Fartlek	Speed	Race	Walk Adjusted Race Pace
To Complete	13:52–15:28	13:52	12:34	11:02	12:36	12:10

Run/Walk Interval = 10 min Running/1 min Walking
Hills are a distance of 600 m

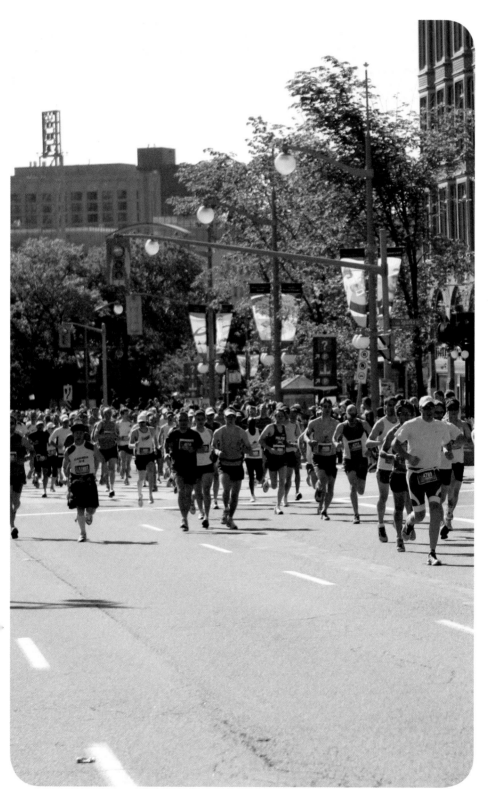

Week	Sun	Mon	Tue	Wed	Thu	Fri	Sat	Total
1	6 LSD Run/Walk	Off	4 Tempo	6 Tempo	4 Steady Run	Off	4 Steady Run	24
2	6 LSD Run/Walk	Off	4 Tempo	6 Tempo	4 Steady Run	Off	4 Steady Run	24
3	8 LSD Run/Walk	Off	4 Tempo	6 Tempo	5 Steady Run	Off	4 Steady	27
4	8 LSD Run/Walk	Off	4 Tempo	6 Tempo	5 Steady Run	Off	4 Steady	27
5	10 LSD Run/Walk	Off	4 Tempo	6 Tempo	5 Steady Run	Off	4 Steady	29
6	10 LSD Run/Walk	Off	4 Tempo	6 Tempo	5 Steady Run	Off	4 Steady Run	29
7	12 LSD Run/Walk	Off	4 Tempo	4 Hills 3 mi	5 Steady Run	Off	4 Steady Run	28
8	14 LSD Run/Walk	Off	4 Tempo	5 Hills 4 mi	5 Steady Run	Off	4 Steady Run	31
9	16 LSD Run/Walk	Off	4 Tempo	6 Hills 4.5 mi	5 Steady Run	Off	4 Steady Run	33.5
10	12 LSD Run/Walk	Off	4 Tempo	7 Hills 5 mi	5 Steady Run	Off	4 Steady Run	30
11	18 LSD Run/Walk	Off	4 Tempo	8 Hills 6 mi	5 Steady Run	Off	4 Steady Run	37
12	18 LSD Run/Walk	Off	4 Tempo	9 Hills 7 mi	5 Steady Run	Off	4 Steady Run	38
13	20 LSD Run/Walk	Off	4 Tempo	10 Hills 7.5 mi	5 Steady Run	Off	4 Steady Run	40.5
14	14 LSD Run/Walk	Off	4 Tempo	6 Fartlek	5 Steady Run	Off	4 Steady Run	33
15	18 LSD Run/Walk	Off	4 Tempo	6 Fartlek	6 Steady Run	Off	4 Steady Run	38
16	20 LSD Run/Walk	Off	4 Tempo	6 Fartlek	6 Steady Run	Off	4 Steady Run	40
17	14 LSD Run/Walk	Off	4 Tempo	6 Fartlek	6 Steady Run	Off	10 Race Pace	40
18	4 Steady Run	Off	4 Race Pace	6 Race Pace	Off	Off	2 Steady Run	16
19	Race - Marathon							26.2

Pace Schedule	Long Run (LSD)	Steady Run	Tempo/ Hills/Fartlek	Speed	Race	Walk Adjusted Race Pace
To Complete 5:00	12:40–14:11	12:40	11:28	10:02	11:27	11:02

Run/Walk Interval = 10 min Running/1 min Walking
Hills are a distance of 600 m

Marathon To Complete in 4:45
(Recorded in Miles)

Week	Sun	Mon	Tue	Wed	Thu	Fri	Sat	Total
1	6 LSD Run/Walk	Off	4 Tempo	6 Tempo	4 Steady Run	Off	4 Steady Run	24
2	6 LSD Run/Walk	Off	4 Tempo	6 Tempo	4 Steady Run	Off	4 Steady Run	24
3	8 LSD Run/Walk	Off	4 Tempo	6 Tempo	5 Steady Run	Off	4 Steady Run	27
4	8 LSD Run/Walk	Off	4 Tempo	6 Tempo	5 Steady Run	Off	4 Steady Run	27
5	10 LSD Run/Walk	Off	4 Tempo	6 Tempo	5 Steady Run	Off	4 Steady Run	29
6	10 LSD Run/Walk	Off	4 Tempo	6 Tempo	5 Steady Run	Off	4 Steady Run	29
7	12 LSD Run/Walk	Off	4 Tempo	4 Hills 3 mi	5 Steady Run	Off	4 Steady Run	28
8	14 LSD Run/Walk	Off	4 Tempo	5 Hills 4 mi	5 Steady Run	Off	4 Steady Run	31
9	16 LSD Run/Walk	Off	4 Tempo	6 Hills 4.5 mi	5 Steady Run	Off	4 Steady Run	33.5
10	12 LSD Run/Walk	Off	4 Tempo	7 Hills 5 mi	5 Steady Run	Off	4 Steady Run	30
11	18 LSD Run/Walk	Off	4 Tempo	8 Hills 6 mi	5 Steady Run	Off	4 Steady Run	37
12	18 LSD Run/Walk	Off	4 Tempo	9 Hills 7 mi	5 Steady Run	Off	4 Steady Run	38
13	20 LSD Run/Walk	Off	4 Tempo	10 Hills 7.5 mi	5 Steady Run	Off	4 Steady Run	40.5
14	14 LSD Run/Walk	Off	4 Tempo	6 Fartlek	5 Steady Run	Off	4 Steady Run	33
15	18 LSD Run/Walk	Off	4 Tempo	6 Fartlek	6 Steady Run	Off	4 Steady Run	38
16	20 LSD Run/Walk	Off	4 Tempo	6 Fartlek	6 Steady Run	Off	4 Steady Run	40
17	14 LSD Run/Walk	Off	4 Tempo	6 Fartlek	6 Steady Run	Off	10 Race Pace	40
18	4 Steady Run	Off	4 Race Pace	6 Race Pace	Off	Off	2 Steady Run	16
19	Race - Marathon							26.2

Pace Schedule	Long Run (LSD)	Steady Run	Tempo/ Hills/Fartlek	Speed	Race	Walk Adjusted Race Pace
To Complete 4:45	12:04–13:32	12:04	10:54	9:32	10:52	10:29

Run/Walk Interval = 10 min Running/1 min Walking
Hills are a distance of 600 m

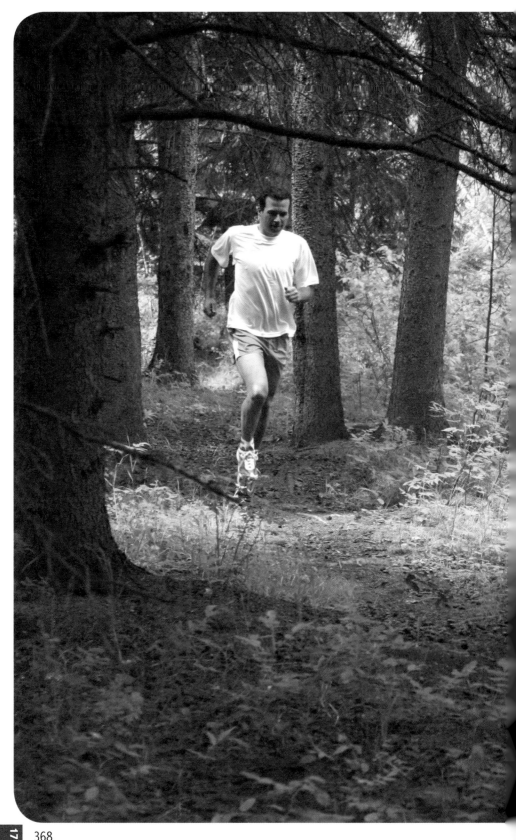

Marathon To Complete in 4:30
(Recorded in Miles)

Week	Sun	Mon	Tue	Wed	Thu	Fri	Sat	Total
1	6 LSD Run/Walk	Off	4 Tempo	6 Tempo	4 Steady Run	Off	4 Steady Run	24
2	6 LSD Run/Walk	Off	4 Tempo	6 Tempo	4 Steady Run	Off	4 Steady Run	24
3	8 LSD Run/Walk	Off	4 Tempo	6 Tempo	5 Steady Run	Off	4 Steady Run	27
4	8 LSD Run/Walk	Off	4 Tempo	6 Tempo	5 Steady Run	Off	4 Steady Run	27
5	10 LSD Run/Walk	Off	4 Tempo	6 Tempo	5 Steady Run	Off	4 Steady Run	29
6	10 LSD Run/Walk	Off	4 Tempo	6 Tempo	5 Steady Run	Off	4 Steady Run	29
7	12 LSD Run/Walk	Off	4 Tempo	4 Hills 3 mi	5 Steady Run	Off	4 Steady Run	28
8	14 LSD Run/Walk	Off	4 Tempo	5 Hills 4 mi	5 Steady Run	Off	4 Steady Run	31
9	16 LSD Run/Walk	Off	4 Tempo	6 Hills 4.5 mi	5 Steady Run	Off	4 Steady Run	33.5
10	12 LSD Run/Walk	Off	4 Tempo	7 Hills 5 mi	5 Steady Run	Off	4 Steady Run	30
11	18 LSD Run/Walk	Off	4 Tempo	8 Hills 6 mi	5 Steady Run	Off	4 Steady Run	37
12	18 LSD Run/Walk	Off	4 Tempo	9 Hills 7 mi	5 Steady Run	Off	4 Steady Run	38
13	20 LSD Run/Walk	Off	4 Tempo	10 Hills 7.5 mi	5 Steady Run	Off	4 Steady Run	40.5
14	14 LSD Run/Walk	Off	4 Tempo	6 Fartlek	5 Steady Run	Off	4 Steady Run	33
15	18 LSD Run/Walk	Off	4 Tempo	6 Fartlek	6 Steady Run	Off	4 Steady Run	38
16	20 LSD Run/Walk	Off	4 Tempo	6 Fartlek	6 Steady Run	Off	4 Steady Run	40
17	14 LSD Run/Walk	Off	4 Tempo	6 Fartlek	6 Steady Run	Off	10 Race Pace	40
18	3.5 LSD Run/Walk	Off	4 Race Pace	6 Race Pace	Off	Off	2 Steady Run	15.5
19	Race - Marathon							26.2

Pace Schedule	Long Run (LSD)	Steady Run	Tempo/ Hills/Fartlek	Speed	Race	Walk Adjusted Race Pace
To Complete 4:30	11:28–12:53	11:28	10:21	9:03	10:18	9:54

Run/Walk Interval = 10 min Running/1 min Walking
Hills are a distance of 600 m

Week	Sun	Mon	Tue	Wed	Thu	Fri	Sat	Total
1	6 LSD Run/Walk	Off	4 Tempo	6 Tempo	4 Steady Run	Off	4 Steady Run	24
2	6 LSD Run/Walk	Off	4 Tempo	6 Tempo	4 Steady Run	Off	4 Steady Run	24
3	8 LSD Run/Walk	Off	4 Tempo	6 Tempo	5 Steady Run	Off	4 Steady Run	27
4	8 LSD Run/Walk	Off	4 Tempo	6 Tempo	5 Steady Run	Off	4 Steady Run	27
5	10 LSD Run/Walk	Off	4 Tempo	6 Tempo	5 Steady Run	Off	4 Steady Run	29
6	10 LSD Run/Walk	Off	4 Tempo	6 Tempo	5 Steady Run	Off	4 Steady Run	29
7	12 LSD Run/Walk	Off	4 Tempo	4 Hills 3 mi	5 Steady Run	Off	4 Steady Run	28
8	14 LSD Run/Walk	Off	4 Tempo	5 Hills 4 mi	5 Steady Run	Off	4 Steady Run	31
9	16 LSD Run/Walk	Off	4 Tempo	6 Hills 4.5 mi	6 Steady Run	Off	4 Steady Run	34.5
10	12 LSD Run/Walk	Off	4 Tempo	7 Hills 5 mi	6 Steady Run	Off	4 Steady Run	31
11	18 LSD Run/Walk	Off	4 Tempo	8 Hills 6 mi	6 Steady Run	Off	4 Steady Run	38
12	18 LSD Run/Walk	Off	4 Tempo	9 Hills 7 mi	6 Steady Run	Off	4 Steady Run	39
13	20 LSD Run/Walk	Off	4 Tempo	10 Hills 7.5 mi	6 Steady Run	Off	4 Steady Run	41.5
14	14 LSD Run/Walk	Off	4 Tempo	6 Fartlek	6 Steady Run	Off	4 Steady Run	34
15	18 LSD Run/Walk	Off	4 Tempo	6 Fartlek	6 Steady Run	Off	4 Steady Run	38
16	20 LSD Run/Walk	Off	4 Tempo	6 Fartlek	6 Steady Run	Off	4 Steady Run	40
17	14 LSD Run/Walk	Off	4 Tempo	6 Fartlek	6 Steady Run	Off	10 Race Pace	40
18	4 LSD Run/Walk	Off	4 Race Pace	6 Race Pace	Off	Off	2 Steady Run	16
19	Race - Marathon							26.2

Pace Schedule	Long Run (LSD)	Steady Run	Tempo/ Hills/Fartlek	Speed	Race	Walk Adjusted Race Pace
To Complete 4:15	10:52–12:13	10:52	9:48	8:33	9:44	9:19

Run/Walk Interval = 10 min Running/1 min Walking
Hills are a distance of 600 m

Marathon To Complete in 4:00
(Recorded in Miles)

Week	Sun	Mon	Tue	Wed	Thu	Fri	Sat	Total
1	6 LSD Run/Walk	Off	4 Tempo	6 Tempo	4 Steady Run	Off	4 Steady Run	24
2	6 LSD Run/Walk	Off	4 Tempo	6 Tempo	4 Steady Run	Off	4 Steady Run	24
3	8 LSD Run/Walk	Off	4 Tempo	6 Tempo	5 Steady Run	Off	4 Steady Run	27
4	8 LSD Run/Walk	Off	4 Tempo	6 Tempo	5 Steady Run	Off	4 Steady Run	27
5	10 LSD Run/Walk	Off	4 Tempo	6 Tempo	5 Steady Run	Off	4 Steady Run	29
6	10 LSD Run/Walk	Off	4 Tempo	6 Tempo	5 Steady Run	Off	4 Steady Run	29
7	12 LSD Run/Walk	Off	4 Tempo	4 Hills 3 mi	5 Steady Run	Off	4 Steady Run	28
8	14 LSD Run/Walk	Off	4 Tempo	5 Hills 4 mi	5 Steady Run	Off	4 Steady Run	31
9	16 LSD Run/Walk	Off	4 Tempo	6 Hills 4.5 mi	6 Steady Run	Off	4 Steady Run	34.5
10	12 LSD Run/Walk	Off	4 Tempo	7 Hills 5 mi	6 Steady Run	Off	4 Steady Run	31
11	18 LSD Run/Walk	Off	4 Tempo	8 Hills 6 mi	6 Steady Run	Off	4 Steady Run	38
12	18 LSD Run/Walk	Off	4 Tempo	9 Hills 7 mi	6 Steady Run	Off	4 Steady Run	39
13	20 LSD Run/Walk	Off	4 Tempo	10 Hills 7.5 mi	6 Steady Run	Off	4 Steady Run	41.5
14	14 LSD Run/Walk	Off	4 Tempo	6 Fartlek	6 Steady Run	Off	4 Steady Run	34
15	18 LSD Run/Walk	Off	4 Tempo	6 Fartlek	6 Steady Run	Off	4 Steady Run	38
16	20 LSD Run/Walk	Off	4 Tempo	6 Fartlek	6 Steady Run	Off	4 Steady Run	40
17	14 LSD Run/Walk	Off	4 Tempo	6 Fartlek	6 Steady Run	Off	10 Race Pace	40
18	4 Steady Run	Off	4 Race Pace	6 Race Pace	Off	Off	2 Steady Run	16
19	Race - Marathon							26.2

Pace Schedule	Long Run (LSD)	Steady Run	Tempo/ Hills/Fartlek	Speed	Race	Walk Adjusted Race Pace
To Complete 4:00	10:15–11:33	10:15	9:14	8:03	9:09	8:45

Run/Walk Interval = 10 min Running/1 min Walking
Hills are a distance of 600 m

17 The Marathon

Week	Sun	Mon	Tue	Wed	Thu	Fri	Sat	Total
1	6 LSD Run/Walk	Off	4 Tempo	6 Tempo	5 Steady Run	6 Steady Run	4 Steady Run	31
2	8 LSD Run/Walk	Off	4 Tempo	6 Tempo	5 Steady Run	6 Steady Run	4 Steady Run	33
3	8 LSD Run/Walk	Off	4 Tempo	6 Tempo	5 Steady Run	6 Steady Run	4 Steady Run	33
4	8 LSD Run/Walk	Off	4 Tempo	6 Tempo	5 Steady Run	6 Steady Run	4 Steady Run	33
5	10 LSD Run/Walk	Off	4 Tempo	6 Tempo	5 Steady Run	6 Steady Run	4 Steady Run	35
6	10 LSD Run/Walk	Off	4 Tempo	6 Tempo	5 Steady Run	6 Steady Run	4 Steady Run	35
7	12 LSD Run/Walk	Off	4 Tempo	4 Hills 3 mi	5 Steady Run	6 Steady Run	4 Steady Run	34
8	14 LSD Run/Walk	Off	6 Tempo	5 Hills 4 mi	4 Steady Run	6 Steady Run	4 Steady Run	38
9	16 LSD Run/Walk	Off	6 Tempo	6 Hills 4.5 mi	4 Steady Run	6 Steady Run	4 Steady Run	40.5
10	12 LSD Run/Walk	Off	6 Tempo	7 Hills 5 mi	4 Steady Run	6 Steady Run	4 Steady Run	37
11	18 LSD Run/Walk	Off	4 Tempo	8 Hills 6 mi	5 Steady Run	6 Steady Run	4 Steady Run	43
12	18 LSD Run/Walk	Off	4 Tempo	9 Hills 7 mi	4 Steady Run	6 Steady Run	4 Steady Run	43
13	20 LSD Run/Walk	Off	4 Tempo	10 Hills 7.5 mi	4 Steady Run	6 Steady Run	4 Steady Run	45.5
14	14 LSD Run/Walk	Off	4 Tempo	Speed 2 X 1 mi 6 mi	5 Steady Run	6 Steady Run	4 Steady Run	39
15	18 LSD Run/Walk	Off	4 Tempo	Speed 3 X 1 mi 7 mi	4 Steady Run	6 Steady Run	4 Steady Run	43
16	20 LSD Run/Walk	Off	4 Tempo	Speed 4 X 1 mi 8 mi	4 Steady Run	6 Steady Run	4 Steady Run	46
17	14 LSD Run/Walk	Off	4 Tempo	Speed 5 X 1 mi 9 mi	4 Steady Run	6 Steady Run	10 Race Pace	47
18	4 LSD Run/Walk	Off	4 Race Pace	6 Race Pace	Off	Off	2 Steady Run	16
19	Race - Marathon							26.2

Pace Schedule	Long Run (LSD)	Steady Run	Tempo/ Hills/Fartlek	Speed	Race	Walk Adjusted Race Pace
To Complete 3:45	9:39–10:52	9:39	8:41	7:34	8:35	8:10

Run/Walk Interval = 10 min Running/1 min Walking
Hills are a distance of 600 m

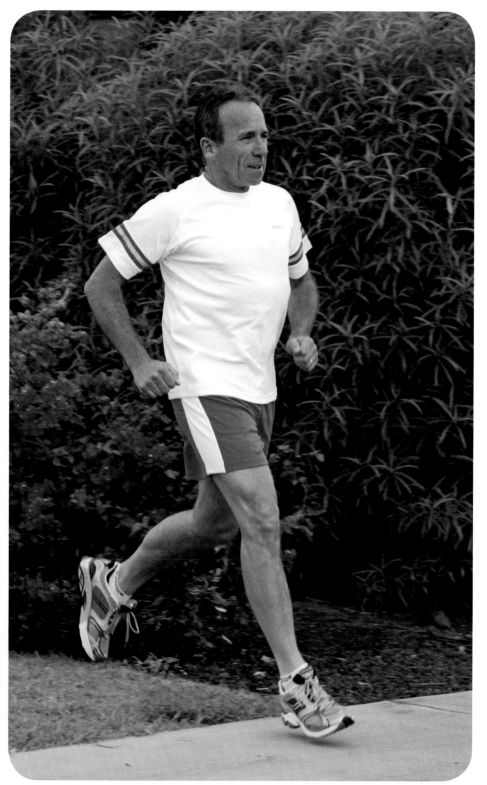

17 The Marathon

Marathon To Complete in 3:30
(Recorded in Miles)

Week	Sun	Mon	Tue	Wed	Thu	Fri	Sat	Total
1	6 LSD Run/Walk	Off	5 Tempo	6 Steady Run	6 Fartlek	5 Steady Run	5 Steady Run	33
2	8 LSD Run/Walk	Off	5 Tempo	6 Steady Run	6 Fartlek	5 Steady Run	5 Steady Run	35
3	8 LSD Run/Walk	Off	5 Tempo	6 Steady Run	6 Fartlek	5 Steady Run	5 Steady Run	35
4	8 LSD Run/Walk	Off	5 Tempo	6 Steady Run	6 Fartlek	5 Steady Run	5 Steady Run	35
5	10 LSD Run/Walk	Off	5 Tempo	6 Steady Run	6 Fartlek	5 Steady Run	5 Steady Run	37
6	10 LSD Run/Walk	Off	5 Tempo	6 Steady Run	6 Fartlek	5 Steady Run	5 Steady Run	37
7	12 LSD Run/Walk	Off	5 Tempo	4 Hills 3 mi	5 Steady Run	6 Fartlek	5 Steady Run	36
8	14 LSD Run/Walk	Off	5 Tempo	5 Hills 4 mi	5 Steady Run	6 Fartlek	5 Steady Run	39
9	16 LSD Run/Walk	Off	5 Tempo	6 Hills 4.5 mi	5 Steady Run	6 Fartlek	5 Steady Run	41.5
10	12 LSD Run/Walk	Off	5 Tempo	7 Hills 5 mi	5 Steady Run	6 Fartlek	5 Steady Run	38
11	18 LSD Run/Walk	Off	5 Tempo	8 Hills 6 mi	5 Steady Run	6 Fartlek	5 Steady Run	45
12	18 LSD Run/Walk	Off	5 Tempo	9 Hills 7 mi	5 Steady Run	6 Fartlek	5 Steady Run	46
13	20 LSD Run/Walk	Off	5 Tempo	10 Hills 7.5 mi	5 Steady Run	6 Fartlek	5 Steady Run	48.5
14	14 LSD Run/Walk	Off	5 Tempo	Speed 2 X 1 mi 6 mi	5 Steady Run	6 Fartlek	5 Steady Run	41
15	18 LSD Run/Walk	Off	5 Tempo	Speed 3 X 1mi 7 mi	5 Steady Run	6 Fartlek	5 Steady Run	46
16	20 LSD Run/Walk	Off	5 Tempo	Speed 4 X 1mi 8 mi	5 Steady Run	6 Fartlek	5 Steady Run	49
17	14 LSD Run/Walk	Off	5 Tempo	Speed 5 X 1 mi 9 mi	5 Steady Run	6 Fartlek	10 Race Pace	49
18	4 Steady Run	Off	5 Race Pace	6 Race Pace	Off	Off	2 Steady Run	17
19	Race - Marathon							26.2

Pace Schedule	Long Run (LSD)	Steady Run	Tempo/ Hills/Fartlek	Speed	Race	Walk Adjusted Race Pace
To Complete 3:30	9:02–10:12	9:02	8:07	7:04	8:01	7:36

Run/Walk Interval = 10 min Running/1 min Walking
Hills are a distance of 600 m

Marathon To Complete in 3:10
(Recorded in Miles)

Week	Sun	Mon	Tue	Wed	Thu	Fri	Sat	Total
1	6 LSD Run/Walk	Off	5 Tempo	6 Steady Run	8 Fartlek	8 Steady Run	5 Steady Run	38
2	8 LSD Run/Walk	Off	5 Tempo	6 Steady Run	8 Fartlek	8 Steady Run	5 Steady Run	40
3	10 LSD Run/Walk	Off	5 Tempo	6 Steady Run	8 Fartlek	8 Steady Run	5 Steady Run	42
4	10 LSD Run/Walk	Off	5 Tempo	6 Steady Run	8 Fartlek	8 Steady Run	5 Steady Run	42
5	12 LSD Run/Walk	Off	5 Tempo	6 Steady Run	8 Fartlek	8 Steady Run	5 Steady Run	44
6	14 LSD Run/Walk	Off	5 Tempo	6 Steady Run	8 Fartlek	8 Steady Run	5 Steady Run	46
7	16 LSD Run/Walk	Off	5 Tempo	4 Hills 3 mi	5 Steady Run	8 Fartlek	5 Steady Run	42
8	16 LSD Run/Walk	Off	7 Tempo	5 Hills 4 mi	5 Steady Run	8 Fartlek	5 Steady Run	45
9	18 LSD Run/Walk	Off	7 Tempo	6 Hills 4.5 mi	5 Steady Run	8 Fartlek	5 Steady Run	47.5
10	14 LSD Run/Walk	Off	7 Tempo	7 Hills 5 mi	5 Steady Run	8 Fartlek	5 Steady Run	44
11	18 LSD Run/Walk	Off	5 Tempo	8 Hills 6 mi	5 Steady Run	8 Fartlek	5 Steady Run	47
12	20 LSD Run/Walk	Off	5 Tempo	9 Hills 7 mi	5 Steady Run	8 Fartlek	5 Steady Run	50
13	20 LSD Run/Walk	Off	5 Tempo	10 Hills 7.5 mi	5 Steady Run	8 Fartlek	5 Steady Run	50.5
14	13.5 LSD Run/Walk	Off	5 Tempo	Speed 2 X 1 mi 6 mi	5 Steady Run	8 Fartlek	5 Steady Run	42.5
15	20 LSD Run/Walk	Off	5 Tempo	Speed 3 X 1mi 7 mi	5 Steady Run	8 Fartlek	5 Steady Run	50
16	20 LSD Run/Walk	Off	5 Tempo	Speed 4 X 1 mi 8 mi	5 Steady Run	8 Fartlek	5 Steady Run	51
17	14 LSD Run/Walk	Off	5 Tempo	Speed 5 X 1 mi 9 mi	5 Steady Run	8 Fartlek	10 Race Pace	51
18	4 Steady Run	Off	5 Race Pace	6 Race Pace	Off	Off	2 Steady Run	17
19	Race - Marathon							26.2

Pace Schedule	Long Run (LSD)	Steady Run	Tempo/ Hills/Fartlek	Speed	Race	Walk Adjusted Race Pace
To Complete 3:10	8:13–9:17	8:13	7:22	6:25	7:15	6:51

Run/Walk Interval = 10 min Running/1 min Walking
Hills are a distance of 600 m

Marathon To Complete in 3:00
(Recorded in Miles)

Week	Sun	Mon	Tue	Wed	Thu	Fri	Sat	Total
1	10 LSD Run/Walk	Off	8 Tempo	6 Steady Run	8 Fartlek	8 Steady Run	5 Steady Run	45
2	10 LSD Run/Walk	5 Steady Run	8 Tempo	6 Steady Run	8 Fartlek	8 Steady Run	5 Steady Run	50
3	12 LSD Run/Walk	5 Steady Run	8 Tempo	6 Steady Run	8 Fartlek	8 Steady Run	5 Steady Run	52
4	12 LSD Run/Walk	Off	8 Tempo	4 Hills 3 mi	8 Fartlek	8 Fartlek	5 Steady Run	44
5	14 LSD Run/Walk	5 Steady Run	8 Tempo	5 Hills 4 mi	5 Steady Run	8 Fartlek	5 Steady Run	49
6	14 LSD Run/Walk	5 Steady Run	8 Tempo	5 Hills 4 mi	5 Steady Run	8 Fartlek	5 Steady Run	49
7	16 LSD Run/Walk	Off	8 Tempo	6 Hills 4.5 mi	5 Steady Run	8 Fartlek	5 Steady Run	46.5
8	18 LSD Run/Walk	5 Steady Run	8 Tempo	6 Hills 4.5 mi	5 Steady Run	8 Fartlek	5 Steady Run	53.5
9	14 LSD Run/Walk	5 Steady Run	8 Tempo	7 Hills 5 mi	5 Steady Run	8 Fartlek	5 Steady Run	50
10	18 LSD Run/Walk	5 Steady Run	8 Tempo	7 Hills 5 mi	5 Steady Run	8 Fartlek	5 Steady Run	54
11	20 LSD Run/Walk	Off	8 Tempo	8 Hills 6 mi	5 Steady Run	8 Fartlek	5 Steady Run	52
12	20 LSD Run/Walk	5 Steady Run	8 Tempo	9 Hills 7 mi	5 Steady Run	8 Fartlek	5 Steady Run	58
13	20 LSD Run/Walk	5 Steady Run	8 Tempo	10 Hills 7.5 mi	5 Steady Run	8 Fartlek	5 Steady Run	58.5
14	13.5 LSD Run/Walk	5 Steady Run	8 Tempo	Speed 2 X 1mi 6 mi	5 Steady Run	8 Fartlek	5 Steady Run	50.5
15	20 LSD Run/Walk	5 Steady Run	8 Tempo	Speed 3 X 1mi 7 mi	5 Steady Run	8 Fartlek	5 Steady Run	58
16	20 LSD Run/Walk	5 Steady Run	8 Tempo	Speed 4 X 1mi 8 mi	5 Steady Run	8 Fartlek	5 Steady Run	59
17	14 LSD Run/Walk	5 Steady Run	8 Tempo	Speed 5 X 1mi 9 mi	5 Steady Run	8 Fartlek	10 Race Pace	59
18	4 Steady Run	Off	8 Race Pace	6 Race Pace	Off	Off	2 Steady Run	20
19	Race - Marathon							26.2

Pace Schedule	Long Run (LSD)	Steady Run	Tempo/ Hills/Fartlek	Speed	Race	Walk Adjusted Race Pace
To Complete 3:00	7:48–8:49	7:48	7:00	6:05	6:52	6:29

Run/Walk Interval = 10 min Running/1 min Walking
Hills are a distance of 600 m

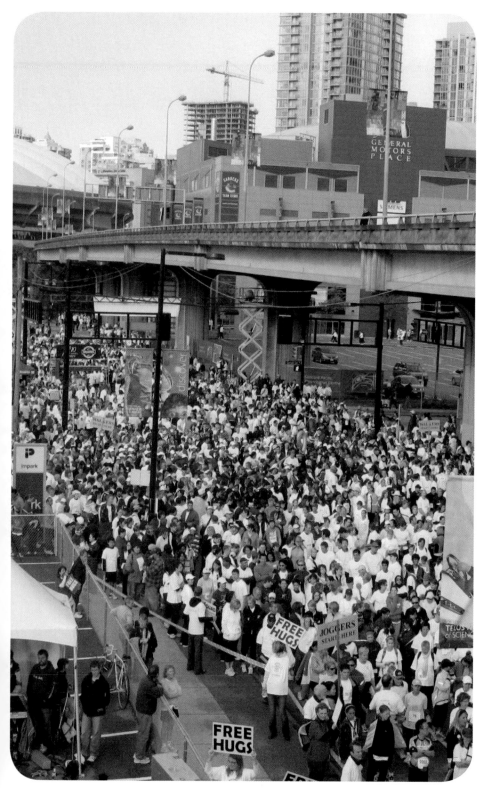

Race Tips

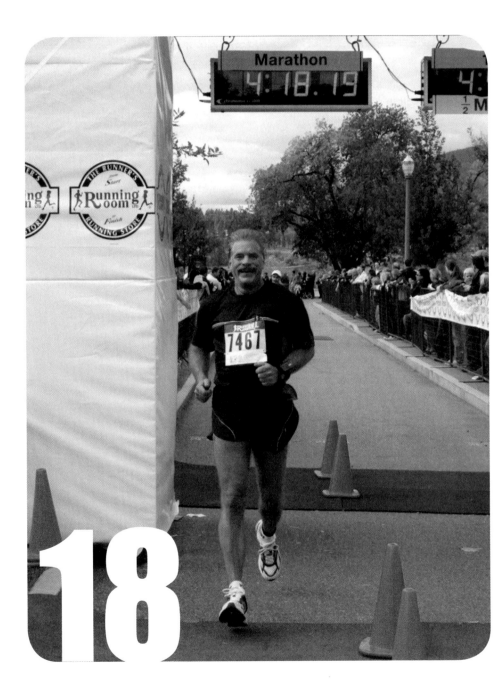

Race Day FAQ

Here are the two most frequently asked questions I get from anxious race participants:

How often should I race?

What is the best method of pacing during the race?

For the most part, the longer the race, the greater the stress endured by the runners. For the trained runner, the rule of one day recovery for every kilometer raced is an intelligent guide. A 5 K requires one week's recovery; 10 K racers can expect to run one every other weekend; half marathons one every two or three weeks; and full marathons one every month or two.

Your recovery time will be dependent on the intensity at which you race. The faster you race, the more recovery you will require.

The deep residual fatigue from racing will leave you heavy-legged and running flat if you attempt to race again after a hard effort.

The less training prior to the event, the more recovery time required by the athlete. Trust and respect your training and respect the distance you are racing. Adapt your training with a longer recovery time for the longer distances.

There are three strategies for race day:

1. Start hard and fast and fade in the later stages of the race.
2. Start slowly and run a faster second half of the race.
3. Run the whole race at a steady, consistent pace.

My recommendation is run the whole race at an even pace. This approach will, in theory, produce the best times for the runner. Start too fast and you will discover an early and deep fatigue created from early oxygen debt. Running the final stages of the race is a challenge because of the deep fatigue. For the best recovery, start slowly and build into the race. Your optimum time may not be achieved, but your post-race recovery will be improved. It makes for the most comfortable race. Even pacing will produce the best race results, which is the reason the Running Room produces race bracelets with even splits that include your walk breaks.

Race Day Preparation

For those of you planning to run a half or full marathon your last quality workout should be on the Saturday preceding the race. This workout should be done at a pace similar to what you will be targeting on race day. This is a high-quality workout that requires your discipline not to run faster than your targeted pace for the event. It is best to concentrate on your form and setting your targeted pace. Do not race or get in a race with one of your training partners. This workout prepares you for race day.

Starting on Monday you will begin to cut back your mileage in the taper phase of the program, some people feel very heavy and their disposition is down during the taper. Concentrate on the joy of less mileage and the fact that you have all this extra time to relax and enjoy the taper phase. This gradual easing up of your mileage allows your body to disperse the residual fatigue products that have been carried from one workout to the other, so that come race day your legs will have that extra snap to ensure your best performance. The most important day is two days prior to the race—take the day off and go to bed early and enjoy as much sleep as possible. Stay in bed, read, relax. Even if you can't sleep, stay in the prone position. It's the best way to get you ready for the race day. Remember, nothing you do in the final week will help you but everything you do can hinder your performance. The key is that quality training takes at least two weeks to improve your performance, but overtraining can affect your next day performance. So the best advice is to relax and enjoy the week and get plenty of rest.

Visualization is a key part of the week as you relax and think about your training and the goals you have set for the marathon. Read and enjoy some of your favorite music to motivate yourself. Relaxation is the key.

Things to Focus On

Principles

- Relaxation
- Efficiency of form
- Economy of effort and motion
- Staying within yourself
- Maintaining a positive attitude
- Staying with a successful program

Moving the Wall?

- The length of your longest run in the last two to three weeks
- Shorten it by running too fast, lengthen it by running slower

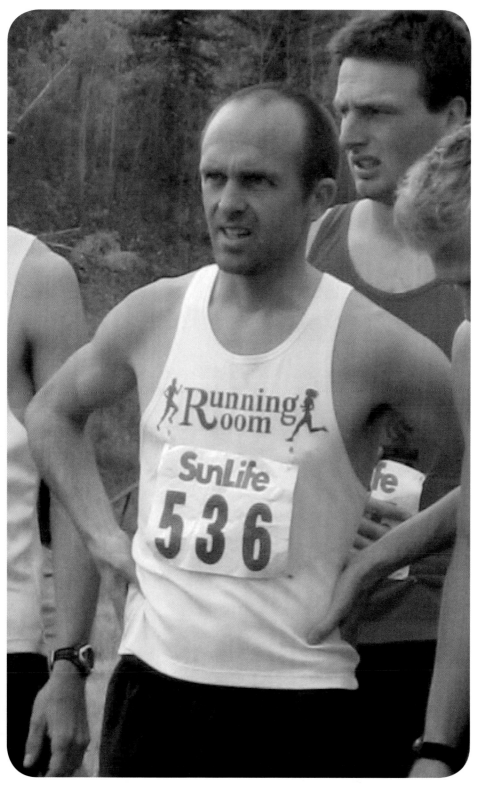

Drinking

- Caffeine and alcohol will dehydrate you
- Small amounts of water (4–6 oz.) every hour you are awake
- Morning of the race: 4–6 oz. every 30 minutes
- Sip water at regular intervals

Eating

- Stay with a program that has worked—don't try anything new for the race
- Last big meal: lunch the day before
- Don't eat too much the night before
- The carbohydrate drinks are easier to digest than solid food

Pacing

- Stay within yourself
- Run an even pace throughout the entire marathon
- Alternate running for 10 minutes with a brisk walk for 1 minute through the entire marathon to maintain an even pace

Striding

- Don't overstride!
- Keep stride short going uphill
- Avoid temptation to overstride going downhill
- As you tire, concentrate on shorter stride, quicker turnover

Be Positive

- Everyone gets negative messages
- Have a strategy for projecting positive thoughts to confront the negative
- Words or phrases relating to the past successes will bring future success
- Learn how to shift into the right brain

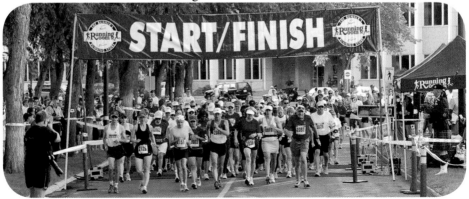

Have Fun!

+ If you enjoy this run, you'll want to do it again, and you'll get better
+ Talk to people, share stories, enjoy the course

Race Day Tip

Rule #1: Relax!

The most important advice we can give to first-time racers is relax. Enjoy yourself. Racing is meant to be a stimulating, memorable experience. It helps to keep things in proper perspective and to use common sense. Even if something goes wrong on your first race— say you get stomach cramps or your shoelaces come untied—it's not the end of the world. You'll live to run and race again.

Race Day Tips for a Great Time

1. Your Goal:

Your goal is simply to finish. Your first race is for the experience, not for the competition. Run it knowing your time will be a personal record.

2. Eating and Drinking:

On race day, don't eat or drink anything out of the ordinary. This is not the time to experiment, no matter what you may have heard about athletic superfoods. Nor do you have to be concerned with the carbohydrate loading you've heard is favored by marathon runners. In fact, for your last meal (taken at least three hours before the race start) you might want to eat less than normal, since nervousness could upset your digestive system.

In warm weather, drink 500 ml of water 1 hour before the start, and continue drinking every 10 minutes during the race. You should practice the same on hot-weather training runs. Don't ever forget: heat can kill. Don't try to be a hero in hot races. Adjust you expectations and drink fluids at regular intervals in relationship to the water loss from your perspiration and breathing.

3. Strategy:

Planning your race strategy in advance will build your confidence. Break the course into small sections, making sure you know where hills and other key landmarks are located. It's particularly important that you know the last half kilometer of the course. On race day, it's a good idea to warm up by running over the last half kilometer of the course to set a few landmarks in your mind.

4. Getting Ready:

When you arrive at the race, don't be intimidated by what you see other runners doing. Many of them are preparing for a hard effort, whereas you want to make sure you save your energy for a more comfortable race. Do some walking, some stretching and some light jogging to loosen up.

5. Lining Up and Starting:

Make your way to the back of the starting pack where you won't get caught in the starting sprint. Many marathons have pacing groups, join the group running at the pace you feel comfortable with. Begin slowly. Don't worry about all the runners who take off ahead of you. It's far better to start slowly and catch up later than to begin too fast and be passed by hundreds of runners after a km or two. Once you get room to run freely, move into your normal, relaxed training pace. Maintain that pace (it should be one that allows you to talk comfortably) at least until you reach the halfway mark. Then if you feel strong and want to pick it up, go ahead—but make sure you do it gradually. If you reach a point of struggle, slow down to regather your strength.

6. Walking:

Run 10 minutes and walk 1 minute. Nowhere on the entry form does it say that you can't walk. So if you feel the need to, take walking breaks, particularly on the hills. But never stop moving forward unless you are hurt. Disguise your walking breaks by calling them water breaks. Since drinking water is so important during a race, many runners stop and drink when they get to the water tables. You can do the same—getting water plus the rest you need—and no one will be the wiser.

7. Finishing:

Keep your pace constant and steady. Don't sprint hard at the finish line. That is not only unwise, but it can be dangerous. Concentrate on finishing with a good, relaxed, strong form.

8. Recovery:

After you finish, be sure you walk around for a cooldown. Drink plenty of fluids, especially if it's a hot day. Change into dry clothes as soon as possible, and when you get home, stretch your muscles thoroughly after taking a cool shower. Don't do any running the next day, although it's OK to swim or bike. You might find it hard to contain your newfound racing enthusiasm, but to run on leg muscles that might be sore would only tempt injury.

Where to go with your training post race

After training meticulously for 18 weeks to a year for your race, many ask, "Now what?" To avoid suffering from post-race syndrome following your big race, set some new goals for yourself. First and foremost, do not lose the new level of fitness you have attained through your recent training cycle.

This is the time to think of maintaining the level of performance your body has reached as an athlete. The key to maintaining your level of fitness is a maintenance program while you contemplate a new goal.

For the 10 K racer, keep your long run in the 8 km (5 mi.) range and use your new level of fitness to race some fast 5 Ks. Your base training is in place, and you can use the 5 K races to improve your overall self-assurance and speed.

Half marathon runners can schedule a long run of 12 km (7.5 mi.) to maintain their endurance. The half marathon runner on the off weekends can schedule in some 10 K races to work on your strength, speed and self-confidence.

The marathon runner can keep their long run in the range of 16 km (10 mi.). In addition to keeping you in shape, 16 km every other weekend can be a great way to abbreviate your training for the next marathon. By maintaining your long run in the 16 km range you can prepare for the next marathon in as little as 12 weeks. Or you can prepare for a half marathon in six weeks.

Give yourself adequate recovery from your race—two weeks for a 10 K race, three weeks for a half marathon and four weeks for a marathon—before you race any distance or do any high-quality running. You can run, but think of your runs as "massage type" running to loosen the legs.

Select your races sparingly and aim for great results. Run some for time goal achievement and run some for fun. A race can provide the stimulation to compete to your very best level of performance or it can awaken you to the joy of running and the fun, camaraderie and festivities of race day.

Mental Preparation

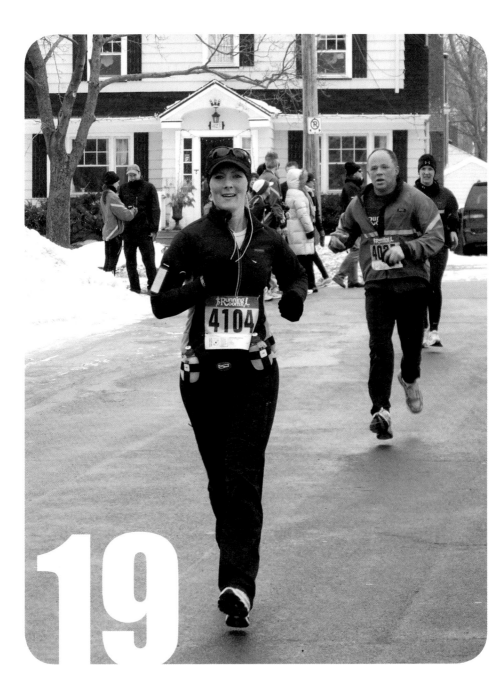

19

What makes elite athletes perform to gold medal standard? What is that motives them to perform better than their peers? If you study their training programs, most are similar to those used by folks they are competing with. Ask most coaches and they will quickly tell you that their primary job is to mentally prepare the athlete for competition.

Not every athlete can have the benefit of an individual coach, but the advice in this chapter can give you a tremendous advantage over your individual competitors. It will increase your personal performance, whether your target is to beat the last time you ran a particular distance or to run a challenging new distance.

Relaxation

To start with, get yourself in a comfortable space. It could be sitting in a big soft chair, lying on your hotel bed or lying on the floor. The key is to spend a few moments just getting comfortable and relaxed. Put on some music that relaxes you. Take your mind off your worries or stress. Close your eyes and listen to the music, to the individual instruments, notes and sounds that make up the music selection. Focus on the music, thinking only of the music and your body lying in the comfortable position.

Think of your body as a fine-tuned musical instrument ready to perform. Think back to all the positive training experiences you have had in preparation for the event. Think only positive thoughts. Relax and listen to your breathing. Breathe in, hold, breathe out. Feel the air filling your lungs that have trained and are now ready for the challenge of the day. Feel your heart rate lowering as you listen to the sound of your own breathing. Turn down the music and focus in on your healthy, fit body.

Start with the top of your head. Relax. Let the stress of the day leave your mind. Breath in, hold, breath out. Feel your forehead relax and the frown line between your eyes relax and disappear. Your eyelids are heavy and relaxed. Feel your jaw grow heavy with the relaxation. Open your mouth in a relaxed yawn. Roll your neck to relax the muscles of the neck and shoulders. If you are right-handed, start to concentrate on the right side of your body. Feel it getting heavy and relaxed. If you are left-handed concentrate on the left side of your body.

Feel your shoulders heavy with the relaxed, peaceful feeling. Think of your body: strong, fit and ready. Your shoulders are now relaxed. Breathe in, hold, breathe out. Feel the air filling your lungs. Feel your abdominal muscles relaxing as you

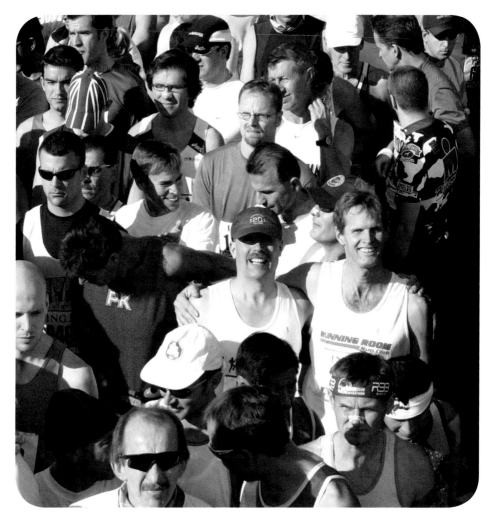

breathe out. Your back is relaxed; you feel the tenseness slowly leave the muscles, leaving them heavy and relaxed. Feel your hips heavy against the floor. Relax. Breathe in, hold, breathe out.

Feel your hamstrings and quadriceps, strong and ready from the months of training, now relaxed and rested. Feel the calf muscles that give you that special leveraged drive in your running, now relaxed and still. Breathe in, hold, breathe out. Roll your ankles and feel the relaxation all through your feet—the feet that are ready to carry you to your goal. Breathe in, hold, breathe out.

Listen to the stillness. Breathe in, hold, breathe out. There is no sound, just the rhythmic breathing of your relaxed body as your mind focuses on your visualization of the race.

IO K Visualization

It is the morning of the race. You see yourself walking to the start area where runners have started to gather. You see the activity throughout the area: the race pick-up area with runners standing in line for their kits; some runners are stretching; some are jogging lightly; others are doing short wind sprints to ready themselves for the competition. You are quiet as you approach. You hear the sound of the race announcer calling for people to pick up their kits in time for the start. You hear the sound of other runners laughing and talking. You sense the excitement in the air, mixed with the early sunrise and the smell of athletic rub. The smell of fresh coffee in the volunteer area reminds you that it is time for you to rise to the occasion.

You know you are ready. You have done your training. You repeat your power words: you are strong, you are in control, you are fit, you feel good.

You see yourself talking to some running buddies as you give your running gear a final check. You smile to yourself as you hear some of the familiar pre-race comments: "I'm only doing this as a training run." "My knee is sore. I think I'll just jog this one." "Haven't been training much—that old Achilles has been acting up." "I had planned on racing this but I think I'll just take it easy, the hip's a little sore." You smile once again because you know all of the minor aches and pains disappear as soon as the start gun goes off. You take that last drink of water as you head to the start line to join the group of people already in position. Runners are now all standing, nervously awaiting the start. Some are quiet; some are laughing nervously; others are staring and holding their wrists, ready to start their watches. All are awaiting the signal to start.

The announcer gives out some last-minute instructions and counts down to the start. The horn goes off and you start running.

You have seeded yourself well, but there is still a little bumping as the occasional runner brushes by you. You get around a couple of runners who are still walking and talking as you breeze by them. You gradually pick up the pace and then settle into your own rhythm. You are fluid and strong. You feel good. It is a good day as the warmth of the sun warms your shoulders and a light breeze cools your forehead.

You pass the 1-km mark and you hear the time being called. You're right on target. You now concentrate on keeping the pace. You remember that the first third of the race you should be holding back; the middle third will feel just right;

you will have to work hard in the final third. The key is an even pace—not even effort, but a modified effort throughout the race. You know your training has taught you the importance of holding back at the start and how to time the extra effort that is needed in the later stages of the race. You remember practicing this in your training.

As you continue past the 1-km mark you are now running in a group of several other runners. The occasional runner passes the group and the group passes a small group of three runners talking and joking to one another that they started a little fast. You know you started in control and are right on target. More importantly, you feel great. You're strong—you have done the training.

You pass the 2-km mark and you do your system check: your breathing is relaxed and controlled, your form is strong, your leg turnover is fast and fluid. You are looking and feeling good. You have settled into a comfortable, rhythmic pace. This is the part of the race that feels good; the pace seems easy as you flow along with the group of runners.

You spot the 5-km mark—halfway there and you are feeling strong and in control. As you pass the 5-km mark, you notice you are pulling away from some of the runners. Your group is growing smaller. You hold your pace, check your time. You are right on target as you enter the second half of the race. You check your form in your shadow on the road and focus on your stride, which is strong. Your breathing is even and you say to yourself: l am strong, I am in control, I am fit, I am focused, I feel good, I am fast.

You come up on the 8-km mark, the point where most runners start to question why they are racing: Why not just run? Who needs to race when you can just run for fun? You laugh and smile as you recognize the familiar negative thoughts that come at this part of the race. You know you are in control and focus on your form. Listen to your footsteps, light on the ground. You say to yourself, Hang in there, you're looking good. Concentrate on shortening your stride and increasing your leg turnover. I feel better already. I can do it.

One mile to go and you are feeling strong. You know you are going to hit your target. You're fatigued but you know you can dig a little deeper and achieve that goal. Your stride improves as you can hear the noise of the finish line. You push yourself, increasing the tempo. You pass one, then two more runners. You're fit. You feel your breathing becoming labored. Breathe in, fill your lungs with energy, breathe out, feel the negative feeling leave, feel the strong sense of well-being.

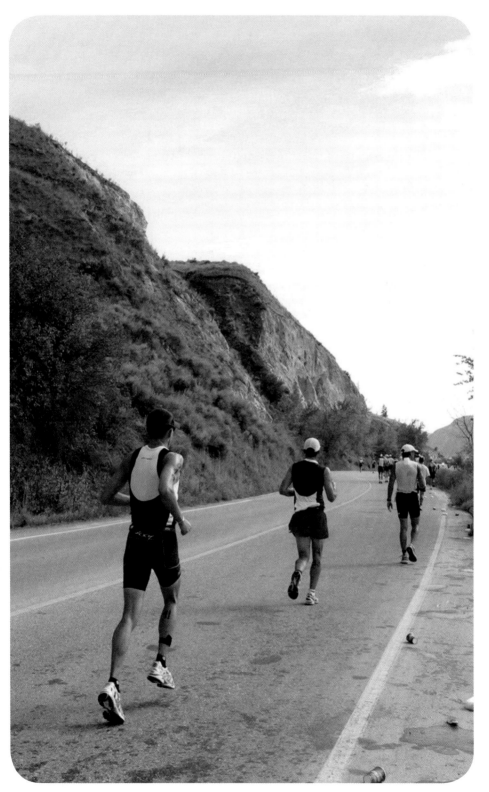

Adrenaline kicks in as you hear and see the finish line. Your stride opens up as you pass a couple of runners accelerating towards the finish line. Your form is fluid and strong. You knew you could do it! Your leg turnover increases rapidly. It is like you are running on hot coals. Your pace continues to quicken. You pass two more runners as you near the finish line. The announcer calls out your name and time. You have done it—you hit your target. You slow to a walk in the finish area, your hands on your hips as you thank your body for the effort. You give thanks to the good health and hard training that has enabled you to complete the race and be rewarded with this euphoric sense of well-being and accomplishment. You know that with the proper physical training and the right mental preparation, you can achieve any goal you set for yourself; that reality is a creation of the way we see ourselves in our own minds.

Positive Self-Suggestions
+ I am in control of my own thinking, my own focus, my own life.
+ I control my own thoughts and emotions and direct the whole pattern of my performance, health and life.
+ I am fully capable of achieving the goals I set for my self today. They are within my control.
+ I learn from problems or setbacks, and through them I see room for improvement and opportunities for personal growth.
+ Every day in some way I am better, wiser, more adaptable, more focused, more confident, more in control.

Marathon Visualization

The day you have been looking for has finally arrived. After months of self-discipline and hard training, it is the morning of the marathon. You are rested and well hydrated. You are making your way to the start/finish area. You know you are ready. You are in the midst of other runners, some talking, some silent and pensive, others laughing and joking. You can feel and sense the excitement in the area. There is a mixture of nervous adrenaline and anticipation as the sun begins to brighten and warm the area. The grass is damp with the morning dew as you set you sports bag down and pull off your sweat top to start your prerace preparation. The music and noise is interrupted with the announcer calling out last-minute instructions to the runners. You take your final drink of water while zipping up your bag to turn it over to the check-in folks.

You make your way into the crowd to seed yourself with the other runner who will be running about the same pace as you plan to run. Suddenly, it is quiet for a

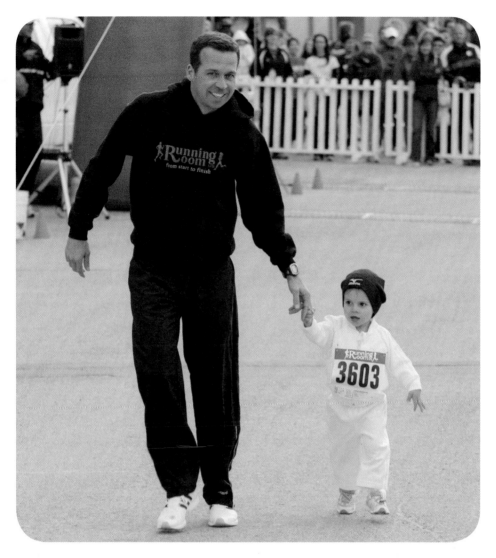

moment as you hear the announcer call, "Five…Four…Three…Two…One…"

The horn sounds and you are off. At first, it is more of a shuffle than a run as laughter and noise again fill the air. You hear a mixture of race chatter, both from the runners and the people lining the course at the start.

Slowly, the crowd around you starts to open up and you start to find that familiar stride. Your breathing is now relaxed and you feel comfortable as you make the first turn on the course and head down the long straightaway. You are passed by a couple of runners who are joking with one another as they find their own pace. Just as you pass a small pack of five or six runners you realize you are already

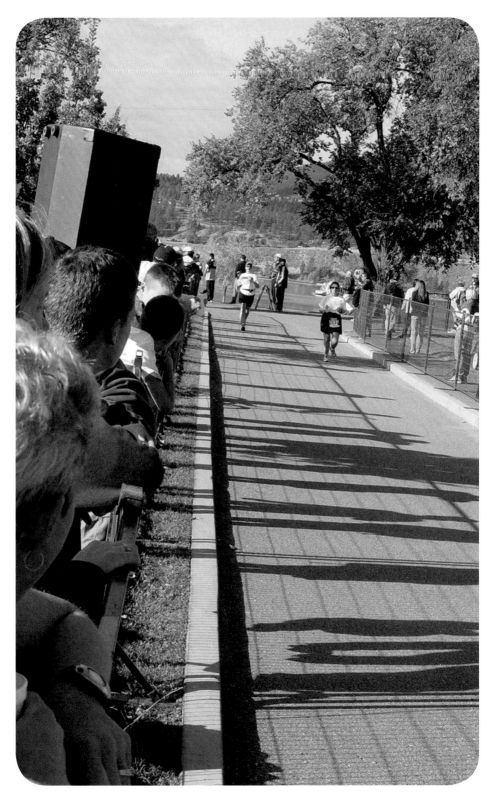

at the 1-km mark. Are you right on target, did you start a little fast, or did the crowd slow you? Either way, this is only a benchmark to adjust your pace. You are feeling good. You think back to the months of training, some of it done with the group but a good portion done on your own. You know that those runs will pay big dividends to you today in your marathon.

At the 2-km mark you do your first systems check. Are you relaxed? Is your breathing relaxed and are you taking deep, full breaths? Is your chest out, hips forward? Have you started to sweat yet? Is your head straight, eyes up the road, spotting a runner ahead? Arms relaxed and in tune with the rhythm of your push off each ankle? You feel good and you are going to do your best.

At the 5 km mark you come out of a park area and start up the hill. You shorten your stride slightly, just like you did in all of those hill repeat sessions. This is a piece of cake; you did 10 to 12 hill repeats on a lot steeper hills than this. You continue with even effort as you head up the hill, passing a runner who appears to be struggling, while you are smooth and fluid. As you near the top of the hill you automatically push through the crest, just like in your training. You are now back on a flat stretch and regain the old familiar rhythm. You think back to those long runs with your training buddies. This is just another long run. Stay relaxed and enjoy the sights and sounds.

As you pass through a water station, there are people dressed in costumes cheering you on. Whoever talked about the loneliness of the long-distance runner? This is fun, this is life! You are getting to experience something less than one tenth of a percent of the population ever has the good health the fitness to accomplish: you are running your marathon.

As you pass the halfway mark, you remember your power words: I am strong; I am in control; I feel good. As you say them to yourself, you feel the power boost they give you, both mentally and physically, as your legs respond to the familiar, comforting words.

You are passing through an older part of the city now filled with character, history and friendly enthusiastic crowds of people calling words of encouragement to you. Someone hands you a cup of water and you drink it in, feeling the cool, clear water on your throat. It is refreshing. It is refilling not only your liquids but you can feel the confidence build as you start to realize you are way past halfway. You repeat your power words. You are strong. You are in control. You are a strong and powerful athlete, well trained and prepared. You feel good, your body and mind are in rhythm with each other. As you repeat your power words, you feel them fill you with confidence and strength. You can do this. You have taken the challenge and you will succeed.

As you pass the 32 km mark, you start down a hill. You feel like you're not doing this by yourself as that old training buddy gravity gives you a little push on the downhill section. You know that this is the tough part of the race, but you also know that you are ready. You think back to some of the long runs when you felt tired and you were not always sure you would make it, but you did, and after completing them you felt great.

You think back to some of the games you played with yourself on the long runs, like the one with the fishing rod where you cast out the line to the runner ahead of you and then ever so gradually started to reel him in. You laugh to yourself as you focus in on the runners ahead and slowly, ever so slowly, you start to gain on them.

You now have less than 5 km to go. You are strong and feeling confident as you start to pass runners. Some of them passed you earlier but you chose to let them go. They are now walking. You pass them and pick up the pace as you realize this is your race—you prepared well and are now ready. You think for a moment of the finish area… Just then you hear the announcer's voice and the cheers of the crowd in the finish area. A feeling of well-being and joy comes over you as you instinctively start to surge ahead and pass a couple more runners who appear to be struggling. You are alone and running strong; you are really in control.

You begin to say your power words one last time: I am strong; I am in control; I am fit and a powerful runner; I am a strong runner; I am fast and fluid.

As you cross over the final bridge and start towards the finish line, you can hear the cheering of the crowd, the screaming of the cheerleaders, the race announcer calling your name...

You cross the line and someone asks you if you are OK. You smile, unable to speak. You feel that special euphoric feeling that is somewhere between joy and the pain of the moment. With your hands on your hips, you walk towards the refreshment area, medal around your neck. You did it! You ran a marathon and you know that the confidence you now have will help in accomplishing any challenge you set for yourself. Even with all of life's speed bumps and challenges, you will achieve success because of the confidence that today has brought to you. You are a marathon runner! You know that any time you set a goal, train and work hard towards it, and dream of it, you will eventually achieve it in reality.

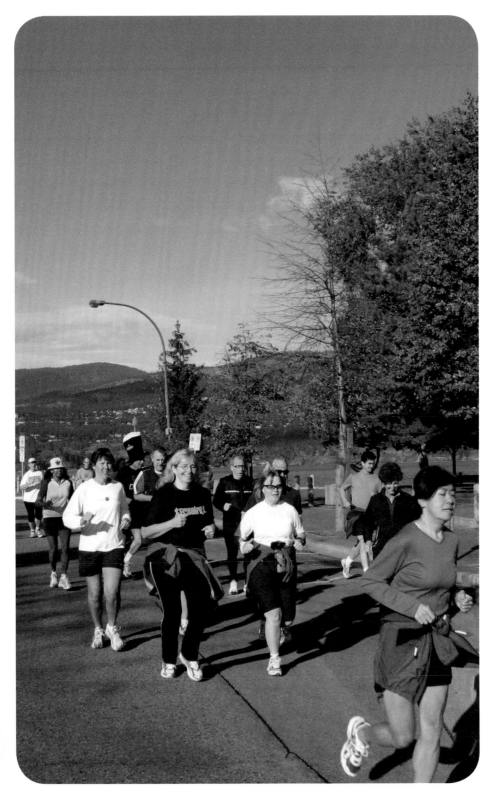

19 Mental Preparation

Last Words

Take a moment now to think of your breathing and gradually come back to the time and place of the moment. Think of the response of all of the Olympians when asked what they thought was their greatest asset: they all said it was mental toughness and confidence. For all of us, we should practice this mental training often and in concert with our physical training.

Positive Self-Talk

+ I am in control of my own life.
+ I can achieve any intelligent goal I set for myself.
+ I believe in myself and the people around me.
+ I treat every day as a new challenge to improve myself in some way.

How to Practice Positive Imagery / Mind-Power

I. Visualization

+ Visualize the first goal of your training. e.g. to run 10 K, to complete the marathon.
+ Next visualize the key elements that get you there.
+ Then fill in as many details as possible.
+ Be positive but realistic.

II. Analyze the Problems

+ Motivation? Determination? Performance?
+ Where are you losing it?
+ What are the causes?

III. Focus on Your Successes

+ List the times when you started to have the problems and then overcame them and went on.
+ Relive the successful experiences and store them in your memory.
+ Your past successes can lead you to future ones!

IV. Power Words

+ Develop a power word for your success with each of your major problems.
+ With each new or recurring problem, use the words and store the successes, e.g., imagining the word "character" as noted in our hill training session.

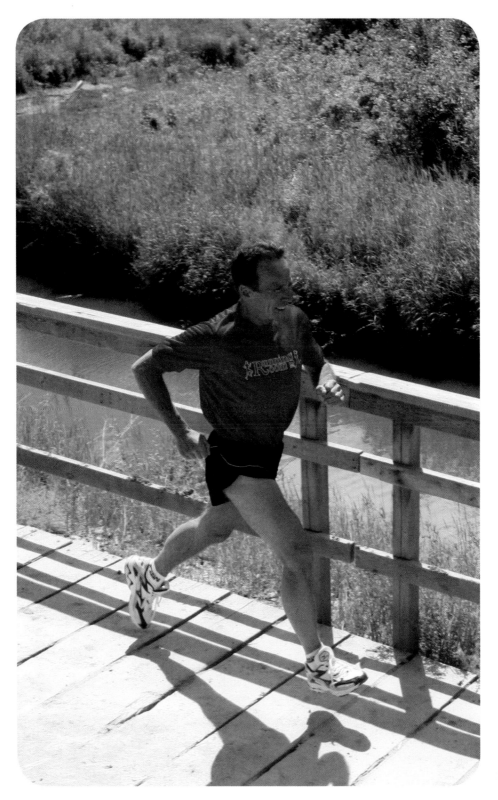

V. Mental Rehearsal

+ Rehearse the experience many times each week.
+ Start with the key elements, problems, successes and goal fulfillment, and then fill in key details.
+ Always be realistic but positive and successful.
+ The more problems you project, the more likely you are to overcome them.

VI. Shifting into the Right Brain

+ The logical left brain has all the excuses.
+ The creative right brain can get the job done.
+ You can train yourself to shift over through Ignoring, Distracting, Projecting, Imaging.
+ Mental rehearsal will help you shift into the right brain so you can "do it."

VII. An Unlimited Bag of Tricks

+ Creativity can overcome almost any problem with time, realism, visualization.
+ If you believe in something, you can make it happen if it's do-able.

Tricks:

+ The rubber band: think of a huge rubber band pulling you up the hill.
+ The fishing rod: you have hooked the person in front of you and now you are slowly reeling them in.

VIII. You Have the Capacity to Overcome Any Problem

+ Work through your problems.
+ Learn from your experiences.
+ Become part of your success.

Psychology and Running

Some final points...

1. Can people be overmotivated?

Overtraining or overstress can be a problem when all these stresses add up. It shows up in our motivational state. For example, not feeling like working out, feeling fatigued, sore, achy, having colds that won't go away, having an elevated resting heart rate in the morning, etc. As suggested above, monitor your "feeling index" and look for patterns. If you feel this way for more than a few days in a row, perhaps go and see your doctor and get it checked out. It may be a virus or something else, but it also may be your system's way of saying "Give me rest!"

Decreases in performance are because our bodies are responding to training stresses. With a bit of rest and time you'll be back stronger than ever. It is part of the training cycle.

2. Dealing with setbacks.

Some people get worried if they miss a workout or two, don't. The key to increasing your performance is to be consistent over the long run (months or years). Therefore, if you miss the odd run, there will be plenty of time to catch up in the future. Rest if you feel tired. This way you will have more energy for the next workout. Rest is as important as exercise. Missing an occasional run is unavoidable owing to other commitments (e.g., work, family). Learn to keep a healthy balance.

3. Dealing with Injuries.

There is a strong tendency for runners to ignore their body's warning signs of stress. Often these are aches and pains which precede major overuse injuries. See a doctor if your symptoms haven't alleviated in two or three days. Running on injuries usually makes them worse. We often put stress on other body parts when we run on an injury. The result...another injury. Just think of things in the big picture. Taking two or three weeks out to heal an injury now with professional help may save you from having to take six months off after trying to run through an injury and trying to cope with it yourself.

Helpful Tips on Keeping Motivated

1. Run with a friend, pet or running group.

Having to meet somebody is a great way of making sure you run, on days when you're unmotivated.

2. How do I know if I'm lacking motivation or if I need a day off?

Try the 10 minute rule. If you start running and feel like you have no energy and are tired, try one of the following tips:

+ A walking warm-up: sometimes you feel more like running once the stresses of the day have been eliminated.

- Jogging for about 10 minutes: if you feel better, carry on; if you do not, it's probably you're body saying "Give me rest."

- Try at another time of the day after you've had some food. You may just be low in energy from being hungry, or just because of our normal daily "bio rhythms."

3. How do I keep going on a run when I'm tired?

One idea is to break down the run into smaller segments and then focus on completing each segment as they come. Think positively; it'll make your goals more attainable.

4. Keep things fun.

Try new runs; perhaps drive to a new training area and explore. Speed or hill training once or twice a week can break up the monotony of long runs. Cross-training can also relieve the monotony. Think of your runs a playtime!

The Last 100 Meters

The highlight of the race comes in the last 100 m. Much has been written about the various stages of a race, in particular the marathon. The famous "wall" has entertained many readers, but the true joy and rewards usually come in the final 100 m or so of any race.

I have seen many a self-professed big tough runner brought to tears of joy as they run the final 100 m. Watch the finish of a marathon, you will see the joy of success mixed with the tears and toil of hard work that has brought the runner to

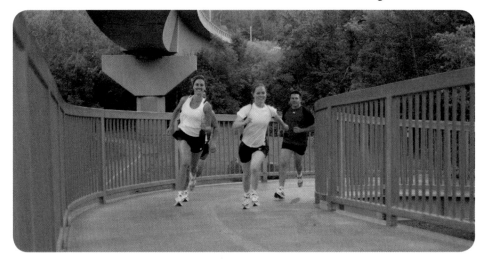

the finish line. The real elation comes from the fact that each runner has pushed and paced themselves though the various difficult stages of the race. They have gone through the high and low points of the race and now can savor the sweet smell of the successful finish. Every runner that crosses the finish line knows that they have achieved success and are all winners in life as well as in the race.

Runners learn that during the race they need to focus on the goals of the day to get through the low points of the race. Experience teaches us that during each race, everyone goes through some low points where they ask, why am I in this race? We think: I like running but I don't like racing. It hurts. Why don't I just quit? Who will know? I'm too old for this; people are asking why is that runner even in the race? I could just drop out and never enter a race again, no one would notice. I could take the bus back and even stop for a muffin and cold juice. I'm too old; I'm too fat.

We have all heard that negative side of our brain nagging away at us during these times. Well, that's when it's important for you to take control of the situation and get the old positive brain—the "I feel great about everything" side—kick-started to take control of things. The best way is to think about something that requires your creative brain. A technique you can use is to run the final 100 m of the race during the warm-up. That way, when you're running in the race and are at a point where you're struggling, focus on that final 100 m, or think of the final 100 m of a previous race. Visualize the race finish banner, the crowd cheering you on and the race announcer's voice. See yourself finishing in control with powerful strides. You are strong; you are fit; your breathing is in control; you are in control. Feel the elation of the finish and savor the moment for future training runs and races. The final 100 m is the self-motivational start of your next goal.

After the Race

The time immediately after a race is a great time to get motivated to train again. Change into some clean, dry clothes and savor the electric feeling that comes after a run. Enjoy the company of the other runners.

Try to keep moving around after the race. It will help flush your muscles of any waste products that can leave you sore. In the evening, a warm bath will help you gently loosen your muscles. If you are visiting a new city, the post-race afternoon is a great time to do some touring and model your new race T-shirt. You have special bragging rights for the balance of the day. You did it.

The day after the race is a good day to take off to allow your leg muscles to

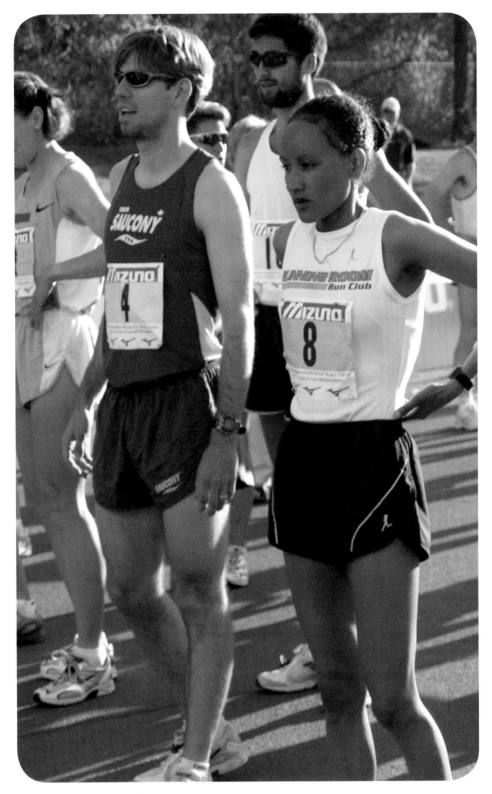

recover from the hard effort. You can swim or bike, if you want, because those activities will help loosen up your legs. I find that a swim after a race or hard training day is like a massage. Depending on the distance and your recovery, you may find that running only every other day during the week after a hard race will help the recovery of tired legs.

Often, after a race in which everything has gone well, you will be left with a new sense of motivation and confidence that will get you right back to your training with some new vigor and enthusiasm.

Marathon Pacing Charts

Want to know at what pace you ran your last race, or what pace you have to maintain to run a goal time? Our pace charts can help.

How to use:
Pace charts are a guide to what pace you race per kilometer (mile) for the most common race distances.

1. Start with a desired pace.
Even pacing: if you want to run a marathon in an even pace of 10 minute miles you can look up your splits to determine the pacing for the whole event - 10K (1:02:06) - 20K (2:04:08) - Half Way (2:11:03) - 30K (3:06:12) - Marathon (4:22:05).

2. Start with a goal time.
You may start with a goal finish time to help determine the pace that you should start at. For example, your goal finish time may be 4:30:00, therefore your goal pace would be 6:19–6:25 min/km (10:10–10:20 min/mi.)

3. Look up your average pace
If you ran a half marathon in approximately two hours you can locate your average pace as 5:42 min/km (9:10 min/mi.).

Marathon Pace Charts

Km	Mile	5K (3.1mi)	10K (6.2mi)	15K (9.3 mi)	20K (12.4 mi)	Half Marathon 21.1K (13.1 mi)	25K (15.5 mi)	30K (18.6 mi)	Marathon 42.2 Km (26.2 mi)
3:06	5:00	0:15:32	0:31:04	0:46:36	1:02:08	1:05:33	1:17:40	1:33:12	2:11:05
3:13	5:10	0:16:03	0:32:06	0:48:09	1:04:12	1:07:44	1:20:15	1:36:18	2:15:27
3:19	5:20	0:16:34	0:33:08	0:49:42	1:06:16	1:09:55	1:22:50	1:39:24	2:19:49
3:25	5:30	0:17:05	0:34:10	0:51:15	1:08:20	1:12:06	1:25:25	1:42:30	2:24:11
3:31	5:40	0:17:36	0:35:12	0:52:48	1:10:24	1:14:17	1:28:00	1:45:36	2:28:33
3:37	5:50	0:18:07	0:36:14	0:54:21	1:12:28	1:16:28	1:30:35	1:48:42	2:32:55
3:44	6:00	0:18:38	0:37:17	0:55:54	1:14:32	1:18:39	1:33:10	1:51:48	2:37:17
3:50	6:10	0:19:09	0:38:18	0:57:27	1:16:36	1:20:50	1:35:45	1:54:54	2:41:39
3:56	6:20	0:19:40	0:39:22	0:59:00	1:18:40	1:23:01	1:38:20	1:58:00	2:46:01
4:02	6:30	0:20:11	0:40:24	1:00:33	1:20:44	1:25:12	1:40:55	2:01:06	2:50:23
4:09	6:40	0:20:42	0:41:26	1:02:06	1:22:48	1:27:23	1:43:30	2:04:12	2:54:45
4:15	6:50	0:21:13	0:42:28	1:03:39	1:24:52	1:29:34	1:46:05	2:07:18	2:59:07
4:21	7:00	0:21:44	0:43:30	1:05:12	1:26:56	1:31:45	1:48:40	2:10:24	3:03:29
4:27	7:10	0:22:15	0:44:32	1:06:45	1:29:00	1:33:56	1:51:15	2:13:30	3:07:51
4:33	7:20	0:22:46	0:45:34	1:08:18	1:31:04	1:36:07	1:53:50	2:16:36	3:12:13
4:40	7:30	0:23:17	0:46:36	1:09:51	1:33:08	1:38:18	1:56:25	2:19:42	3:16:35
4:46	7:40	0:23:48	0:47:38	1:11:24	1:35:12	1:40:29	1:59:00	2:22:48	3:20:57

4:52	7:50	0:24:19	0:48:40	1:12:57	1:37:16	1:42:40	2:01:35	2:25:54	3:25:19
4:58	8:00	0:24:50	0:49:42	1:14:30	1:39:20	1:44:51	2:04:10	2:29:00	3:29:41
5:04	8:10	0:25:21	0:50:44	1:16:03	1:41:24	1:47:02	2:06:45	2:32:06	3:34:03
5:11	8:20	0:25:52	0:51:46	1:17:36	1:43:28	1:49:13	2:09:20	2:35:12	3:38:25
5:17	8:30	0:26:23	0:52:48	1:19:09	1:45:32	1:51:24	2:11:55	2:38:18	3:42:47
5:23	8:40	0:26:54	0:53:50	1:20:42	1:47:36	1:53:35	2:14:30	2:41:24	3:47:09
5:29	8:50	0:27:25	0:54:52	1:22:15	1:49:40	1:55:46	2:17:05	2:44:30	3:51:31
5:36	9:00	0:27:56	0:55:54	1:23:48	1:51:44	1:57:57	2:19:40	2:47:36	3:55:53
5:42	9:10	0:28:27	0:56:56	1:25:21	1:53:48	2:00:08	2:22:15	2:50:42	4:00:15
5:48	9:20	0:28:58	0:57:58	1:26:54	1:55:52	2:02:19	2:24:50	2:53:48	4:04:37
5:54	9:30	0:29:29	0:59:00	1:28:27	1:57:56	2:04:30	2:27:25	2:56:54	4:08:59
6:00	9:40	0:30:00	1:00:02	1:30:00	2:00:00	2:06:41	2:30:00	3:00:00	4:13:21
6:07	9:50	0:30:31	1:01:04	1:31:33	2:02:04	2:08:52	2:32:35	3:03:06	4:17:43
6:13	10:00	0:31:02	1:02:06	1:33:06	2:04:08	2:11:03	2:35:10	3:06:12	4:22:05
6:19	10:10	0:31:33	1:03:08	1:34:39	2:06:12	2:13:14	2:37:45	3:09:18	4:26:27
6:25	10:20	0:32:04	1:04:10	1:36:12	2:08:16	2:15:25	2:40:20	3:12:24	4:30:49
6:31	10:30	0:32:35	1:05:12	1:37:45	2:10:20	2:17:36	2:42:55	3:15:30	4:35:11
6:38	10:40	0:33:06	1:06:14	1:39:18	2:12:24	2:19:47	2:45:30	3:18:36	4:39:33
6:44	10:50	0:33:37	1:07:16	1:40:51	2:14:28	2:21:58	2:48:05	3:21:42	4:43:55
6:50	11:00	0:34:08	1:08:18	1:42:24	2:16:32	2:24:09	2:50:40	3:24:48	4:48:17
6:56	11:10	0:34:39	1:09:20	1:43:57	2:18:36	2:26:20	2:53:15	3:27:54	4:52:39
7:03	11:20	0:35:10	1:10:22	1:45:30	2:20:40	2:28:31	2:55:50	3:31:00	4:57:01
7:09	11:30	0:35:41	1:11:24	1:47:03	2:22:44	2:30:42	2:58:25	3:34:06	5:01:23

Marathon
Pace Charts

Km	Mile	5K (3.1mi)	10K (6.2mi)	15K (9.3 mi)	20K (12.4 mi)	Half Marathon 21.1K (13.1 mi)	25K (15.5 mi)	30K (18.6 mi)	Marathon 42.2 Km (26.2 mi)
7:15	11:40	0:36:12	1:12:26	1:48:36	2:24:48	2:32:53	3:01:00	3:37:12	5:05:45
7:21	11:50	0:36:43	1:13:28	1:50:09	2:26:52	2:35:04	3:03:35	3:40:18	5:10:07
7:27	12:00	0:37:14	1:14:30	1:51:42	2:28:56	2:37:15	3:06:10	3:43:24	5:14:29
7:34	12:10	0:37:45	1:15:32	1:53:15	2:31:00	2:39:26	3:08:45	3:46:30	5:18:51
7:40	12:20	0:38:16	1:16:34	1:54:48	2:33:04	2:41:37	3:11:20	3:49:36	5:23:13
7:46	12:30	0:38:47	1:17:36	1:56:21	2:35:08	2:43:48	3:13:55	3:52:42	5:27:35
7:52	12:40	0:39:18	1:18:38	1:57:54	2:37:12	2:45:59	3:16:30	3:55:48	5:31:57
7:58	12:50	0:39:49	1:19:40	1:59:27	2:39:16	2:48:10	3:19:05	3:58:54	5:36:19
8:05	13:00	0:40:20	1:20:42	2:01:00	2:41:20	2:50:21	3:21:40	4:02:00	5:40:41
8:11	13:10	0:40:51	1:21:44	2:02:33	2:43:24	2:52:32	3:24:15	4:05:06	5:45:03
8:17	13:20	0:41:22	1:22:46	2:04:06	2:45:28	2:54:43	3:26:50	4:08:12	5:49:25
8:23	13:30	0:41:53	1:23:48	2:05:39	2:47:32	2:56:54	3:29:25	4:11:18	5:53:47
8:30	13:40	0:42:24	1:24:50	2:07:12	2:49:36	2:59:05	3:32:00	4:14:24	5:58:09
8:36	13:50	0:42:55	1:25:52	2:08:45	2:51:40	3:01:16	3:34:35	4:17:30	6:02:31
8:42	14:00	0:43:26	1:26:54	2:10:18	2:53:44	3:03:27	3:37:10	4:20:36	6:06:53

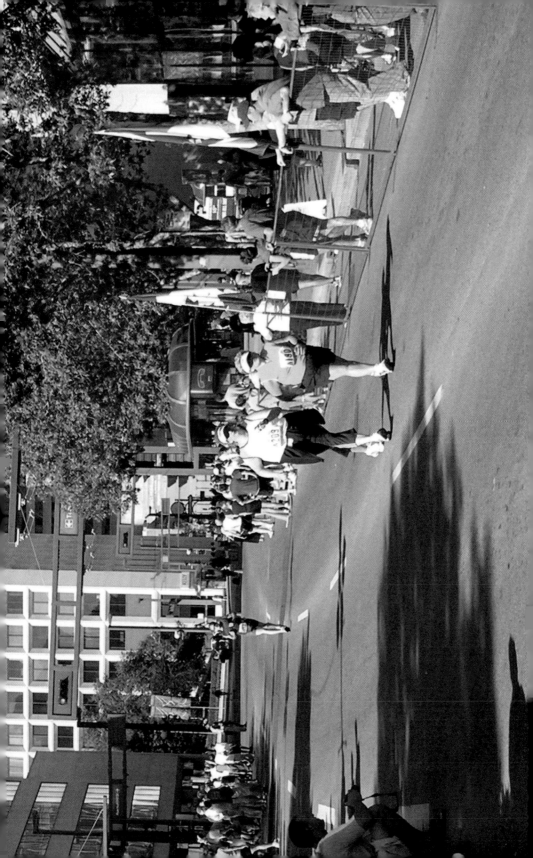

Testimonials

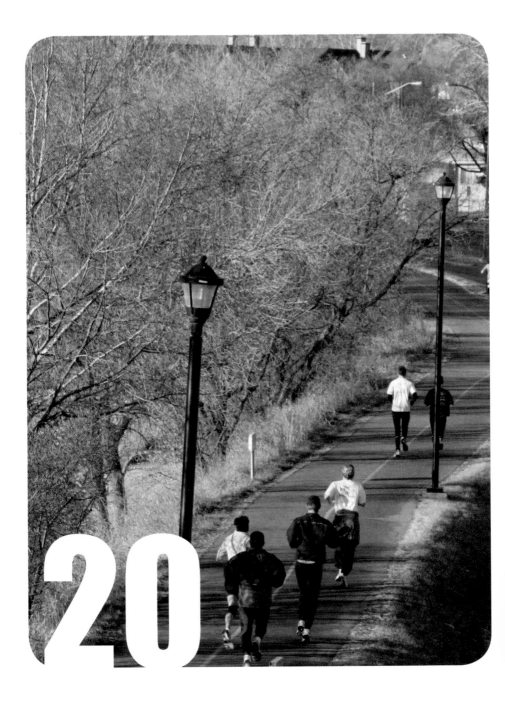

20

Dear John,

I expect that it is never tiresome to hear from people who have taken your book and "run with it." I'll add my note to your inbox today!

Four years ago a friend mentioned that she was going to learn to run. I had just turned 40 and realized that I needed to be fit (not thin) in order to live the quality of life I had in mind. I've always liked a project, so I decided to join her. For many weeks we met on my front step at 5:30 a.m. for the prescribed run/walk combination of the day. My husband thought we were crazy. I remember wondering if three minutes could possibly be any longer once we worked up to running for that incredible amount of time. We figured out how to use our Timex watches and felt good about our ever so slight "negative splits." My goal was to complete an 8 K race, and although my time was nothing special (just over 50 minutes), it felt tremendous. Still excited by the Shaughnessay 8 K, I asked a marathon-running friend about her training program and she recommended Running:Start to Finish so highly that I bought a copy the next day. One thing has certainly led to another. I trained for my first half marathon alone, completed the Royal Victoria and then joined a Running Room clinic at the Alma Street store to prepare for the next one. I've just outlined my race and training plans for the future, intending to tackle my first full marathon (yikes!) in the fall. I have a dog-eared copy of your book, and refer to it just about every day to ponder where I am in training and to see where I'm going. My half marathon time has improved from 2:22:21 to 2:06:04, and I'm in better shape that I've been at any age. I give your book as a gift to anyone who expresses the slightest interest in getting started.

I think that Running Room clinics, entry fees to races and at least one pair of running shoes should be tax deductible each year. (OK, so we may all need to work on that!) I have not had a day of injury (yes, I'm touching wood) since I started running regularly, and by following sound 10/1 advice I ran 20 km yesterday morning, then spent the afternoon cleaning house and cooking for a dinner party. I feel great today.

Running is no longer a special event but an ordinary part of my life. I am thankful for my good health, a beautiful Vancouver beach to run on and for each day. Thank you for the inspiration.

—Corinne, Running Room Supporter

Hi John,

I met you at the Quebec City Marathon just before you opened the Moncton store. Six of us from Moncton went to Quebec City, and you gave us a pep talk at the Running Room booth when we went to register. I will always remember that because I was really nervous about attempting my first marathon. Your encouraging words made me think I could do it, which is what I needed! Thanks again, I am still running and love it!

—Susan, Running Room Supporter

I run for the enjoyment of it and my health. I had always wanted to run a marathon, but thought I would never be able to do it. Last year I met John Stanton. He showed me the program for the 10 and 1's and it opened up new possibilities for me. On July 26, I ran 16 mi. in training, the longest by far that I had ever run. This year I volunteered to be a street marshal at the Twin Cities Marathon so I can hug my running group as they cross the finish line. Next year, I will run it. Thanks Running Room for looking beyond my health situation, my age and the fact that I was the slowest and probably oldest runner in the group, and seeing the marathoner in me.

—Jan, Running Room Supporter

A Rookie's Take on National Capital Race Weekend

I am an athlete. At least that's what Running Room founder John Stanton told me when I picked up my National Capital Race Kit the day before my first 5 K on May 29.

Greeting my faithful running partner and me with as much enthusiasm as he did the team of experienced marathoners in the line ahead of us, Stanton encouraged us to recite power phrases to ourselves during our first race, such as "I am an athlete who is in control of my body. I have trained for this and today I am ready."

And oh how we trained! Could it really be just 10 weeks ago that I meekly walked into the first session of the Women's Learn to Run Clinic, worried that I wouldn't be able to run for a minute straight, let alone consider a 5 K? Many a time my friend Magda (whom I "strenuously volunteered" to join the clinic with me) wondered what we'd gotten ourselves into. Imagine thinking we could keep up with all these 20-year-olds and ever look like we belonged in those tiny running shorts!

Each week I'd toss and turn with anxiety the night before the clinic, hoping this week's extra minute of running wouldn't be the one to do us in. But something magical began to happen. We'd take a deep breath as we headed out as a group to do our run/walks along the beautiful Ottawa canal and suddenly we'd find ourselves doing it. Yes, we were running! (OK, so in the beginning it was a bit more like trudging, but we weren't at home on the couch, and that was a minor miracle in itself.)

By mid-clinic, we admitted we were actually enjoying ourselves. We got used to our sleepy families giving us funny looks as we jumped out of bed for our group runs on Sunday mornings. Little did they know that we really weren't insane, just hooked on the thrill of having a group of marathoners wave "good morning" and "keep it up" as we all practiced our various distances along the canal before most of the city was even awake.

The next week I bought new running shoes (who knew there was more to consider than just matching the outfit?!) and the difference in comfort and cushioning made it feel like I'd strapped two pillows to my feet. I cursed myself for waiting so long to get fitted with the right gear and felt I owed it to myself to also buy one of the famous Running Room "cult" jackets. Now I actually looked like a runner as opposed to some schlep who accidentally found herself on the track after a wrong turn at the supermarket.

But while I was improving each week, the thought of entering (much less finishing) a 5K was daunting. By the time we realized that our distance wouldn't actually get up to a full 5K during our clinic we were in a downright panic. Surely our instructors had over-estimated us? Didn't they realize we were over 35 and that on Wednesdays and Sundays we pretended to be runners but the rest of the week we were mere mortals with kids, jobs and a secret love of all things fried and fatty?

We decided to grit our teeth and enter anyway. Meeting John Stanton was our first clue that we'd made the right decision. I think he was even more thrilled that we were taking the plunge than we were! We held out our race bibs for him to sign like groupies at a rock concert and felt truly blessed by the running gods to have his autograph. His parting advice was typically sage: "Enjoy your first 5 K race. Look around you and take it all in—hear the crowd, feel the energy. It will be something you never forget." He was so right.

When we finally lined up at the start there were runners up and down the route as far as the eye could see. Magda and I looked at each other with a grin—surely in this sea of thousands there were other rookies we could keep up with! After about a dozen trips to the bathroom (10 of which were false alarms—classic "race day bladder syndrome") we were as ready as we were going to be.

Suddenly the crowd surged ahead and we were off! The sun was shining, the music was blaring and the roar of the crowd was almost deafening. Forget worrying about the fact that the first 500 m was uphill, I could get used to the throngs of adoring fans! We'd barely gone three minutes and I already knew this 5 K wouldn't be my last.

All along the route strangers cheered us on from bridges and doorways while fellow runners beamed at each other with pride. It was race day and for the first time in my life I was in the middle of the action instead of on the sidelines.

I was even more determined to complete my first 5 K because 10 days earlier, my father had tragically passed away and he was the kind of man who believed in finishing the goals you set for yourself. I ran to honor his memory, and because I recently discovered he was quite the track star in his day, I carried his picture in my shoe under my timing chip for inspiration.

He didn't let me down. I figure it must have been his spirit that carried me over the finish line because the last 200 m were a euphoric blur. I'm quite sure my feet never touched the ground. Out of nowhere I got this incredible burst of energy, and I heard the announcer say, "If anyone wants to finish under 40 minutes, you've got six seconds!" Adrenaline washed over me and I was off like a rocket.

The next thing I knew it was over and a race official put a medal around my neck as sweet to me as any handed out in Athens this summer. My goal was to finish the 5 K "upright and smiling" in under an hour. Despite the doubts, stress and grief of recent weeks, I had managed to do it in 37 minutes.

So, thanks, John Stanton. Thanks, Magda. Thanks, Running Room instructors Jeanne, Cathy, Nicole and Josée. And last but definitely not least—thanks Dad

—Betsy, Learn To Run Clinic Participant

Hi,

I simply wish to thank you. For many years I used to run a 10 K each day. Last year I got injuries over injuries to the knees and back. I had decided to stop running, having reached the age of 40 and thinking that my body couldn't take it anymore.

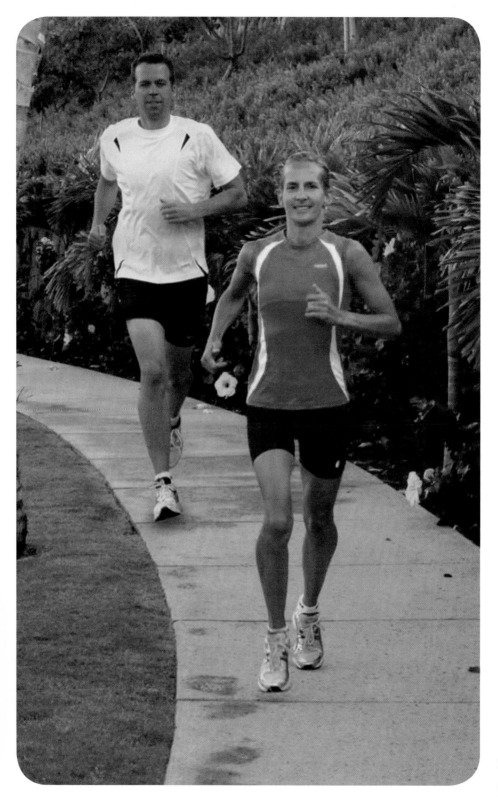

Lately I have been to a Running Room store. They sold me new running shoes. What a difference from my old ones bought in a usual sport store where the sales staff do not know much about running. Those old running shoes caused all my injuries during the last year.

I restarted my training, and despite having gained a few pounds because I stopped running, I was able to run a 10 K again without problems because of your sound advice on how to buy new shoes. Many thanks!

—Yves, Running Room Supporter

In the past I'd always viewed people who run as a completely different species. I thought that running was boring and couldn't grasp why on earth people would go out and run for the apparent enjoyment of it, and in all kinds of weather! I decided early in the year to sign up for some courses that would get me out of the house and to meet people. A coworker suggested Learn to Run. I nodded and said I'd think about it, all the while going through in my head all the reasons I couldn't run: bad knees, asthma, joint problems. But as the year progressed I found myself thinking about it more and decided to go ahead and give it a try. A friend was going to sign up with me, so at least when we hated it we could hate it together. Three weeks in and I can't believe it took me this long to see what fun running can be. I find myself sitting at my desk at work waiting for it to be time to go home so I can strap on my shoes and start my intervals. I'm running everyday, sometimes twice a day, rain, snow, cold winds and sunshine.

The Running Room's Learn to Run clinic is fantastic in its approach to beginner runners. Starting us out slowly with two minute walking intervals and one minute running allowed me to feel on the very first night that, wow, I can do this. Having a group leader stay at the back with us slow ones and tell us that it's the pace she normally runs at, true or not, is a great moral booster. There is always encouragement from the group leaders and fellow runners, not to mention from more experienced runners at the Running Club on Sunday mornings! The Run Club is something I very much look forward to, enough to haul myself out of bed bright and early on a Sunday morning no matter what time I got to bed the night before, or what the weather is.

The staff in the store are very friendly and patient. Four different staff members put up with me and my shoe purchase that took three weeks and the return of one pair. And the shoes I ended up with are fantastic. I noticed the difference the first time I wore them running.

I like the Running Room clinic so much that I'm already looking into signing up for the 10 K clinic in June and am trying to convince all my friends to do it too.

Thanks, Running Room!

—Learn To Run Clinic Participant

I joined my first 10 K Running Room clinic in Sudbury. I have to thank Stephanie (another clinic member) for introducing me to the Running Room; I had no idea it existed until I met her, so we joined the clinic together. I was very nervous about starting the clinic and really didn't know what to expect. I have to say, what a wonderful environment. It was so friendly, and open and not intimidating. I have learned so much about myself, and of course about running, that I never would have learned if I didn't join this clinic.

The Running Room is not just about running, but about friendships, encouragement, motivation and the list goes on. The group atmosphere makes running a lot more enjoyable and helps you get through the training period and the tough times. Without them it would have been difficult to do this one on my own. The instructor was amazing: she was there to make sure all our needs were met, gave us a lot of encouragement and taught us about "character!"

Now that the training is almost over, I am ready for the challenge of the half marathon! I want to thank the Running Room for deciding to spread its wings to Sudbury. I would definitely recommend a clinic to anyone; whether you are a beginner or advanced there is always something to learn, whether it is from an instructor, speaker or group member. I think the Running Room rocks!

—Ellena, 10 K Clinic Participant

This has been a fantastic experience! I never thought I would be able to run, and I certainly never thought I would enjoy it! The instructors (Ben and Paul and the others who join us sometimes) are so friendly and positive and encouraging. I love the group atmosphere and how we feel like a team. The pace and the steady increase in time and distance has been much more doable than I thought it would be. I have been pleasantly surprised by the whole experience. I really don't feel that anything could be done to improve it. (I know criticism is helpful, but I don't have any!) It's great that there's always an instructor up ahead with the fastest and someone at the end with the slowest. No one gets left out. Thanks so much for this wonderful experience, I will be back for the 5 K clinic in the fall! Keep up the good work!

—Learn To Run Clinic Participant

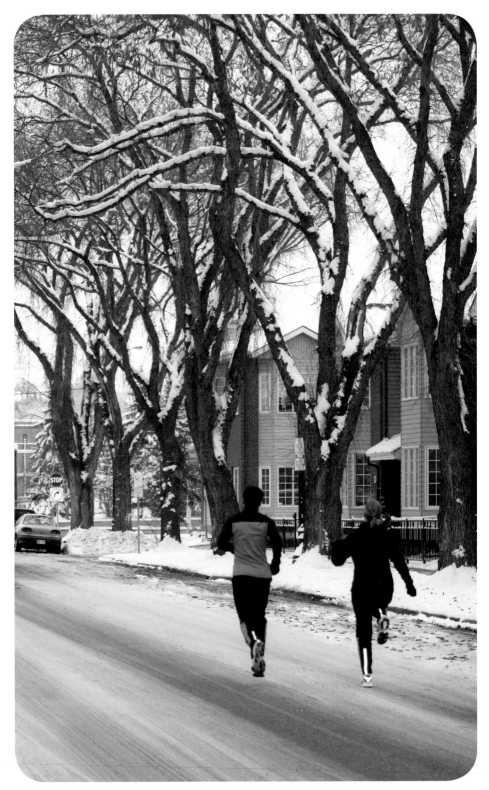

This running clinic has been a lifeline for me! I am truly enjoying every minute of this experience, from the challenge to the support! We have a great group, and Joanne is an excellent leader and one of the most "real" people I know! Thanks so much, you guys! Wish me luck!

—Half Marathon Clinic Participant

The instructor was exceptional and the staff at the store were great! This was the most fun I have had running. I have also been able to improve my time and distance while meeting new friends and new running mates. Thanks so much Clara and Kim and the Running Room York Mills.

—10 K Clinic Participant

Thanks, Running Room, for an excellent, well-organised program. It's a great format that promotes distance running, injury-free!

—Marathon Clinic Participant

This group had a really great camaraderie. Everyone seemed extremely supportive of each other. Our instructor Sonya also participated in the run clubs with us on Wednesdays and Sundays, which was extremely motivating, as well as helping us improve with more confidence. I would really recommend this program to anyone who was thinking of taking up running. I had tried to run on my own before, without any success. The "group" is most definitely the way to go. Our ages stretched as far as the distance between the first and last runners. Everyone was encouraged to run at their own speed. No one ran alone.

—Sonya, Marathon Clinic Participant

I found the program to be excellent, and really cannot make any suggestions for improvement. I struggled through the first three weeks, and then found it getting easier and easier. It is a well-planned program, and the gradual increases each week make it possible for the middle-aged person to complete the program. Stephanie is a great instructor: very energetic, very positive. One of the most enjoyable programs that I have enrolled in. Keep up the good work!

—Learn To Run Clinic Participant

I love it! It is a great structured support with daily (almost) e-mails that keep me on track. I use what I need in terms of the online services and intend on signing up for the 10 K class. It has helped me gain an understanding of myself as a runner and my needs. The instructors are accessible, knowledgeable, supportive and friendly. They are there when you need them and do not smother you. I will recommend this to others.

—5 K Clinic Participant

Your leadership, guidance and endless encouragement and motivation got me over the finish line again this year. Before the Running Room I couldn't run to the end of the street. Now, after your Learn To Run, 10 km and Half Marathon clinics, I completed my fourth half marathon this calendar year. I couldn't do it each time without you and the Running Room clinic. The training schedule, speaker topics and camaraderie are second to none and I plan to run another half with you next year.

I have a success story to share. A coworker of mine was training for his first full this year. Each week after his long run he would complain of aches and pains and was going to give up and quit. I convinced him to join us at the Pembina store that next Sunday and try 10 and 1s with his pace group of choice and try it "the Running Room way" before totally giving up. That Sunday made a 10 and 1 believer out of him and he crossed the finish line for his first full marathon yesterday.

You touch so many lives by making runners, dreamers and believers out of all of us. Thank you so much! I look forward to training with you for another half marathon next year!

–Half Marathon Clinic Participant

This clinic was fantastic! It was exactly what I needed and definitely exceeded any expectations that I had. I am running farther and longer than I ever thought I could, and the support within our group made it easy to stay motivated. I can't say enough good things about this clinic and I would highly recommend it to anyone!

Special thanks to Erin our instructor. Her enthusiasm and encouragement was motivating and contagious!

—For Women Only Clinic Participant

The Running Room provides what every marathoner needs: community spirit, running pals to help you make it up those hills on cold, rainy mornings and experienced sales staff eager to provide you with top-flight equipment.

—Julian, Marathon Clinic Participant

The Running Room group is not just about running, it's a complete social and emotional experience. When I signed up for the marathon group I never fully believed I would run a marathon, since all I had run in my life was two 10 km races (one with a lot of difficulty).

There is an instant bond that gets created as you share every increase in mileage on the long runs. The instructors are always there making sure your personal needs are met. Yes, the group gets you through the whole training experience. Alone I could not of done it.

Now that the training part of the marathon is done I have started "celebrating" the whole experience, doing the actual marathon is icing on the cake.

—Ann, Marathon Clinic Participant

As a former runner who was plagued by injuries and had to hang up her shoes, I was looking to the Running Room program to ease me back into my favorite sport. The steady progression approach to building time and distance helped me to control my injuries and listen to my body better. At the end of the 10 weeks I realized that I still do love running and the euphoria of a great run still lives in me. I credit the Running Room for getting me out of my rut and back onto the pavement.

—Alisa, Clinic Participant

Training and running with the Running Room Team transformed me. At the end of my training program, Learn to Run, I realized I could run a 5 K for a charity event, which was the Run for the Cure. It was such a good feeling to accomplish such a challenging run, understanding this was the biggest endeavor of my life. I loved the experience right up till the end (so did the other runners). I will never forget my run. What I learned most of all was the people at the Running Room are service oriented towards their customers. They help you sincerely achieve your goals whether it is for weight loss, for health reasons or personal reasons.

—Debbie, Clinic Participant

Running and training with the Running Room has opened up a whole new world for me. By the time you get to the end of the session, you realize that you can run your first marathon. By the time I got to the end of my Learn to Run clinic, I realized that I would be able to run my first 5 K run for charity. I chose the Run for the Cure. The sense of achievement is amazing, especially because I found the race itself to be the toughest thing I've ever done. I enjoyed the experience right up to the last minute (along with all the others) and left feeling tremendous! The most important lesson I learned was that the Running Room staff are "people" oriented—sincerely helping you achieve your goals, whether it's for weight loss, health reasons or personal goals.

—Betty, Learn To Run Clinic Participant

There is no doubt that this training program provided me with the challenges, instruction and motivation I needed. I thought the pace of the clinic was good, and although the hill and speed training were tough, they did pay off! Sandi's weekly e-mail communications were always much appreciated, and I looked forward to reading her words of encouragement. I think the choice of guest speakers were always on point to what was important to me: nutrition, injury-prevention, etc. The social aspect of the program was wonderful and I believe I have made a few new friends. Overall I am really happy with the Running Room training program, and I know I'll continue to take training programs because the fitness and social benefits are wonderful!

—Marathon Clinic Participant

This is the third clinic that I have taken, and they just get better and better. Every week I still find it hard to believe that I'm going to make the distance, but every week I do. The combination of an excellent schedule and great instruction/ motivation have gotten me to a point where I never believed I could be a year ago. Thanks especially to Kris for not only teaching our clinic, but creating an environment at the store that makes everyone want to come back every Sunday. Well done!

—Marathon Clinic Participant

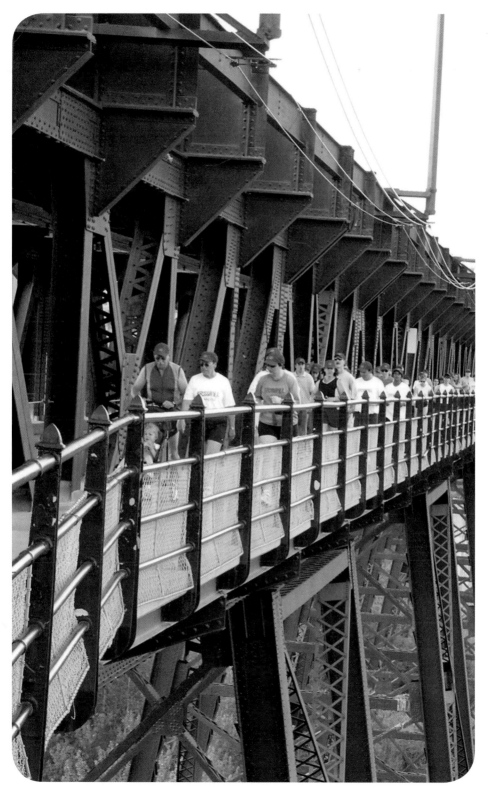

I had tried many times, without success, to establish a consistent exercise program, but no matter how slowly I tried to begin an activity, it always was too much for my body and I would become very ill. In January, I was lucky enough to try a Learn to Run program at the Running Room. We began by running only one minute and walking two minutes 10 times. I would have never thought you could start that slowly, but I could do it. And it felt great! Now eight months later, I run/walk five days a week, 2–10 mi. at a time. I feel so much better. I am so thankful for the knowledge and support the Running Room staff of professionals have given me. Thank you very much!

—Cory, Clinic Participant

My Running Story

I was introduced to running back in the early '80s when I was in my late 20s with two very small children. It was a program called OWLS (Overweight Ladies) at Carleton University and was a wonderful program instructed by some very inspirational "senior" ladies who taught us all how to lead a healthy lifestyle through proper nutrition and exercise, which just happened to include running. I was certainly never an athlete, but I quickly became hooked on running. I loved the camaraderie on nights where we ran together, the quiet "time for myself" moments when running alone and my first taste of that feeling of accomplishment that comes from pushing yourself just a little and being amazed at what you can actually achieve!

For many reasons I slipped back to the old unhealthy lifestyle of sedentary living. Fast forward quite a few years and I am told at a doctor's appointment that my cholesterol level is through the roof and I had better get it under control or the consequences could be serious. This was the wakeup call that you hear everyone talk about. I was referred to the Lipid Clinic at the Heart Institute, where I worked with Beth Mansfield, a nutrition and exercise specialist. I started getting physically active again, joined a gym and started walking every day. Within a year I had lost 60 lb. and my cholesterol levels were down to normal range without having to resort to any medication. The good news was that I found I was wanting to run instead of walk, and it felt great! The bad news was I felt so great that I pushed it and did too much too fast, resulting in an ITB injury. Oh, if only I had attended a Running Room clinic to begin with, I wouldn't have made that mistake!

The Running Room clinics were recommended to me by a couple of friends who had taken them, so I decided to join the Learn to Run program. What a wonderful group of instructors and leaders at the Merivale Running Room! Hilda and Linda were so welcoming, and if anyone had any trepidation it was certainly short-lived. We were all encouraged and supported every single week, and I cannot say enough good things about the program. Pretty soon my youngest daughter Jessica started to come along on my practice runs. She was in third year university and found running a great stress reliever. Our clinic goal race was the St. Patrick's Day 5 K run. It was a freezing cold day in March, but boy did we enjoy that run. Jessica and I ran our first 5 K race together in 35 minutes. I can remember being all smiles that day.

Jessica then decided to join me in the 10 K clinic. Cara and Jim, the instructors, were a perfect complement to each other: Cara has a terrific sense of humor and always has some great tips and Jim was so totally inspiring. We had fun in the clinic and worked hard. Jess and I even managed to keep on the training schedule during a visit to Vancouver. (We dropped by the Alma Street Running Room and got maps of runs by the sea!)

Our goal race for the clinic was the 10 K run in the National Capital Race Weekend. Even though we knew it was a huge event, we were overwhelmed by the sheer volume of runners downtown that evening, somewhere over 5,000! Truth be told, I was a bit nervous, but I knew the clinic had well prepared us for the race. We knew we could do the distance (we had run up to 13 K in the clinic) and just wanted to savor the experience.

What I wasn't prepared for were all the spectators cheering the runners on. If we experienced any fatigue during the race, the sounds of all the people shouting, "You can do it. Not much farther," was just so encouraging that it still brings tears to my eyes. I remember reaching the 9 K point and thinking, "We did it, we are almost there." My daughter reached for my hand just as we were approaching the finish so that we could cross the line together. We did it in 69 minutes and our goal had been to come in at under 70 minutes! What a moment—and an unbelievable feeling to be able to share it with my one of my daughters—absolutely awesome!

I was thinking back to all those years ago when I started running at OWLS with the idea that I was doing it for my children so that I could be healthy and fit and watch them grow up. And 21 years later here I was crossing the finish line with my 22-year-old daughter. How incredible!

John Stanton signed our bibs at the Sports Expo—mine reads "You can do it," and I remember thinking about that all through the race. Also I kept thinking about what John had said: "You are fit; you are strong; you can do it." Jessica's was

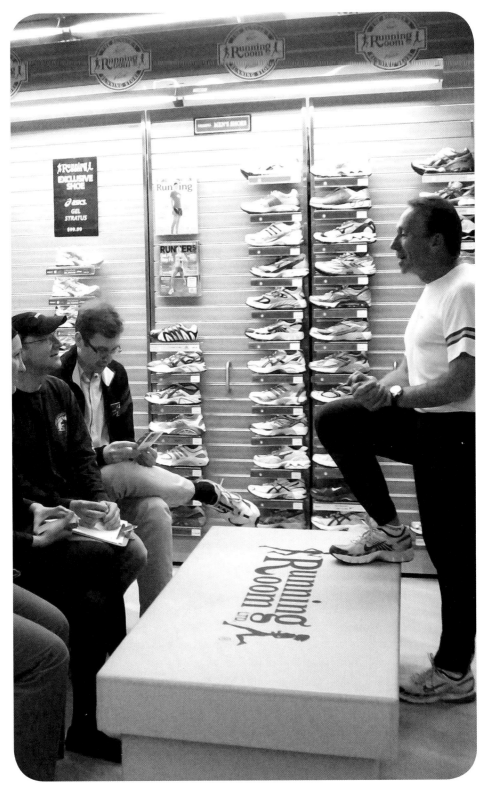

signed "Keep the family running!" The next goal for me and Jessica is to run a half marathon together after I turn 50 in December. We're even going to try to coax Kelly, my oldest daughter and self-confessed couch potato, into joining us!

—Joanne, Clinic Participant

Dreams are born in a single moment!

About 25 years ago, while riding my bike along the canal in Ottawa, I witnessed my first view of a marathon runner. I remember the sense of awe, thinking that these people were of a different ilk, surely light years from what I would ever be capable of doing. I admired them, yet thought the idea of running for 26.2 miles, also known as 42.2 km, was something akin to madness.

Fast forward a few years, when I walk into the Bank Street Running Room store to take my first Learn to Run clinic. At the end of the clinic, I find myself running with our instructor, Emily Gildner. I am having a difficult time; I am running the longest distance I have run in my life. I ask Emily if her first 5 K was as difficult. She admits that her first race was not a 5 K race, but a marathon. I cannot not believe my ears. Later I would learn that she likely had been running in that marathon I had watched many years ago. Much later, her friendship would prove to be instrumental in my development as a runner. She had the body a 20-year-old would envy, and she still does.

I wanted to now run faster—anything this difficult had to be done in a speedier fashion. Phil Marsh, the area manager, took the time to formalize a plan of action for me. I still have that e-mail, and have been known to read it from time to time. I am still amazed at the amount of counsel and education he imparted, freely, giving much of his expertise and time so I could meet my goals. I listened and registered for a 10 K clinic for the fall. Again, Emily would be my instructor. She made running up hills look like a work of art.

The group leader inspired me to challenge that distance, and the following year I registered for the Half Marathon clinic. Phil Marsh would teach, motivate and inspire, not to mention put us through the paces. Two weeks before race day, unexpected emergency surgery set me back. My training for this 21 km race was not to be, but Phil ran for me that day. I would heed his counsel and return six months later to run my half marathon. The half marathon distance was long and made harder by brutal, incessant winds. I would never want to take my body farther. The other part of me innately knew that messing with fate was pointless.

I was lucky enough to run with John Stanton at the opening of yet another store in Ottawa. He mentioned that he would be at the New York City Marathon the following weekend. Dreams are born in a single moment. The words he used to describe running this particular marathon—the picture he created—did it. I knew then, that in November, I would run my first marathon.

This Running Room clinic junkie would now run her first marthon. My instructor, Wendell, had us believe in ourselves, changing many of our habits in order to mold us into marathon machines. My training runs had me planning my next marathons. I crossed the finish line in my head more times that I could count. I became a marathon runner along the banks of the Ottawa River, the Canal, the paths and the wooded trails I have the privilege of running along, during one of Ottawa's warmest summers on record.

Nothing stopped me from running, or crossing that finish line in New York City. Next time I do the marathon in this city, I won't forget to wear my name on my shirt. One learns from every race.

John Stanton's book, Running: Start to Finish was also instrumental in my training, especially for my second marathon a year later in September. Along with being prepared, the trick of putting a sponge inside my cap came in handy. Thanks, John. Sometimes, Mother Nature is in charge, so the more tricks up your sleeve, the better, especially if you can keep yourself cool in 30°C temperature with skyrocketing humidity. Yes, I had become insane with joy as I completed my journey, along with the Kenyans, in beautiful Montréal, albeit more slowly than my training predicted. I was proud to be able to sustain the conditions, and my body was not letting me down. I was a marathoner, and I was very much where I wanted to be. I did not forget to wear my name on my shirt. One learns from every race.

Last summer, I had the privilege of learning that raising money for a good cause can help you not only heal, but also help honor life in a way that might never had been possible had I not been a runner. For me, this race celebrated life as I hope to know it for as long as I can. It reminded me of the importance of staying healthy and my role in doing so. Life is short, better make it healthy. One learns from every race.

In July 2004, the Running Room celebrated 20 years. Twenty years of changing lives like my own, 20 years of recruiting people, much like the ones who have crossed my paths, to make me a healthier, more fulfilled individual. As with most successful companies, the people who work for this company continue to empower people to change lives, one at a time. I suspect we have but seen the tip of the iceberg with respect to the success of this company. Happy birthday and many more! I will run on your birthday, and be proud to be a part of your celebration. I will quietly celebrate my own four years of running, hopefully with my running partner Cori—need I say I met her at a running clinic! I learn a lot from her, too.

—Linda, Clinic Participant

A die-hard runner and Running Room customer/fan who is a bit too humble to "toot" her own horn!

I am excited to tell you the story of my wife, Jill, who in my opinion should be the poster child for the Running Room clinics and the running "addiction." In December, Jill was confronted by our 9-year-old daughter that she was concerned about her mom's health because she smoked. Although she was relatively healthy, Jill had not formally exercised since her early or mid teens. It was around the same time that I had told Jill about my idea of trying out one of your running clinics. Certainly not that intrigued, Jill showed no interest in running with me until I jokingly suggested to her that maybe she couldn't handle it. Luckily, her pride and competitive spirit kicked in!

Of course both of us were apprehensive that first night, not knowing what to expect when we sat in that first clinic. We learned a couple important lessons the first time we attended the clinic. Firstly, although it is difficult, running for a minute and walking for a minute will not kill most people of standard build and attitude. We were welcomed and quickly made comfortable amongst people of all shapes, sizes and motivations. Secondly, it was interesting to learn that people actually went outside in Edmonton in January, and ran!

Since that time Jill's progress has been nothing short of amazing. There is no question that the Running Room clinics were the exact formula that we needed to give us the confidence to finish the 5 K fun race at the end of the clinic. In fact, it was so well designed that anyone, us included, could go from never running to finishing a 5 K run.

What happened next was fantastic. I had my fill of challenge; Jill was just getting started.

Not pleased that she had just completed the Learn to Run clinic, she enrolled again, this time in the 10 K clinic with a goal of "to complete." In six months, she had not only become considerably more fit, but Jill also made several new friends along the way. Jill quickly decided to become a clinic volunteer, and while she was running in her second 10 K clinic, she was also helping others begin their quest for their first 10 K.

Jill was now a transformed running addict. Obviously the next step was the half marathon clinic! Just over a year later, Jill successfully ran in the "Hypothermic" half marathon, and topped off her first year of exercise in almost 15 years by completing the race. More than that, however, she had done it with her new friends and new confidence, all of which began from the day she attended her first clinic.

Since then there has been another half marathon in Vancouver and after much hard work, training and guts Jill completed the Liberty Marathon in Normandy, France. Only 18 months from when she started running, Jill crossed the finish line in her first marathon. She had made the commitment to run in this marathon, which signifies and recognizes the sacrifices of the men who stormed the beaches of France on D-Day 1944.

I can't say enough about her efforts, or about how the Running Room made it easier for her. She is a different person and has many accomplishments, memories and new friends to be thankful for. I would be insulting her to suggest that it was easy, because she worked so hard, but I am sure she would agree that without the design and assistance of your running programs and the simple formula of support and steady progress, she would not have been able to do it.

Be as proud of your formula, as I am for Jill.

—Clinic Participant

Time to Get Fit!

Last summer I had my first "wake-up" call to get back into fitness. My brother, a marathoner and exceptional runner, asked me if I had ever thought of going back to running. Before my eyes, seven years had gone by and 30-odd pounds had crept up on me. It was so obvious to my family that I wasn't taking the best care of myself—I was not the picture of health! In that moment I replied, "Yes, I'm going out this week to get some new shoes." What a nice and gentle approach my brother had to let me know he cared. Over the next few weeks I started to think about how my body looked years ago when I was a runner and just how great I used to feel. Then of course, in my usual style, I wondered how the heck I got so unfit and fat.

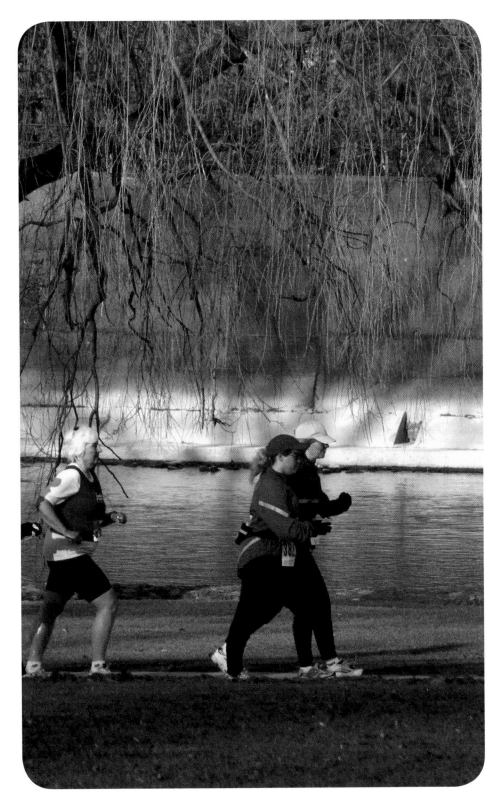

By September I started walking almost daily. I would watch runners go by me and tell myself that I would begin running once I shed a few pounds. I finally made up my mind to start running and not wait a day longer when my 7-year-old daughter (God bless her!) innocently asked me "if there was a baby in there." Talk about an eye opener right out of the mouths of babes. Truly, this was not what any single mother over 40 would ever want to hear. My daughter's words never left my mind and further inspired me to go check out the new Running Room in Waterloo I had driven by a few times. Obviously I needed to get some running gear and really just "get moving."

At that time, I really didn't have a game plan of how to get back into running, but I knew that I wanted to join a group for support and running company, as well as get some great running tips and techniques from the pros. When I finally ventured into the Running Room store, not only did I find the staff to be helpful, I found them so wonderfully encouraging to the new runner that I had become. Wow! I finally joined a clinic that was into its third week. At that moment, I figured it was best for me to start right away and not wait until the next session was beginning. As I said to this instructor, I had already put off running for seven years and did not want to put it off any longer.

Through the fall, winter and spring, I progressed through the Learn to Run and 10 K clinics. Since October, I have continued to run faithfully and follow the programs. For the first time in my life, I have also gone to fitness classes and started lifting weights. Even the fitness instructor encouraged me to run to lower my body fat. I learned the value of cross-training. I told myself that if I could run through the winter (and yes, I had the icicles on my eye lashes), I could run through anything! I am also the proud recipient of two Running Room medals for two 10 K events. Races somehow get me to "pick up the pace." Funnily enough, my daughter proudly wore my medals to school, telling even her teacher that I was medal winner.

Since October, I have lost just over 20 pounds, put on some muscle, and reduced my body fat ratio from 35% to 26%, all without a day of dieting! Just altering my summer work clothes was a small fortune, but how good it felt to see those inches taken away! By accomplishing what I have thus far, I know that I can reach my new goals by doing what I have been doing since I began the first clinic.

I have a whole new appreciation for runners, for their efforts and hard work, and mostly for their commitment to a healthy lifestyle. Thank goodness I got a wake-up call. Mentors are champions who may not even be aware of how much they inspire folks like me. I celebrate the good health I have by running regularly, obviously for more than just the fun of it.

Becoming a runner and improving my fitness level has improved by life tremendously. It feels so good to be taking such good care of myself. I have met lots of great people through the Running Room (including John Stanton) who continue to inspire me and help me reach my goals.

—Marg, Clinic Participant

Debt of Gratitude!

Nine years ago I was diagnosed with type I diabetes, or insulin-dependent diabetes. I've never been fond of exercise, except the occasional hike or cross-country ski, and so even though my first endocrinologist is a runner and strongly advised that I do some sort of exercise to keep my blood sugar levels in the acceptable range (to prevent long-term complications like kidney failure, amputation, etc.), I kidded myself into thinking I could manage my diabetes with insulin and watching my diet alone.

For seven years I saw my blood sugar levels continually rise, and then two years ago my left foot went partially numb and was occasionally painful. I thought at that time that I had diabetic neuropathy, which is one of the complications of diabetes, and this scared me into action. I began testing my blood sugars in between meals, as well as at mealtime, which meant that I sometimes gave myself seven needles per day. I started walking nearly every day, but it was January, and the temperatures were around -20°C for two weeks. Needless to say, I didn't enjoy walking in the dark and the cold.

As it happened, I needed to get bigger running shoes to make my numb foot feel more comfortable, and my doctor suggested going to the Running Room. While there, I saw posters for a Learn to Walk class, and I decided to sign up. The leaders were great, and when the class was over I wanted to stay involved, and I nervously signed up for the Learn to Run class.

The group leader, Tiffany, was an inspiration to us all, having lost so much weight and run marathons in such a short period of time. By the time I completed the advanced level, I was running 5 km non-stop, although I was slower than most people in the group and decided for that reason to just continue to train on my own. But I really enjoyed the group support while there, thought all the leaders were great motivators and learned a lot.

Because exercising while taking insulin presents challenges, I decided to go on

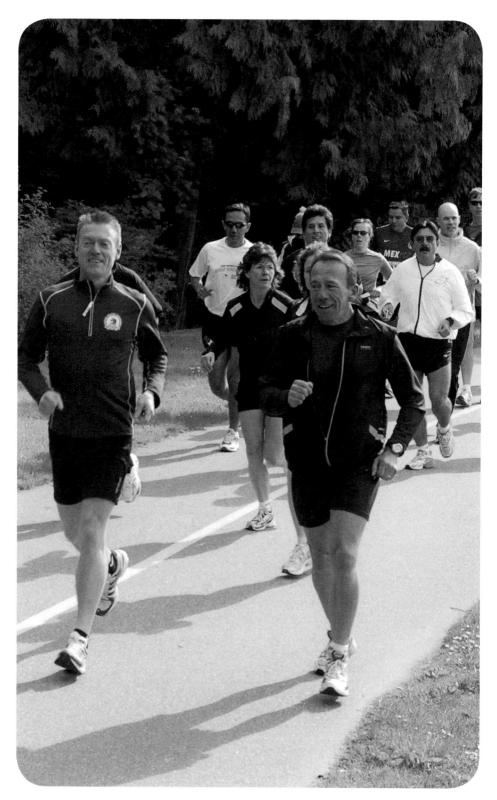

the insulin pump, and this made things a lot easier, although it's still a challenge to keep my levels from dropping too low and passing out before completing the run. However, exercising has definitely been worth it, because the running alone dropped my blood sugar levels from 9.5 to 8.4, and after going on the pump and continuing to run, I've dropped further down to 7.3. (Blood sugar levels below 8.4 reduce your chances of getting long-term complications by 40%.) As it turns out, the numb foot is not related to diabetes, and with specially made insoles, I no longer have pain in that foot.

I managed to run 10 km, and I did the Santa Shuffle run in December, but after some time away from running, owing to a fall and moving house, I'm back to 5 km again. However, I realize that it's not the speed or the distance that matters, but rather the fact that I'm regularly exercising. I know that I look better since I started running (I lost 12 lb.), I generally have more energy (except immediately following a run!), and I now have a much better chance of having a healthier and longer life. If it wasn't for the classes at the Running Room, I never would have had the courage or the knowledge to try it on my own, and for that, I owe them a debt of gratitude.

—Karen, Clinic Participant

Caution: the Running Room can be addictive!

There were no warning signs posted at the door as I innocently wandered in, looking for some running shoes on a cold Calgary day in January. They had exactly what I was looking for and a whole lot more. As I was making my exit I was stopped short by the brochures for upcoming races, clinics and a spring fitness weekend in Canmore, Alberta (like Banff but way better). I took almost one of each pamphlet to peruse later. The fitness weekend sounded too good to be true—I could walk or run, it had an excellent location, and it was super cheap—so I signed up. What a blast! Did you know that those Stanton guys are all regular, real life nice people (and so are their wives)? Whoever said success will go to your head was way off here. Anyway, the bug was planted because, like they say, anybody can use John's plan to move from couch potato to athlete.

By December I had decided to move up from walking to running, and I signed up for Women's Only Learn to Run clinic in March. We split into three groups: Group A (those who could already run for 5 minutes), Group B (those who would start at running one minute and walking one), and Group C (those who would start at running for 30 seconds and walking for one minute). My hand shot up for Group C! I didn't want to overdo it on the first try, especially with all the snow and ice on the ground. Well, by the next week I had bumped myself up to Group B to see if I could do it. A few weeks down the road I was routinely running at the front of the pack. I missed the final class because we moved to Guelph, Ontario, which is also blessed with a Running Room. I toyed with the idea of taking the 10 K clinic, but after some soul searching I took a huge leap of faith in myself and the Running Room clinic instructors and joined the half marathon clinic! How do I summarize the year? I started learning to run in late March, ran my first half marathon in late September, my second in mid-October and completed 11 other races of various length, placing third in my age category twice!

This year I decided to take up power/race walking and focus on the marathon distance using the program from John's book Running: Start to Finish. There is some kind of giddy mystic bonding that happens when you pass the 38 K sign and say out loud, "I've never been this far before," and complete strangers around you are saying "Ya, me neither." Or when you pass the 40 K and say, "We can do 2 K in our sleep. This is the home stretch now," and hear the chuckles and see the broadening smiles as everybody realizes that they are going to conquer this marathon. The next marathon is going to be conquered in less than two weeks, with a few more planned for the fall, as well as some much shorter races sprinkled in between.

Next year I'm considering either running a marathon or taking a triathlon clinic with the Running Room; or maybe both.

This will sound cliché, but if I can do it so can you. I don't look like a stereo-typical athlete—sleek, fast and muscular—in fact, I am overweight, but I am an athlete, and the Running Room has played a colossal roll in helping me get there with their training skills and encouragement.

It's easy to see why the Running Room has been around for 20 years and is still growing strong. While there are scores of athletes out there who appreciate it just for the excellent stuff they sell, there are also the masses—myself included—that went from inactive to athlete thanks to John and his excellent Running Room team, who get us across the finish line smiling and upright. Thanks guys!

—Carolynn, Clinic Participant

Learn to Run clinic was my first success

Imagine running an errand to purchase fish for a family supper and you end up running a marathon! Well, believe it or not this is not a fish tale because it happened to me! Three years ago, on a September evening, I became a member of the Running Room located in Churchill Square, St. John's, Newfoundland.

I noticed a sign posted in their window offering a clinic titled "Women's Learn to Run." As I had no experience with running, and did not even own a pair of sneakers, I decided to see what it was all about. It was autumn, and although running at night did not really appeal to me, I asked myself "What have I got to lose?" I then thought "Well, if I don't like it I'll give it up. No big deal." After a little deliberation I took the first step and joined, realizing that the only thing I was truly certain about was that I indeed did not know how to run!

I learned from the store manager, Bruce Bowen, what I had actually gotten myself into. He informed me that a 30-minute clinic was being offered on Friday evenings and that each weekly clinic would offer presentations and talks, followed by a question and answer period and concluding with a short run. I thought one run a week couldn't hurt. Little did I know that that would be one of four runs a week.

The presentations would be given by guest speakers, who would provide information on areas such as nutrition, sports medicine, running techniques, etc. I became more curious, but I was also uncertain of my fitness level.

Upon arriving at my very first clinic, I scanned the room and quickly noticed that perhaps I was out of my element—most of the women in the clinic were the same age as my children! Two weeks into it, I quickly realized that age was not an issue. We were all there to learn how to run. It didn't matter the age or fitness level; we all came from different backgrounds. I was the oldest and the one with the least experienced in physical activity. Completing the Learn to Run clinic was my first success. I was in my 60s and was never an athlete or had even participated in sports on a recreational level. So, as you can imagine, running 5 K, experiencing no injuries and loving every minute was a real unexpected thrill for me! My excitement continued to grow with every run, and as I progressed I came to realize that I had truly found a passion. You might say I hit the ground running!

I became involved with many more clinics, meeting fellow runners from all over the province and becoming involved with community-sponsored activities. Sticking to the program step-by-step helped me prepare both mentally and physically, as well as handle the demands of my daily runs. The many benefits of running and the sheer thrill of completing marathons, along with becoming a member of the Running Room, has enabled me to achieve goals I never thought possible. The tremendous support I received from the members of the club allowed me, with great success, to complete a half marathon and the 10 mile "Tely-Ten" race in St. John's, the NYC Marathon and also the National Capital Marathon in Ottawa—all within one year! Without the encouragement from my running mates and my family this feat would have been totally impossible.

Thank you, Running Room, running mates and instructors for this. A special thanks to my family who, by the way, never got fresh fish for dinner on that September evening!

—Rosemarie, Clinic Participant

My true passion—Running!

When I was born my mother was diagnosed with breast cancer. She was treated and has been cancer free for 17 years! When I was four my mom's sister was diagnosed with breast cancer and passed away the same year. When I was 10 my father was in a severe explosion. He was hospitalized for a month and a half in the burn unit at Foothills Hospital. He made a tremendous recovery! Despite having 21% of his body burned and being rehospitalized the following month because of a blood clot from having skin grafts, he has come out a stronger man than I could ever imagine. For the next three years, members of my dad's side of the family passed away. This was a horrific downfall for my father's well being. In 1999, my father's mom was diagnosed with lung cancer and passed away. I was incredibly close to her and spent many weekends with her. I went through a hard time for the next four years because of her death and my own personal problems. But in May of this year, my other grandma lost her life as well. She fought a very couragous battle with Parkinson's disease. Since I can remember, she had a very difficult time moving around.

Despite my family's setbacks, they have come out on the other side! I've been in a slump for four years with severe clinical depression. Recently, I met a young lady who is very involved in running. She completed the half marathon in Winnipeg in June. When I heard that and saw the look in her eyes, I sensed a feeling of true accomplishment. That is something I think I have been lacking for a long time. I started looking into a running club near my house to just give it a try. I've been going to drop in runs for about three weeks now, and I feel like another person. I've recieved many compliments about my appearance, not my figure, but my eyes and my smile. They're more loving and accepting of life. Just over the past three weeks, I have been able to stick with my goals and achieve them. Even if they are just little, they're still a spirit lifting project.

Since joining the Running Room, I look forward to getting out of bed, and I enjoy meeting people and being sociable. I am allowing myself to do the activities I enjoy as well as challenging myself. I still have days where getting out of bed seems just out of the question, but then I reflect back on how good I felt after my run with the Running Room or my daily routine that the Running Room has allowed me to do—that alone gets me out of bed!

I have since discovered my true passion: running. I'm planning on doing a marathon next year. Because of everyone in my life and at the Running Room, the support is tremendous and greatly appreciated!

—Charley, Running Room Club Member

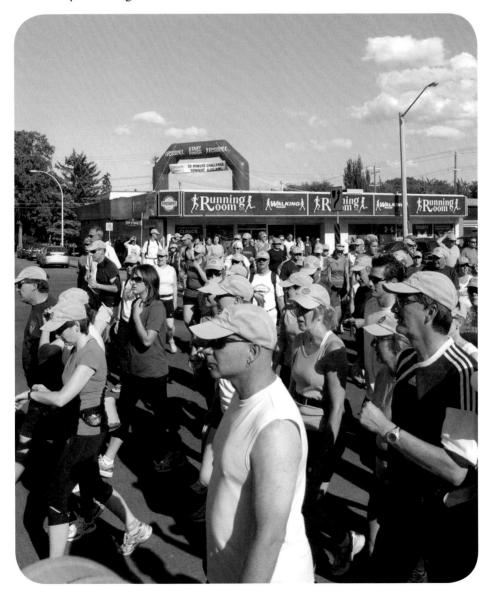

Hats off to you, John Stanton, and all your staff!

I was first introduced to the Running Room when I participated in a Nike Survivor Clinic three years ago in preparation for the Run for the Cure that fall. I am a breast cancer survivor and I can say that these clinics need to continue to encourage women going through the disease or treatment. It's uplifting, and people who walk or run are ultimately surprised and even shocked to find out they can run or walk long distances. I was one of the first to finish in our group that first year, and while my wonderful husband Nigel went back to run with the incoming members of our team, encouraging them, I was shouting at the finish line waving them in. What a feeling to see the expression on their faces when they cross that line. It's just amazing.

I had basically never run before, I was more of a power walker, I even resisted the running until about the fourth week because I was walking but passing many of the people running—needless to say, I walk pretty fast. Then all of a sudden I started running with the group and I've kept going ever since. We run all year, and if someone had told me I'd be running on cold winter days three years ago, I would have said they were crazy.

The Running Room is a wonderful organization: helping people get fit; organizing so many runs for charitable organizations; their staff volunteering their time for clinics; great, professional help at the store for purchasing the shoe; information sessions; you name it, they do it. I'll be there on the 14th to commemorate their 20th year. Hats off to you John Stanton and all your staff across North America.

—Elaine, Clinic Participant

What an accomplishment for me!

I've been at the track and field and road races for over 12 years watching my boys run. I really never thought I could do it, but I have always wanted to run. I joined the Running Room Learn to Run for Women Only in March. Not only did I find out that I could do it, but I found some very lasting friendships.

I've done three clinics in total, and I think the one that I value the most is the half marathon. Who would have thought that I could run a half marathon. I went to Ottawa for the National Capital with the normal jitters, but on the morning of race day I felt very calm. What an accomplishment for me! Something else that really made that day very special is that Matthew, one of my sons that I've watched running for the past 12 years, was living in Ottawa for the summer.

Well, Matthew ran me in the last 3 km and that was a very emotional experience for me.

Thanks, Running Room. It proves that if you try to do something you can.

—Diane, Clinic Participant

Thank you for inspiring me! Congratulations on 20 years of inspiring Americans and Canadians to get, and stay, fit!

Because of a Running Room program, I was able to walk a marathon for the Arthritis Society, a month before my 55th birthday! I still use the techniques that were taught to me, and I am still living an active lifestyle. My latest adventure is Dragonboat racing. Thank you so very much for inspiring me to stay in shape. God bless you.

—Margaret, Clinic Participant

Running Room has changed my life!

When I walked into the Running Room store in Kingston, Ontario, to sign up to walk the Run for a Cure course, little did I know that my life was about to change. Derrick Spafford, the store manager, suggested I might consider signing up for the For Women Only Learn to Run Clinic. I laughed at this suggestion— I was 49, and although not overweight, I had been fairly inactive for 20 years. Besides, I was one of those kids who hated gym class—I was always the weakest, the smallest, the clumsiest—the last chosen for a team. For some reason I went back to my office and gave some thought to what Derrick had said, and I did sign up for the clinic. I was really nervous before the first clinic morning—What had I done? Was I about to be humiliated again—childhood memories flooded back, but I made myself go. Guess what? It was okay!

Not only did I finish this clinic, but I went on to do the Intermediate 5 K clinic, the 10 K clinic and the Half Marathon clinic. I ran my first half marathon this spring in Ottawa, and I finished in the top 20% for my age category at the age of 51.

Now running is such a natural part of my life I can hardly remember what life was like before! I am a runner, I am an athlete, and those childhood memories of being miserable in gym class are just a distant memory.

Thank you, Running Room, you've changed my life!
—Joanne, Clinic Participant

Running Room made me what I am today!

In 1994 I was a Yukon-Gold coach potato ready to be deep fried. The Running Room's marathon clinic changed me from a sweaty, wheezy, panting rambler into a sweaty, wheezy, panting runner. Hooked on stopping every 10 minutes for a break (my boss doesn't like that too much), I went on to complete several marathons and then Ironman USA and Ironman Canada a year later. Today I am a professional speaker specializing in using humor to motivate people to change. I use running and triathlon as examples and show people that if I can do it then everyone possesses the courage to change. Oh yes, I also now teach marathon courses for the Running Room and gently help those coach potatoes become baked potatoes.

–Dave, Clinic Participant

My next marathon!

I don't know where to begin to share my story. I have taken part in four clinics since the spring. I have always been a walker, but I decided to join a walking group to meet people who have a passion for walking as I do. I started losing weight in November and lost 13 lb. to date. I attribute a lot of the weight loss to the extensive exercise since I have been with the Running Room.

I have had two heart open heart surgeries. One at an early age and the second one 11½ years ago. I plan to enter the half marathon/walking in October in Toronto. I see a cardiologist annually and can hardly wait to tell him next year about the marathon.

The Running Room offers an opportunity to meet new and inspiring people to enjoy walking with. Thank you for fabulous services. I brag about the store and the people who run it all of the time.

—Jane, Clinic Participant

Two years ago I was 45 lb. heavier than I now am. I felt much older than I was and knew that my weight was interfering in every aspect of my life. I joined Weight Watchers just before my 30th birthday because I knew I had to do something. I was too overweight to run, but it was something that was in the back of my mind. Once I had lost about 15 lb., I joined the 10 km clinic in January. Learning to run when it was that cold was quite the challenge, but everyone was always supportive and I soon began to really enjoy it. I began to look forward to those Wednesdays and Sundays and to increasing the distances.

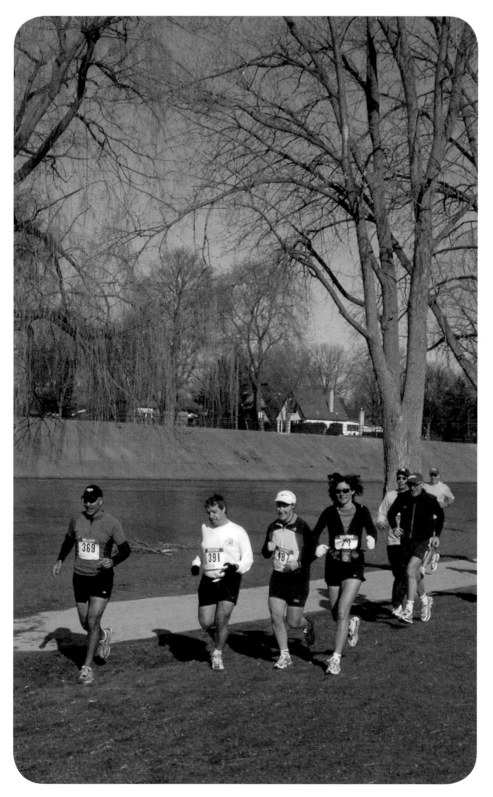

I have never in my life been athletic, in fact, I always thought that it would be impossible for me to be athletic in any way at all. Running gave me confidence physically, but more importantly it gave me confidence emotionally as well. I joined the half marathon clinic, which overlapped the last 10 km clinic meeting. I was completely pumped up to run my first half marathon. I ran in Ottawa and finished with a decent time of 2:04:35. That was in May the same year. I went on to run the Toronto half marathon in October and finished with 2:01:59—painfully close to my goal of under two hours! I will begin to prepare to run the half-marathon in Chicago this September at the end of June, and I feel confident I will finally break that two hour mark.

Running has taught me that you can really only compete against yourself—there will always be people much faster than you and there will always be people slower than you. It has taught me that I can do absolutely anything as long as I put my mind to it and prepare for it! A dream is a goal with a long-term plan (or something like that, right?).

I love telling people I'm a runner. It's something that took me at least seven or eight months to be able to say and believe it, but I do believe it now. I can't tell you how huge a role the Running Room played in my transformation. I'd like to thank all your staff and wish you the happiest of anniversaries! And many more.

—Mariel, Clinic Participant

My first marathon

I first got the idea to take part in the Montreal Marathon this past June. I had begun training, inside on a treadmill, in January of 2009. As I am a fervent cyclist, I wanted to maintain if not increase, my cardiovascular capacity.

After running approximately 200 K in the gym, I began to run outside. I had never imagined how different this would be, much harder and more demanding, especially on the muscles of the legs. This was now April. It was at this time that a work mate said to me "you should go and run a Marathon, one of these days!" The seed had been sowed. Where, when and how would this be possible? I began to look for reference material, which I discovered in the Yellow Pages under the sports heading, and it read: RUNNING ROOM. Why not start with them? They should know what they are talking about?

Upon my arrival at the Laval store, which shall remain nameless, I was asked "how can we help you?" They answered all my questions, gave me invaluable advice, like changing my shoes and signing up for the upcoming Marathon training program. As I was not available on training program days, they suggested a purchase which would change my way of training, and my perception of the effort which awaited me, to reach new goals. This purchase was The Running Room's Book on Running.

I began my training, armed with my new shoes and the excellent tips which I found in Mr. Stanton's book, both of whom were of great help. No more pain in my feet, in my shins or my heels. All was wonderful, and my shoes gave me wings.

I followed the tips and the training schedule in the book, for a first time Marathon in 4h15. This was May 11, 2009. A few hundred kilometers later, I signed up for a Half Marathon in the Boucherville Islands, which I was able to complete in 2:03, obliterating the 2:15 I was aiming for. I was absolutely thrilled by my first ever race, and that is when I signed up for my first Marathon, Montreal.

On that long awaited morning, I was very relaxed and quite confident, considering it was my first Marathon. The starting gun went off after a 16 minute delay and I took off like a rocket. I was running at a much faster pace than I had planned on, and a little voice whispered to me "you should slow down if you want a photo finish and especially if you want to finish this Marathon". I would say it took me about 3 K to settle on the pace I had worked so diligently on during my workouts. The race went as planned, no surprises, no injuries, my resolve was good and so was my form. Coming into Olympic Stadium was magical. I had a spurt of adrenalin which enabled me to generate a final kick, for a 4:08:01 finish.

A heartfelt thanks to John Stanton for his excellent book, I have already recommended it to several people, to the Laval and Brossard Running Rooms, to Annie my wife, my family and friends, for all the support.

PS: it would seem as though my wife also caught the bug, as she has now started running. I would like to take this opportunity to congratulate Pierre, my brother-in-law, who recovered from a by-pass operation last winter, and who will be running his first Half Marathon next spring. I will be honoured to run with him

Thank you!
—Alain, Training Program Participant

John Stanton
Founder of the Running Room and Walking Room

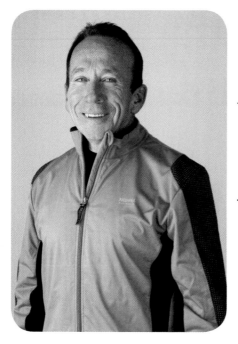

A best-selling Canadian author of four books on running and, most recently, Walking: A Complete Guide to Walking Fitness, Health and Weight Loss, John Stanton was named to Maclean's magazine's 2004 Canada Day Honour Roll as one of 10 Canadians making a difference in our nation for his contribution to health through fitness. John has been featured in the National Post and The Globe and Mail, and has appeared as a guest on CBC, CTV's Canada AM, CHUM Television, Global Television, A-Channel, Rogers, the Weather Channel and numerous radio and television programs across Canada and the United States.

A three-kilometer fun run with his sons in 1981 was the catalyst for the then out-of-shape, overweight John Stanton to realize he had to change his lifestyle. A food industry executive who smoked two packs of cigarettes a day, Stanton began running secretly before dawn because he felt self-conscious about having his neighbors see "this chubby little guy" who could only run from lamppost to lamppost before having to take a walk break. In 1984 Stanton opened a store and meeting place for runners in an 8×10 foot room of an old house shared with a hairdressing shop in Edmonton. Twenty years later, the Running Room is one of North America's most recognized names in running and walking. In 2004, to be more inclusive, the Walking Room was launched—a mirror of the Running Room concept. The store caters specifically to the needs of walkers. His sons John Jr. and Jason are now partners in the family business, which boasts over 100 stores in Canada and the United States.

John Stanton has run more than 60 marathons, hundreds of road races and numerous triathlons, including the Canadian Ironman and the Ironman World Championship in Kona, Hawaii. His pre-dawn runs would ultimately become John Stanton's 10:1 run/walk combination that has helped well over 600,000 Canadians do everything from learn to run to complete marathons, upright and smiling. An Honorary Lieutenant-Colonel of The Loyal Edmonton Regiment (4th Battalion, Princess Patricia's Canadian Light Infantry), John Stanton was the recipient of the 2009 Dr. Harold N. Segall Award of Merit, which recognized his significant contribution to the prevention of cardiovascular disease and the promotion of cardiovascular health in Canadians.

John Stanton, C.M., is a Member of the Order of Canada. He works with many charitable organizations and boards and is a vice president of the Commonwealth Games Association of Canada.

Thousands of people have lost weight, improved their health and fitness levels and truly changed their lives as a result of one man who was determined to change his own life by losing weight and getting fit.

Index of Select Terms

This index lists pages where you will find descriptions of various concepts and terms in the book. (It is not meant to be a comprehensive list for every time a word appears.)